'This is a text that child therapists have long needed. It brings together understandings which have historically been too separate, of the effects of complex trauma on children, alongside psychodynamic, attachment and developmental science, integrated into a deep but user-friendly and effective way of working not only with the child but also with the significant adults and systems around them. Clinicians, from the most experienced to newer therapists, will breathe a sigh of relief that this is available'.

Dr Graham Music, *Consultant psychotherapist, Tavistock Clinic,*
Author of Nurturing Children *(2019) and* Nurturing Natures *(2016)*

'The present volume is much needed as communities around the world face more strife and conflict and complex trauma in children is increasingly common. The authors offer a concise and invaluable integration of clinical theory with insights into how therapists create a safe space to facilitate children's recovery and growth. In language accessible for students as well as parents, the authors provide a vivid portrait behind the scenes of experienced therapists working with great skill with traumatized children and their families'.

Linda Mayes, *Arnold Gesell Professor Child Psychiatry, Pediatrics,*
and Psychiatry, Yale Child Study Center, Yale School of Medicine

'Child psychotherapists working in the psychodynamic tradition have always worked with children and families struggling with the effects of complex trauma. Yet there has been a lack of an integration of longstanding psychoanalytic clinical experience with contemporary ways of working with trauma emerging from other fields, including neuroscience, developmental psychology and mentalization-based work. Nicole Vliegen and her colleagues have produced an approachable and inspiring practice guide, which will be useful for any child psychotherapist working with traumatised fostered and adopted children. Especially useful is the three-track treatment approach: direct therapy with the child has to be combined with active work with the parents/carers and the wider network for the work to have a lasting impact'.

Maria Papadima, PhD, *Editor of the* Journal of Child Psychotherapy;
Senior Child and Adolescent Psychotherapist in the NHS Service
for Adolescents and Families in Enfield (SAFE)

Therapeutic Work for Children with Complex Trauma

Therapeutic Work for Children with Complex Trauma offers a contemporary three-track psychodynamic treatment model to mental health professionals working with traumatised children and their caregivers.

The book provides a contemporary and comprehensive approach to working with traumatised children by integrating knowledge and skills from traditional psychodynamic child psychotherapy and more contemporary trauma-informed and mentalization-based frameworks. It advocates three tracks of work, involving direct work with the child, work with the child's primary caregivers and work with the network. The book is divided into two parts: Part I of the book covers the theoretical background and Part II discusses the core components and phases of the trauma-informed and mentalization-based treatment approach. The authors bring out the specific dynamics of the psychotherapeutic work through four composite cases woven through the book.

Written in accessible language this treatment guide is primarily aimed at psychodynamically trained psychotherapists, mental health professionals and professional caregivers working with traumatised children.

Nicole Vliegen, PhD, is Professor of Clinical Psychology at KU Leuven, Belgium, where she heads the postgraduate training programmes in Psychodynamic Child Psychotherapy and Infant Mental Health. She is a licensed psychodynamic child psychotherapist and heads the team of psychodynamic child psychotherapists at PraxisP, the clinical centre of KU Leuven.

Eileen Tang, PhD, is a postdoctoral researcher in Clinical Psychology at KU Leuven and Professor in Psychology at Vrije Universiteit Brussel, Belgium. She is a licensed psychodynamic child psychotherapist and is part of the team at PraxisP.

Nick Midgley, PhD, is a child and adolescent psychotherapist and Professor of Psychological Therapies with Children and Young People at UCL/the Anna Freud Centre, UK. He has edited and co-authored several books, including *Mentalization-Based Treatment with Children: A Time-Limited Approach* (2017).

Patrick Luyten, PhD, is Professor at the Faculty of Psychology and Educational Sciences, KU Leuven, Belgium and Director of the PhD in Psychoanalysis Programme at University College London, UK. He heads a treatment service for patients with depression and functional somatic disorders at PraxisP.

Peter Fonagy is Head of the Division of Psychology and Language Sciences at University College London; Chief Executive of the Anna Freud Centre, UK; Consultant to the Child and Family Programme at Baylor College of Medicine and visiting professor at Yale and Harvard Medical Schools. He has received Lifetime Achievement Awards from several national and international professional associations.

Therapeutic Work for Children with Complex Trauma

A Three-Track Psychodynamic Approach

Nicole Vliegen, Eileen Tang,
Nick Midgley, Patrick Luyten
and Peter Fonagy

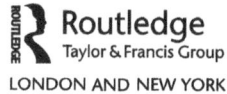
Routledge
Taylor & Francis Group

LONDON AND NEW YORK

Designed cover image: © Street artwork by Achilleas Michaelides
(Paparazzi Art Studio, Karaoli & Dimitriou, Larnaka, Cyprus).
Photograph taken by Lieve Van Lier

First published 2023
by Routledge
4 Park Square, Milton Park, Abingdon, Oxon OX14 4RN

and by Routledge
605 Third Avenue, New York, NY 10158

*Routledge is an imprint of the Taylor & Francis Group, an informa
business*

British Library Cataloguing-in-Publication Data
A catalogue record for this book is available from the British Library

ISBN: 978-0-367-49177-2 (hbk)
ISBN: 978-0-367-49175-8 (pbk)
ISBN: 978-1-003-04491-8 (ebk)

DOI: 10.4324/9781003044918

Typeset in Times New Roman
by Apex CoVantage, LLC

Contents

Acknowledgements

Writing a book like this is always the result of exchange, collaboration, thinking and writing together. Many children, parents, network partners and colleagues have contributed each in their own way to this book. We first and foremost wish to acknowledge the many children and adoptive parents and foster carers we have been fortunate to work with and from whom we have learnt so much. It is because they allowed us to be part of their life and to share in their sorrows and longings, their confusion as well as their growth, that we have been able to develop our psychotherapeutic approach to children who have experienced complex trauma and their carers. In this book, we have called them 'Jemal', 'Lisa', 'Mei-Lan' and 'Youri', each representing the many children referred to PraxisP, the practice centre of the Faculty of Psychology and Educational Sciences at KU Leuven, Belgium. Furthermore, we are indebted to the many teachers, foster care workers, residential care workers and psychiatrists with whom we have worked collaboratively and from whom we learnt so much in the process of our joint efforts to support and foster psychological growth in often severely traumatised children.

In line with the mentalizing approach that is central in this book, the clinical work we do with children, their parents and other adult carers is per definition a 'joint venture'. Therefore, we are extremely grateful to the psychodynamic team at PraxisP for the many years of working and thinking together, which has enabled us to improve the mental health care we provide to these vulnerable children and their carers. Eva Bervoets, Annabel Bogaerts, Orfee Callebert, Ilse De Clippeleer, Simon Fiore, Stefanie Hesemans, Karolien Hobin, Astrid Lauwereins, Saskia Malcorps, Patrick Meurs, Let Moustie, Lise Robeyns, Hilde Seys, Lisa Vanbeckbergen, Ann Van de Vel, Camille Van Havere, Lieve Van Lier, Yannic Verhaest, Sus Weytens – thank you, all, for your mentalizing presence and contributions!

We are also immensely indebted to our many collaborators and colleagues at University College London and at the Anna Freud National Centre for Children and Families in the UK, who have contributed so much to our thinking about this work. Similarly, we are immensely grateful that we have been able to participate in a network of like-minded colleagues around the world, whose thinking about psychodynamic and mentalizing approaches to working with children and families has been so inspiring.

Finally, we wish to acknowledge the Fund Dr. Pierre Vereecken for the opportunities it has afforded us to develop our thinking on trauma and its impact on children's development.

**NICOLE VLIEGEN AND EILEEN TANG, NICK MIDGLEY,
PATRICK LUYTEN AND PETER FONAGY
SEPTEMBER 2022**

Introduction

Meeting the children

 Ten-year-old Jemal had a difficult start in life, and although he now lives with two very caring adoptive parents, he shows severe behavioural and educational problems, impacting his functioning and performance at school. His adoptive parents also report eating and sleeping difficulties at home. In an intake session, they tell the therapist that Jemal decided one day that he no longer wanted drawings on the wall in his room, and removed all the stuffed animals from his bed, claiming to be 'too old for such childish stuff'. Mother exclaims in desperation that he also hates her food and barely eats. 'And when he goes to bed, he insists on going by himself without a hug or a kiss, but then he can't sleep, gets really fussy and keeps us up all through the night', Father adds. The first term that comes to Jemal's adoptive parents' mind when the therapist invites them to describe him, is 'hard to reach'.

 Lisa's foster carers seek help when she is nine years old. They ask for a psychiatric assessment, being convinced that she meets the criteria to be diagnosed with an 'attachment disorder'. They began to read everything they possibly could on the internet about the disorder, trying to find more information and particularly tips as to what they could do to help Lisa. When they read a post by one parent, saying her son is 'a child whose needs are un-ending', they instantly feel that this describes the way they often feel about their foster daughter perfectly, namely that whatever they do for this 'attachment disordered' child, it never will be enough.

 Seven-year-old Mei-Lan often misbehaves inexplicably, in a way that exhausts her adoptive parents. In these moments, she seems to be in a kind of blind rage, kicking and biting, seemingly without any reason causing these outbursts. In other moments, she acts like a needy infant, wanting to be dressed by her adoptive mum, or crying inconsolably

DOI: 10.4324/9781003044918-1

when Mum is not there. Although her adoptive parents believe that Mei-Lan is quite an intelligent child, she doesn't do very well at school, and fails to establish and maintain friendships with other children. Her adoptive parents are extremely concerned about her future and increasingly believe that Mei-Lan has some form of autism.

Youri's foster mother seeks help when Youri has just turned eight, because even after being in their family from his first year of life, he doesn't seem to be able to 'settle'. His biological mother died shortly after his birth after years of being addicted to drugs; his father suffers from mental illness and is unable to care for him. Youri's foster mother first hoped that the loving home environment she and her husband provided would be enough, but now she's worried that it's not.

Jemal, Lisa, Mei-Lan and Youri are all children with an history of complex trauma, as typically referred to psychodynamic child psychotherapists. We will tell their stories throughout this treatment guide, in an attempt to help understand the problems these children face and the ways we try to help them and to explore how their foster carers or adoptive parents can deal with the developmental issues their families are struggling with. Their stories are composite cases of real children's and families' stories that have been compiled and adapted so as to protect children's and families' privacy.

The previous brief vignettes illustrate typical problems which traumatised children present with when referred for treatment. Jemal and Mei-Lan are internationally adopted children; Lisa and Youri are children who have been placed in (long-term) foster care. As is evident from the vignettes, children like them form a somewhat heterogeneous group in terms of reasons for referral. The fact that their symptoms and observable behaviour show similarity to other, more commonly known disorders often complicates the clinician's assessment and diagnostic task. However, a common thread through these children's stories is the extreme level of behavioural problems they exhibit and the intense arousal they tend to evoke in the people around them. Their intense, often rapidly shifting and difficult-to-manage behaviour is an energy-guzzler for all those who try to support them – whether family, friends, teachers or other professionals. As a result, their carers typically struggle with feelings of exhaustion as well as with being able to keep thinking about what lies behind the child's 'incomprehensible' behaviour (e.g., intense anxiety), thereby compromising their ability to provide the child with the growth-promoting responses needed to foster developmental recovery. This ability of parents and other caregivers to be curious about the thoughts and feelings that shape our behaviour and to reflect on the often complex mental states behind these children's challenging behaviours has been termed 'mentalizing', and the temporary loss of this capacity under stress or high levels of arousal has been described as 'mentalizing breakdowns' (Bateman & Fonagy, 2019). Such mentalizing breakdowns are to a large extent inevitable in carers of children presenting with these problems. They also frequently occur in professionals working with these children. One of the main aims of this treatment guide is to present professionals and carers with tools to prevent such mentalizing breakdowns and to restore their capacity to provide a genuinely understanding, caring and mentalizing context for these children.

Which children is this treatment guide (not) about?

It is important to note that we do not consider every foster or adopted child at risk for severe or even mild developmental problems. Research suggests that about a third of foster and adopted children follow typical developmental trajectories; a further third develop mild mental health problems at a certain time during their development, for which relatively brief treatment may suffice to get these children back on track; however, the other third of foster and adopted children have been shown to be at increased risk for multiple complex and pervasive developmental impairments (Barroso et al., 2017; Juffer et al., 2011; Palacios & Brodzinsky, 2010; Palacios et al., 2014; Vasileva & Petermann, 2018).

In this regard, research has also consistently shown that foster care or adoption may result in a substantial developmental catch-up in the majority of children with a history of early adversity (Fisher, 2015; Palacios & Brodzinsky, 2010; Welsh et al., 2007). Fostering and adoption, in this respect, are profound therapeutic interventions in their own right. However, this catch-up does not appear to be complete across all developmental domains, and neither do all children show the same extent of catch-up (Fisher, 2015; Palacios & Brodzinsky, 2010; Welsh et al., 2007). A substantial minority of looked after and adopted children suffer from developmental vulnerabilities that may well have longer-term impact on their health and wellbeing. For these children, the stable and loving environment of their new foster or adoptive family does not seem to suffice to buffer the deleterious effects of adversities suffered earlier in their life.

Evidently and unfortunately, complex trauma is not unique or exclusive to children in foster or adoptive placements; however, this is the group of children that clinicians often encounter in clinical practice. In Flanders (the Dutch-speaking part of Belgium), adoption mainly concerns international adoption, in accordance with the 1993 Convention on Protection of Children and Co-operation in respect of Intercountry Adoption. The group of domestically adopted children is very limited in Flanders (about 5% of all adoptees), as domestic adoption is only rarely part of a child protection measure. Rather, foster care is typically seen as indicated when biological parents are considered to be (temporarily) unable to take care of their children. However, unlike in other countries such as the UK, it is not common for children to be adopted from long-term foster care. In Flanders, foster care only exceptionally moves on to adoption, for instance, for orphaned children. Foster care may comprise different measures, ranging from foster care in crisis situations to longer-term foster care. The present treatment approach has been developed for the following children: (internationally) adopted children and children in long-term foster care who have a history of severe relational difficulties in their early years but who presently live in a stable family environment.

Adopted children and children in long-term foster care have in common that they have suffered at least one experience of major loss, as they cannot grow up in their family of origin. More often, these children have had to face multiple losses of caregivers as well as of familiar surroundings – and all aspects of 'culture' that belong to it. Moreover, by the nature of having been in need of a foster or an adoptive family, they went through less or more other early adverse experiences. Jemal and Mei-Lan, for example, were foundlings, abandoned between birth and about one year of age, and they spent some time in an orphanage prior to being adopted. Mei-Lan was adopted from an orphanage in China at the age of eight months. Jemal was adopted from Ethiopia at the age of three, after having lived in two different orphanages. Lisa and Youri were placed in foster care by child protective services. Lisa suffered severe abuse and neglect from her biological parents. Youri was taken into care after his drug-addicted mother died of an overdose and his mentally ill father was unable to take care of him. As stated by Steele and Steele (2015, p. 429), there is something uniquely damaging to the human character in spending the first years of life in an environment devoid of typical parental care. As such, from the earliest beginnings, children like Jemal, Lisa, Mei-Lan and Youri have had to face 'the greatest threat in life, that of being deserted and left alone' (Bettelheim, 1976, p. 145).

Attachment failures and exposure to other adverse experiences in early childhood have unfortunately been all too common to many of these children's life histories (Ensink et al., 2019). Prior to being placed in a foster or an adoptive family, some children have grown up with caregivers with severe social and/or psychiatric problems and have gone through experiences of neglect, rejection, role reversal and physical or psychological abuse at the hands of their primary caregivers. Most of these children subsequently spent some time in residential or foster care, some of which was of questionable quality. Whether at the hands of the biological parents or family members or in low quality institutional or foster care, many of these children have experienced 'simultaneous or sequential occurrences of child maltreatment – including emotional abuse and neglect, sexual abuse, physical abuse, and witnessing domestic violence – that are chronic and begin in early childhood' (Cook et al., 2003, p. 5). All this constitutes 'complex trauma'. In such circumstances, the early caregiving system, the very social environment that is supposed to be the primary source of safety and stability in a young child's life, has been a source of stress, danger and traumatic events. 'The earliest and possibly most damaging psychological trauma is the loss of a secure base' (van der Kolk, 1987, p. 32). This is why a subgroup of adopted as well as fostered children suffer from difficulties that can be summarised as constituting complex trauma. Undoubtedly, there are also differences between internationally adopted children and children in long-term foster care – we have attempted to discuss these differences in this book when these have relevant implications for the therapeutic work conducted.

These children are the focus of this treatment guide: children who have been unfortunate to have accrued cumulative adverse experiences in the context of their primary attachment relationships, which overwhelmed their coping capacities.

Their subsequent development, often on different domains simultaneously, is paying the price to date. In other words, this book is about children who have experienced and are struggling to recover from complex trauma. Their problems are often persistent and unlikely to respond swiftly to treatment. Therefore, these children and their families may benefit from specialised psychosocial interventions targeting their particular difficulties. Brief treatments, although these may be helpful in the short run or may lower the threshold to seek more extensive treatment, are typically insufficient and may even be harmful (e.g., because they may lead to parents feeling disappointed in mental health professionals because they are unable to help their child or because their child quickly relapses after a brief course of treatment).

For reasons of readability, we will sometimes refer to children who have experienced complex trauma as 'children suffering from/with complex trauma' or 'traumatised children'. Similarly, we will use the term 'parent' and 'caregiver' interchangeably when it is clear that it refers to the child's primary caregiver, i.e., in the Flemish context, adoptive parents and foster carers. When it is important to differentiate between biological parents on the one hand and adoptive parents or foster carers on the other hand or between adoptive parents and foster carers, we have attempted to do so.

Whom is this treatment guide for?

The present treatment guide is primarily intended for child psychotherapists with a psychodynamic training who encounter children who have experienced complex trauma and their families in their clinical practice. This guide integrates 'traditional' psychodynamic, more contemporary mentalization-based approaches and developmental psychopathology approaches to the understanding of the impact of trauma on child development, including the burgeoning research on the neuroscience of trauma. As such, this treatment guide can also be of interest to other mental health professionals who do not necessarily have a background in (psychodynamic) psychotherapy but who are interested in this approach because of their work with this group of children, such as clinical psychologists, child psychiatrists and family therapists, special needs education teachers, social work professionals or foster care workers. In this regard, we have attempted to explain and frame relevant psychodynamic concepts in concise and accessible language.

This principle-based, rather than protocol-based, treatment guide aims to provide a contemporary psychodynamic approach to the understanding and the treatment of foster and adopted children with a history of complex trauma and the parents and other adult carers living and working with these children. A psychodynamic approach, perhaps different from some other kinds of psychotherapeutic approaches, lends itself less to be captured in purely behavioural terms (what a therapist *does*). Rather, it is, in our opinion, a thought process, an active way of being present with and thinking about the child or the carer, which subsequently needs to translate into specific interventions (what a therapist *thinks and* how this informs therapeutic *action*). In line with this, this treatment guide aims to provide the reader insight into this thinking process of the psychodynamic psychotherapist in working with traumatised children and their carers, by providing structure, delineating guiding principles and outlining interventions and specific techniques that therapists can apply flexibly based on clinical judgement. To this end, clinical vignettes with accompanying commentaries have been integrated throughout the book in order to illustrate theoretical concepts as well as specific treatment interventions and techniques. Following Lemma et al.'s (2011) apt statement that 'knowledge of therapeutic strategies and techniques does not guarantee that a therapist will be competent' (p. 23), we contend that the therapist's competence in considering the timing and the choice of interventions as well as in flexibly applying these interventions is regarded as a prerequisite of good practice (Fonagy & Luyten, 2019). Flexible use of theoretical understanding and therapeutic interventions is considered a key meta competence in effectively delivering psychodynamic psychotherapy (Lemma et al., 2011), and this applies to an even greater extent to the work with this particular group of children and their carers. Therefore, individual and group supervision are important components of training in the proposed treatment approach.

Yet, it is important to note that successful implementation and delivery of the treatment approach outlined in this volume not only involves training and individual and group supervision but also requires support at the team and organisational levels. Studies have amply shown that the implementation of psychosocial treatments in routine clinical care should not only focus on the individual therapist level but also on the team and organisational levels. This is particularly the case with regard to the implementation of more complex, longer-term treatments such as the present treatment approach. For instance, lack of support and lack of implementation planning at the organisational level have been shown to be associated with resistance to change in mental health professionals, communication problems and lack of an adequate supervisory structure at the team level and a lack of competence and adherence to the treatment model at the therapist level, as well as with higher dropout rates and critical incidents in patients during the treatment, resulting in the treatment effects being more than halved (Bales et al., 2017; Hutsebaut et al., 2012). Hence, implementation of the current treatment approach is only likely to be successful when the conditions necessary for the successful implementation of this approach at the level of therapists, teams and the organisation or service in which it is implemented are met. This also implies that we do not support training and implementation of the current treatment approach in clinical settings where these conditions are not met or cannot be guaranteed for at least five years. We are currently conducting a pilot feasibility study to further investigate these assumptions and a larger pragmatic clinical trial is planned.

Finally, it is also important to note that the present treatment approach was originally developed for elementary school-aged children living in Flanders, exhibiting complex trauma symptoms due to a history of early adverse experiences. These ideas were then shared and expanded on in discussions with colleagues from University College London and the Anna Freud Centre in London. Yet, the principles outlined in this treatment guide are also relevant for those working with infants and pre-school children who exhibit problems related to complex traumatic experiences and can be adapted to work in other cultural contexts. Similarly, mental health professionals working with adolescents will recognise many of the issues discussed in this treatment guide. The therapeutic approach outlined will need to be adapted when working with younger or older children and young people or in other settings or contexts.

Outline of the treatment guide

This book consists of two main parts. In Part I, we outline the theoretical approach that underpins the proposed treatment approach, described in Part II. In Chapter 1, we describe the theoretical background underlying the present treatment approach. In Chapter 2, we aim to provide a contemporary comprehensive framework to understand traumatised children's inner world by outlining the specifics of their developmental impairments. In Chapter 3, we discuss how these children's developmental impairments continuously and pervasively challenge the mentalizing capacities of the parents and other adult carers living and working with these children.

Part II of the book discusses the principles of the contemporary psychodynamic treatment approach for adopted and foster children with complex trauma. In Chapter 4, we outline the three-track conceptualisation of the present treatment model as well as the basic principles, including principles underlying the therapeutic stance. In the following chapters, we describe how the basic principles and attitudes of the treatment approach take shape and are applied in the assessment phase, which we see as a central and integral part of the treatment (Chapter 5), the direct work with the child (Chapter 6), the work with parents/carers (Chapter 7) and the work with the network (Chapter 8). Finally, Chapter 9 covers the ending phase of the treatment.

References

Bales, D. L., Timman, R., Luyten, P., Busschbach, J., Verheul, R., & Hutsebaut, J. (2017). Implementation of evidence-based treatments for borderline personality disorder: The impact of organizational changes on treatment outcome of mentalization-based treatment. *Personality and Mental Health, 11*, 266–277. https://doi.org/10.1002/pmh.1381

Barroso, R., Barbosa-Ducharne, M., Coelho, V., Costa, I.-S., & Silva, A. (2017). Psychological adjustment in intercountry and domestic adopted adolescents: A systematic review. *Child and Adolescent Social Work Journal, 34*(5), 399–418. https://doi.org/10.1007/s10560-016-0485-x

Bateman, A., & Fonagy, P. (Eds.). (2019). *Handbook of mentalizing in mental health practice*. American Psychiatric Publishing.

Bettelheim, B. (1976). *The uses of enchantment. The meaning and importance of fairy tales*. Vintage Books.

Cook, A., Blaustein, M. E., Spinazzola, J., & van der Kolk, B. A. (2003). *Complex trauma in children and adolescents: White paper from the National Child Traumatic Stress Network Complex Trauma Task Force*. National Center for Child Traumatic Stress

Ensink, K., Borelli, J. L., Roy, J., Normandin, L., Slade, A., & Fonagy, P. (2019). Costs of not getting to know you: Lower levels of parentel reflective functioning confer risk for maternal insensitivity and insecure infant attachment. *Infancy*, *24*(2), 210–227. https://doi.org/10.1111/infa.12263

Fisher, P. A. (2015). Review: Adoption, fostering, and the needs of looked-after and adopted children. *Child and Adolescent Mental Health*, *20*(1), 5–12. https://doi.org/10.1111/camh.12084

Fonagy, P., & Luyten, P. (2019). Fidelity vs. flexibility in the implementation of psychotherapies: Time to move on. *World Psychiatry*, *18*, 270–271. https://doi.org/10.1002/wps.20657

Hutsebaut, J., Bales, D. L., Busschbach, J., & Verheul, R. (2012). The implementation of mentalization-based treatment for adolescents: A case study from an organizational, team and therapist perspective. *International Journal of Mental Health Systems*, *6*, 10.

Juffer, F., Palacios, J., Le Mare, L., Sonuga-Barke, E. J. S., Tieman, W., Bakermans-Kranenburg, M. J., Vorria, P., van IJzendoorn, M. H., & Verhulst, F. C. (2011). II. Development of adopted children with histories of early adversity. *Monographs of the Society for Research in Child Development*, *76*(4), 31–61. https://doi.org/10.1111/j.1540-5834.2011.00627.x

Lemma, A., Target, M., & Fonagy, P. (2011). *Brief dynamic interpersonal therapy. A clinician's guide*. Oxford University Press.

Palacios, J., & Brodzinsky, D. M. (2010). Review: Adoption research: Trends, topics, outcomes. *International Journal of Behavioral Development*, *34*(3), 270–284. https://doi.org/10.1177/0165025410362837

Palacios, J., Román, M., Moreno, C., León, E., & Peñarrubia, M.-G. (2014). Differential plasticity in the recovery of adopted children after early adversity. *Child Development Perspectives*, *8*(3), 169–174. https://doi.org/10.1111/cdep.12083

Steele, M., & Steele, H. (2015). Attachment disorders. In P. Luyten, L. C. Mayes, P. Fonagy, M. Target, & S. J. Blatt (Eds.), *Handbook of psychodynamic approaches to psychopathology* (pp. 426–444). The Guilford Press.

van der Kolk, B. A. (1987). The separation cry and the trauma response: Developmental issues in the psychobiology of attachment and separation. In *Psychological trauma* (pp. 31–62). American Psychiatric Publishing.

Vasileva, M., & Petermann, F. (2018). Attachment, development, and mental health in abused and neglected preschool children in foster care: A meta-analysis. *Trauma, Violence, & Abuse*, *19*(4), 443–458. https://doi.org/10.1177/1524838016669503

Welsh, J. A., Viana, A. G., Petrill, S. A., & Mathias, M. D. (2007). Interventions for internationally adopted children and families: A review of the literature. *Child and Adolescent Social Work Journal*, *24*(3), 285–311. https://doi.org/10.1007/s10560-007-0085-x

Part I

Theoretical background

Psychotherapeutic work with children who have experienced complex trauma requires a flexible theoretical framework that allows therapists to tailor their treatment to the specific needs and vulnerabilities of each child and their environment. In Part I, we outline the theoretical background underpinning the contemporary psychodynamic treatment approach set out in the second part of this book. Specifically, in Chapter 1, we first present a contemporary psychodynamic approach to complex trauma that offers a dynamic and integrative understanding of the profound and pervasive impact of complex traumatic experiences on the child themselves in terms of developmental impairments but also on the adults caring for such children on a daily basis. In the next chapters, we elaborate on these two aspects, as a profound understanding thereof is crucial to informing an effective treatment approach. In Chapter 2, we discuss four domains of child development that are central in understanding the profound disruptions in social-emotional and behavioural development that typically result from complex trauma experiences. In Chapter 3, we outline the particular challenges to parents' and other carers' resources in general – and mentalizing capacities in particular – in caring for traumatised children.

DOI: 10.4324/9781003044918-2

Chapter 1

A contemporary psychodynamic perspective on and approach to complex trauma

In this chapter, we outline the theoretical background underpinning a psychodynamic treatment approach to children with complex trauma. We briefly define complex trauma and discuss what this means in terms of the mental health needs these children and their families present with. We then explain the four basic assumptions underlying psychodynamic treatment approaches to children with complex trauma.

Complex trauma and implicated mental health needs

Complex trauma, also known as attachment trauma (Allen, 2013; Schore, 2009) or developmental trauma disorder (van der Kolk et al., 2009), refers to negative experiences occurring early in life in the context of unsafe and unreliable primary attachment relationships. As such, complex traumatic experiences have a tremendous detrimental impact on the child's subsequent development, often in multiple domains. In this introductory section, we first briefly define complex trauma, relative to other types of trauma. We then discuss its consequences for child development, as well as how it impacts upon the people living and working with children who have experienced complex trauma. Finally, we elaborate on what this means in terms of these families' – often complex – mental health needs.

Complex trauma defined

Trauma in general is defined as an event or a series of events that exceeds an individual's resources and skills to cope with the event itself and the accompanying physical and emotional consequences. By and large, traumatic experiences can be situated on a continuum, ranging from impersonal trauma (e.g., being involved in a car accident resulting in severe injury or losing a sibling or grandparent), to interpersonal trauma committed by people other than one's primary attachment figures (e.g., being bullied by peers or being abused by a sports coach) and complex trauma, committed in the context of the child's early attachment relationships (Luyten & Bateman, in press; see Table 1.1).

For children, the impact of traumatic experiences is mostly intense (at least initially), not only because of the impact on the developing child themselves but also

DOI: 10.4324/9781003044918-3

Table 1.1 Types of trauma and their impact on child development

	Type I trauma Impersonal One-off incident by a non-human agent	**Type II trauma Interpersonal** Recurrent incidents by a human agent	**Type III trauma Attachment figure** Multiple incidents within the caregiving environment
Examples	A tsunami, a car accident, a major loss (of a sibling, a grandparent whom one was close to)	Maltreatment, exploitation, sexual abuse (in child care, school, leisure environment)	Neglect, maltreatment, abuse, unpredictable parental care due to (mental) illness, loss of a primary caregiver
Possible consequences	Overwhelming thoughts and feelings, excessive anxiety, nightmares, trauma triggers	Overwhelming thoughts and feelings, excessive anxiety, nightmares, trauma triggers	Fundamental disruptions in multiple developmental domains
Impact on caregiving environment	Involved in trauma, loss of availability Existing care is source of resilience	Involved in trauma, loss of availability Existing care is source of resilience	Is (or has been) source of fear/ threat/danger/ stress Lack of 'safe haven'

Source: Adapted from Vliegen et al. (2023)

because in some situations, parents are themselves involved in the traumatic experiences, which may understandably result in a (temporary) loss of their availability and ability to help their child cope. On the other hand, in cases of Type I or Type II trauma, parents can be supported to regain access to their resources or skills, or other important caregivers can step in, to help the child to cope with the trauma and its consequences. This is fundamentally different in case of complex trauma, where a positive and growth-promoting caregiving environment is lacking from early on in life, thus impacting the earliest and deepest layers of development, starting at the neurobiological level.

Accumulating knowledge from neuroscience suggests that particular problematic behavioural patterns originate from trauma-induced, often pervasive, alterations in neurobiological systems and circuits that are implicated in, for instance, arousal and stress regulation (e.g., hypothalamic-pituitary-adrenal axis, i.e., the main human stress response system), emotion regulation and social-cognitive capacities, such as mentalizing (for recent reviews, see e.g., Koss & Gunnar, 2018; McCrory et al., 2017). These alterations have occurred in order to accommodate the adverse circumstances the child has been subjected to. In this regard, Blaustein and Kinniburgh (2010) have aptly described how two salient factors shape behavioural responses in children affected by complex trauma. First, the chronic presence or threat of danger has resulted in safety-seeking or danger-avoiding behaviours. Second, the absence of sufficient fulfilment of physical, emotional, relational and environmental needs has resulted in these children's frequent reverting back to need-fulfilment strategies. Moreover, these behavioural strategies are prioritised above and thus interfere with other developmental tasks, such as the development of regulatory, neurocognitive, interpersonal and intrapersonal competencies (Blaustein & Kinniburgh, 2010). This implies that 'even the most seemingly pathological of children's behaviours may make sense, when understood in light of the purpose they serve for the child' (Blaustein & Kinniburgh, 2010, p. 25). For instance, a child who has a tantrum when a teacher praises them for their good work may be responding to this apparently benign behaviour with a fighting response, because any act of kindness is experienced as a potential indicator that something dangerous is about to happen. Such a 'fight' reaction may have been highly adaptive to a dangerous and unpredictable environment but now prevents the child from making good use of the benign care being offered. As such, insights from a developmental psychopathology perspective (Cicchetti & Toth, 2009), including neurobiological findings, are highly informative for understanding how complex traumatic experiences have shaped – and continue to shape – both the content and the process a traumatised child brings into everyday life as well as the therapeutic encounter. These neurobiological changes and their accompanying developmental vulnerabilities have been shown to persist into adulthood (Leve et al., 2012; Palacios & Brodzinsky, 2010; Welsh et al., 2007). This, of course, comes at a high cost to the individual child, their family, and society as a whole (Caspi et al., 2016).

The impact of complex traumatic experiences on child development

The quality and stability of a child's relationships in the early years lay the foundation for a wide range of later developmental outcomes that really matter – self-confidence and sound mental health, the motivation to learn, achievement in school and later in life, the ability to control aggressive impulses and resolve conflicts in non-violent ways, knowing the difference between right and wrong, having the capacity to develop and sustain friendships and intimate relationships and ultimately to be a successful parent oneself (National Scientific Council on the Developing Child, 2004). There is little doubt about complex trauma conferring vulnerability to a range of negative developmental outcomes, ranging from physical growth delays to cognitive and behavioural problems to vulnerabilities in the social-emotional realm, typically with impairments in multiple developmental domains co-occurring (Anda et al., 2006; Cicchetti & Banny, 2014; Esposito & Gunnar, 2014; Juffer et al., 2011). Many of these negative outcomes and risks can be understood as arising from core developmental deficits in intrapersonal competencies (i.e., sense of self and self-development), interpersonal competencies (i.e., the capacity to form and engage in relationships with others), regulatory competencies (i.e., the capacity

Table 1.2 Impact of complex trauma on child development

Domain of development	Possible clinical symptoms
Development of stress and affect regulation	Functioning in states of fluctuating or chronic dysregulation Falling prey to fight/flight/freeze states Falling prey to trauma triggers, flashbacks, nightmares Concentration and learning difficulties Sleeping problems Eating problems Irritability and aggressive behaviour (often to achieve a sense of coherence or to protect against anxiety and pain)
Attachment development	Insecure or disorganised attachment patterns, leading to strong destructive templates of relationships (heightening the risk of retraumatisation) Hyperactivating or deactivating attachment strategies or getting caught in an approach-avoidance conflict Profound distrust, making it extremely difficult to establish and maintain healthy relationships
Development of representational and mentalizing skills	Poor capacities to represent (by talking, drawing or playing) what is going on in one's mind Poor capacities to think and feel about an inner world (of self and of others) underlying own and others' behaviour Lacking introspection and self-awareness Lacking empathy
Identity development	Lack of vitality and a sense of self Lacking connection with own longings, interests and talents Negative self-image Inflated positive self-image masking more fundamental insecure and negative self-representation

to recognise and modulate emotional and physiological experience) and neurocognitive competencies (i.e., the capacity to engage executive functions and other cognitive abilities to act meaningfully on the world; Blaustein & Kinniburgh, 2010).

The model on which the present treatment approach is based delineates four domains of development implicated in complex trauma (see Table 1.2). As complex traumatic experiences interfere with the development of stress and affect regulation while these systems are still fully developing, as well as with the development of secure attachment representations, the consequences for emotional and relational functioning are huge. When the early development of regulatory skills and relational capacities is taxed heavily, with the child growing up in an enduring or even a chronic state of dysregulation and attachment insecurity, the related challenges of developing mentalizing capabilities and representing and communicating inner experiences may be compromised, as well as the development of an adaptive sense of self and identity. The theoretical underpinnings of the impact of complex trauma on these four domains of development will be elaborated on in Chapter 2.

The impact of complex trauma on primary caregivers and the network

Complex trauma is not only a problem of the individual child but deeply affects parents and other adults caring for the child. Due to the immense impact of complex trauma on multiple domains of development and functioning, traumatised children tend to draw their caregivers into reacting in non-thoughtful ways and thus into negative interactions. Their unpredictably fluctuating behaviour and way of relating can tax parents' and other caregivers' intuitive caregiving skills, interrupt spontaneous gestures, challenge 'mentalizing capacities' (see later) and thus strain the relationship with the child. Even well-intentioned new caregivers, such as foster carers or adoptive parents, are likely to be challenged to a much greater extent – and for much more extended periods of time – than those caring for a child who has not experienced complex trauma. Such chronic strain often negatively impacts caregivers' problem-solving capacities, caregiving skills and feelings of acceptance and love towards the child. It may pave the way for a vicious cycle of negative – and even retraumatising – interactions with the child, characterised by a lack of reciprocal trust and an atmosphere of hostility (see Figure 1.1). This

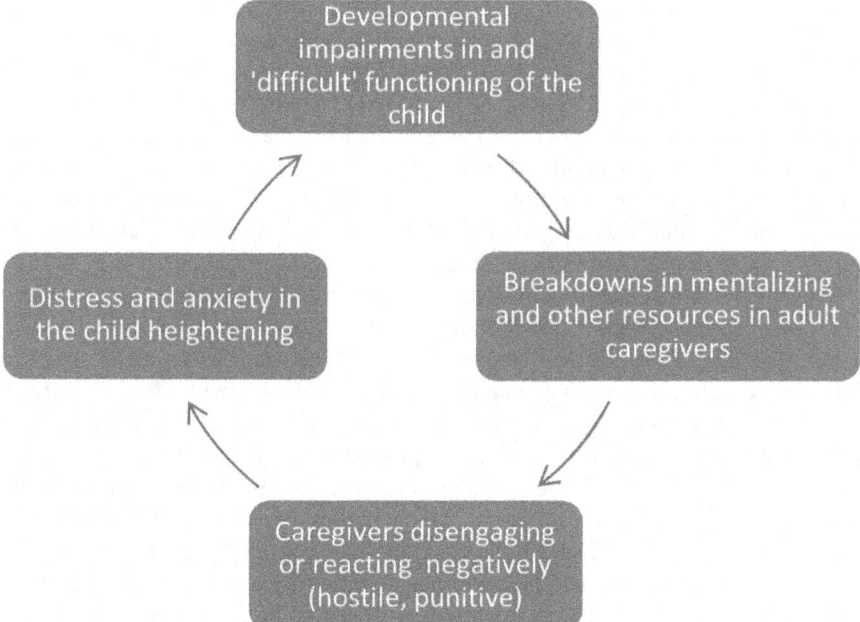

Figure 1.1 The vicious cycle among traumatised children's 'difficult' functioning and their adult carers' mentalizing abilities and well-being.

can lead to an increase of negative interactions and a decrease of shared positive and joyful moments. Caregivers' mentalizing skills may be profoundly challenged, leaving them with a feeling of being stuck in an action-reaction mode (e.g., 'We have to stop this behaviour', 'We cannot tolerate him being so rude') and with no space for thinking, communicating or interacting thoughtfully. The problem with this is that it keeps traumatised children from receiving what they so direly need in order to get back on a more adaptive developmental trajectory: parents and other caregiving adults who are willing and able to remain thoughtful even in the face of complex arousal-provoking situations.

Such difficulties may occur in the context of caring for any child who has experienced complex trauma, even with skilled and reflective caregivers. The risk of getting entangled in negative cycles is even greater for parents struggling with personal vulnerabilities due to unresolved negative or traumatising experiences in their own history. We will elaborate on the theoretical underpinnings of the impact of complex trauma on the child's environment in Chapter 3.

The diverse and complex mental health needs of traumatised children and their families

As discussed earlier, the development of children who have experienced complex trauma is hugely impacted, as are the well-being of and the relationships with important caregiving adults around these children. Moreover, these children's clinical presentation is often diverse and complex, with them being referred with different emotional, social and/or behavioural symptoms and, consequently, running the risk of being diagnosed with one or several 'symptom disorders', such as conduct disorder, attachment disorder, ADHD (Attention Deficit Hyperactivity Disorder), ASD (Autism Spectrum Disorder) and perhaps even (emerging) antisocial or borderline personality disorder. However well-intentioned, these labels seldom succeed in capturing the full picture of these children's developmental impairments – which we have come to understand as a response to complex traumatic experiences. Although the various 'symptom disorder' labels may at times be helpful to make sense of some aspect of the child, our and others' experience is that they do not always explain enough to inform an appropriate treatment approach (DeJong, 2010; Tarren-Sweeney, 2013). The main assessment challenge with these children is that their manifest behavioural problems often obscure the core issues underlying their developmental impairments. At the heart of many of these children's manifest behavioural problems lies an incapacity to regulate arousal and affect, as well as to engage in reciprocal and mutually satisfying relationships with adults and/or peers, which renders everyday life an emotional rollercoaster for the child and their environment. Similarly, their unpredictably fluctuating way of emotional and relational functioning leads to them often being considered as 'hard to reach' in treatment. They often belong to the proportion of children that easily drop out of therapy or are unable to make use of the available treatments (Fonagy et al., 2015).

Basic assumptions of a psychodynamic approach to the treatment of complex trauma

Since Boston and Szur's (1983) publication on psychotherapy with severely deprived children, a vast body of psychodynamic writings on aspects of therapeutic work with these children has emerged (Alvarez, 1992; Alvarez, 2012; Briggs, 2012, 2015; Emanuel, 2002; Hindle & Shulman, 2008; Kenrick et al., 2006; Lanyado, 2004, 2018; Lieberman & Van Horn, 2005; Music, 2019; Nathanson et al., 2022). This treatment guide thus draws on a long tradition of psychodynamic child psychotherapy literature and integrates it with contemporary mentalization-based principles and neuroscientific and other developmentally informed knowledge about the impact of trauma. In the following section, we discuss the four basic assumptions of a psychodynamic approach to the treatment of complex trauma in children (see Table 1.3).

Developmental perspective

Psychodynamic approaches are fundamentally developmental, in that they acknowledge and take into account the formative role of early life experiences and later psychic structures and behaviour (Luyten et al., 2015; Luyten et al., 2008). As such, psychodynamic approaches aim to understand as well as to explain both normal and disrupted development, with a focus on factors explaining developmental disruptions (Luyten et al., 2015). As alluded to in this chapter and elaborated on in Chapter 2, such a developmental psychopathology perspective (Fonagy et al., 2006; Freud, 1973; Lyons-Ruth & Jacobvitz, 2008; Mahler et al., 1975; Midgley, 2011) is of particular relevance in treating children who have experienced complex trauma. A profound understanding of the

Table 1.3 Basic assumptions of psychodynamic work with children with complex trauma

Developmental perspective	A developmental understanding of the impact of complex trauma on the child is central and forms the basis of a model of recovery and growth
Facilitating environment through mentalizing relationships	A context of positive, thoughtful adults, approaching the traumatised child as a subject, whose behaviour is rooted in an inner world of emotions, thoughts and experiences, is core to recovery and growth
Intervening at the level of both process and content	Effective treatment requires flexible and adequate balancing of interventions focused on process as well as on content
Play and playfulness at the heart of recovery	Playful interaction and play are considered the cardinal vehicles to therapeutic progress and change

multi-faceted/-layered and complex impact of adverse experiences early in life that have shaped the child's development – and how this interacts in complex ways with current environmental factors – is to be considered key to inform an effective treatment approach.

Scaffolding mentalizing relationships as the environment conducive to developmental recovery

One major insight about resilience and coping with trauma is the power of healthy relationships to protect from and heal following stress and trauma (Perry, 2009). The decision to place a child who cannot grow up in their family of origin in a new foster or adoptive family is not taken lightly. It is by definition the result of societal consideration and decision-making, family discussion and preparation. Evaluation and preparation of prospective foster carers and adoptive parents – however different in different countries – often constitute a period of intense inquiry. Rooted in the idea that these children, who have gone through adverse experiences in the early years of their life, are in high need of positive family experiences through which they can recover and develop in the best possible ways, society often sets high standards for foster carers and adoptive parents. For instance, research has emphasised the importance of a secure attachment state of mind in parents if they are going to manage the conflicting and vulnerable representations that these children bring with them into their new families (Levy & Orlans, 2003; Schofield & Beek, 2005). Moreover, due to underdeveloped mentalizing capacities and/or trauma-induced mentalizing breakdowns (Midgley et al., 2017c), children who have experienced complex trauma often feel unsure about their own world of feelings and intentions and misread others' intentions. As a result, moments of 'confusion, misunderstanding, and difficulties in interpersonal relating, contributing to escalating conflict or bottled up anger or fear' (Midgley et al., 2017a, p. 18) are common in families caring for these children. Therefore 'high quality parenting' (Pace et al., 2012, p. 47), as is required in an adoptive or foster family, may be understood as parents who can make use of a capacity to think about their own and their child's internal reality, i.e., who can keep their mentalizing capacities 'online', even in the face of arousal- and anxiety-provoking situations (Pace et al., 2014; Sharp et al., 2006; Steele et al., 2009).

As alluded to earlier, parenting a child who has experienced complex trauma severely challenges foster carers' and adoptive parents' mentalizing capacities. Beyond the normal fluctuations in mentalizing that all parents go through in ordinary family life (Midgley et al., 2017c), these parents are faced with behavioural problems, are searching for growth-promoting responses to difficult-to-understand behaviour and are often drawn into high-arousal and high-stress situations. As a consequence, they will frequently experience mentalizing breakdowns (Midgley et al., 2017c), which in turn may prove anxiety-provoking for parents who are highly aware of the importance of being able to remain curious about their child's – and their own – behaviours and experiences. This is often compounded by the fact that adoptive parents and foster carers have generally been through a preparation process before taking children into care and often have been selected for their parental skills. Finding themselves phantasising about 'simply' getting rid of their adopted or foster child, because this will 'free' them from all difficulties at once, may raise feelings of anxiety, shame or guilt. Other parents feel it is their responsibility to manage any issues or problems that may arise, rendering them more hesitant about reaching out for professional help. Such parents will almost try anything on their own before coming to consult. By the time they do consult, they are often exhausted or desperate and/or they face lengthy waiting lists. Hence, a key element in being able to maintain positive caregiving relationships in service of the child's developmental recovery and to refrain from getting caught in destructive experiences (Schechter & Willheim, 2009) is the creation of a mentalizing and trauma-informed network around parents of and families with children who have experienced complex trauma. Such a context will constitute the crucial backdrop against which a psychotherapeutic treatment of the individual child and their family can be delineated (see Figure 1.2). Therefore, the treatment model set out in this book involves a three-track approach, which will be introduced in Chapter 4 and discussed in depth in the remaining chapters of Part II.

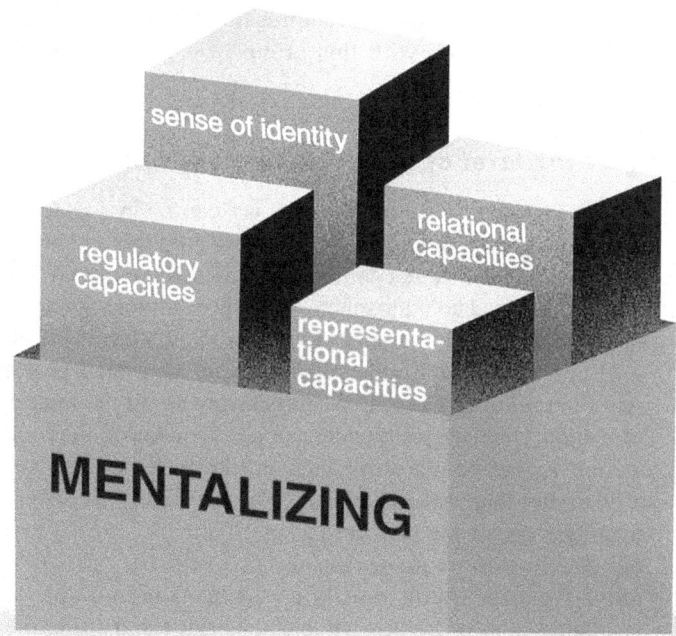

Figure 1.2 A mentalizing environment as a crucial backdrop for the child's developmental recovery.

A particularly considerate approach to relationships is needed when working with internationally adopted children and children placed in foster care. As people and systems coming from different (sub-)cultural backgrounds try to live and work together, a particular sensitivity and competence towards cultural differences and diversity seems warranted (Davis et al., 2018). For internationally adopted and foster children, their placement in a substitute family is inherently accompanied by the loss of continuity not only in their primary caregiving relationships but also in their culture of origin. Internationally adopted children find themselves in a strange country, with a different sensory world of smells, colours and tastes and with unknown cultural habits that seep through in every aspect of their new daily life. As such, they are often confronted with 'being different', for example, in skin colour from their adoptive parents and their peers at school but often also from the mental health professionals they encounter; in being the only adopted child in the family; in having to learn a new language and adapt to new cultural habits. Similarly, foster children are moved from one family, with its way of living, relating to one another and handling things, to another family, with expectedly its very own and different subculture of values and norms. Moreover, the consequences of early adverse experiences (e.g., having learning difficulties, lack of emotional and behavioural control) often make such children 'stand out' even more, compounding their struggle of feeling different, weird, mad or bad. This has major implications for these children's development of a sense of self and identity and thus requires the therapist to explicitly address issues of diversity in working with this group of children and the caregiving adults who surround them.

Intervening at the level of both process and content

 In the early phase of treatment, Lisa comes into a session with her jacket on, stating that she is 'not feeling cold though' and immediately walks over to the trunk containing the dress-up material and starts looking through it. The atmosphere is restless, almost agitated. Lisa refers to 'protection'; the therapist responds: 'You seem to be needing some protection today, I wonder who or what you need protection from'. After ten minutes or so, Lisa starts throwing all the material back into the trunk. The therapist ponders aloud: 'You know, the thing about protection is that people can't look in that well because you're kind of hidden, but then again, you can't look out that well either'. Following that, Lisa decides to take her jacket off and uses a cape to dress up as a bat. She moves around and speaks at a very fast pace. Lisa's play narrative twists and turns rapidly as she takes on multiple and suddenly switching roles of a bat, a witch and a princess, inciting the therapist to follow her lead.

Bervoets et al. (2021)

Child therapists might wonder what Lisa is trying to show here and what to focus their interventions on. Is Lisa trying to show what she thinks and feels about being in need of safety and protection, possibly linked to experiences in her life? Is she showing how her self-image can shift rapidly between a (bad) bat or witch and a (good) princess? Does Lisa then need help to explore her ideas and feelings and to understand where they stem from? Or is she still very much absorbed in a process of trying to think and express experiences about feeling unsafe and unprotected, which is so difficult to bear, as well as about being a bad bat girl or a good princess? Or still, is she falling prey to fragments of experiences, which she needs to 'rid' herself of without really knowing what is happening to her? And does she then primarily need help to bear the turmoil and withstand the undifferentiated and stormy agitation that makes up her inner world, not yet puzzled by the question what is happening to her and why? From a psychodynamic treatment approach, such as the one presented in this book, the answer would, uncontestably, be: all of the above, namely in a dynamic manner that is attuned as much as possible to 'where the child is at' at any one moment.

Since Mary Boston and Rolene Szur (1983) published their insights on psychodynamic work with severely deprived children, the complexity of working with traumatised children in psychodynamic psychotherapy has been well described by several authors (Alvarez, 1992; Alvarez, 2012; Briggs, 2012, 2015; Emanuel, 2002; Hindle & Shulman, 2008; Kenrick et al., 2006; Lanyado, 2004, 2018; Lieberman & Van Horn, 2005; Music, 2019; Nathanson et al., 2022). Much of this complexity stems from the immense impact complex traumatic experiences have on the themes that occupy these children's minds (content) as well as on the way they experience and process themes, events and relationships (process). In a psychodynamic approach, understanding the dynamics of a child's inner world of feelings and thoughts, both conscious and less conscious, as well as their relations to behaviour and symptoms is considered to be of major importance to be able to find new, more adaptive ways of feeling, thinking, behaving and relating. As such, psychodynamic treatment approaches have traditionally been focused on understanding and 'uncovering' what is at stake in the child's inner world. The content of traumatised children's thoughts and feelings may be about unsafety and the need for protection, or about being a bad or a good person, like in Lisa's case. More contemporary psychodynamically inspired perspectives, such as the mentalization-based framework, both build on and complement this body of knowledge, by explicitly adding a more process-oriented focus. A process focus with traumatised children involves the (in) ability to keep thinking, feeling and processing the content that often is hard to bear (e.g., keeping on a jacket, fluttering around in the room, experiencing fleeting thoughts and feelings). Balancing intervening at the level of the process and the content is a major principle in psychodynamic work with traumatised children (see Figure 1.3).

Mentalization-based frameworks define mentalizing as the ability to understand one's own and others' behaviours in terms of mental states, such as thoughts,

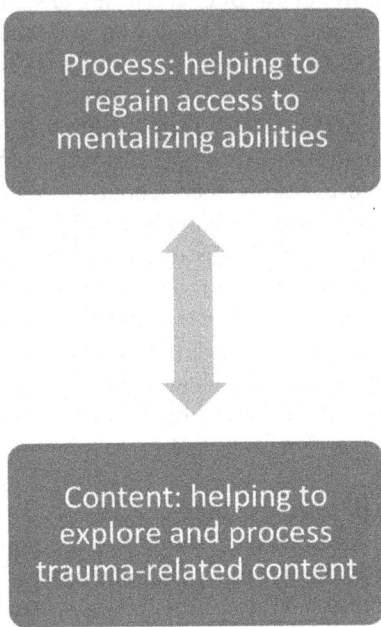

Figure 1.3 Balancing process and content in psychodynamic work with traumatised children.

desires, beliefs and anxieties and the capacity to guide one's own behaviour and predict others' behaviour accordingly (Fonagy et al., 2002). They contend that deficits or breakdowns in mentalizing are at the core of diverse severe developmental disturbances in affect regulation, attentional control and self-control, as manifested perhaps most clearly in trauma-related developmental psychopathology (Allen et al., 2008). As introduced earlier and discussed more in depth in Chapter 2, mentalizing capabilities in children with complex trauma are taxed in two ways. First, the development of mentalizing capacities has often been compromised, as it is impacted by the quality of the early caregiving environment (Camoirano, 2017; Kim, 2015; Luyten et al., 2017; Midgley et al., 2017a; Slade, 2005). The primary caregivers' capacity to accurately read the infant's mental states based on their bodily and behavioural signals and to communicate this understanding back to the infant in a timely and containing manner has consistently been shown to be key to healthy psychological development (Kim, 2015; Midgley et al., 2017a; Slade, 2005). Through processes of interpretation in the caregiver's mind and the subsequent containing communications from the caregiver to the infant, a sense of self in the young child can emerge, which forms the basis for the later development of mentalizing capacities. Being able to connect with who one is and what one feels or needs starts in such early caregiver-infant interactions. By definition, circumstances of complex traumatic experiences are situations of enduring or chronic breakdowns in the mentalizing attunement of a caregiving environment to a young child (Midgley et al., 2017c). Second, going through life with under-developed mentalizing capabilities, traumatised children often face intense, anxiety-provoking and overwhelming trauma-related thoughts and feelings that challenge these vulnerable mentalizing capabilities much more than most normatively developing children ever go through. The most vulnerable minds often live with the most challenging inner dynamics.

As mentalizing is a form of imaginative mental activity, crucially important for humans to successfully navigate our inherently social world (Fonagy et al., 2002), it is at the heart of psychotherapy. Processes of growth and change can only emerge in a mind that is able to open up to what is happening inside one's own mind as well as to what others (e.g., the therapist) bring to the fore. Therefore, a psychodynamic, mentalization-based treatment approach is based on the premise that fostering the (re-)emergence of mentalizing capacities – a clearly process-oriented focus – constitutes a fundamental mechanism in psychotherapeutic treatment (Allen et al., 2008) for two reasons. First, a mentalizing mind enables the child to focus in life, to benefit from growth-promoting relationships and thus to live a more construc-tive life. Second, a mentalizing mind is a prerequisite to experience and process traumatic experiences (content) without the risk of retraumatisation.

Because of the 'predictable unpredictability' of traumatised children's function-ing, expressed in rapidly fluctuating behaviour, effective treatment thus requires the therapist to flexibly and adequately adapt their interventions to the most press-ing needs of the child at any given time in therapy, whether it be process issues or content issues (Bervoets et al., 2021).

Play and playfulness at the heart of recovery from complex trauma

Additionally, and unique to psychodynamic work with children, is the central role of play and playfulness as a port of entry to the child's inner world and as a vehicle for processes of therapeutic change (e.g., Alvarez & Phillips, 1998; Slade, 1994). Win-nicott's (1971) work has been seminal in the acknowledgement of play as an impor-tant catalyst in and of development. In play, children express aspects of their inner worlds, processing and trying to gain control and mastery over their experiences; in play, children practise with roles in relation to others and to rules and values (Alva-rez & Phillips, 1998; Gaskill & Perry, 2014; Tessier et al., 2016). In this context, a child's inability to enter into a playful interaction or to play in an imaginative way is considered to be a sign of developmental disruption (Winnicott, 1971).

In psychodynamic child psychotherapy (Alvarez & Phillips, 1998) and more contemporary Mentalization-Based Treatment for Children (MBT-C; Midgley et al., 2017b), therapists capitalise on the range of opportunities for psycho-logical growth and transformation that play processes provide. In play-based ther-apy, children can practise or experiment with being in the presence of an adult and experiencing safety versus threat, experiencing positive and playful versus controlling and harsh interaction. In play, experiences can be played out in repetitive actions, session after session, while experiencing feelings of anxiety, pain or anger, as well as feelings of control within the safe and controllable relationship and environment offered by the therapist. Moreover, while playing, the child can imagine alternative plots to these experiences in a 'better' world, giving rise to a more positive view of oneself and the outside world. Observing the child's play, the therapist may learn to better understand how the child uses their mind to represent life events and transform them into emotional events, a personal version of the truth (Rustin, 1999).

In this regard, traditional psychodynamic approaches have considered 'pretend play' the place par excellence to discover the representational and symbolic aspects of inner experiences. What can be expressed in play or represented in visual or verbal symbols can be thought about and thus modulated. For instance, the unwanted extra spoon of food that would otherwise have been spat out can suddenly be perceived very differently and ingested when the caregiver pretends it is an airplane or 'a bite for Daddy'. Or in pretending to bake a cake, a two-year-old child discovers imagination and the power of make-believe. Similarly, a more contemporary mentalization-based perspective awards 'pretend play' a particularly important 'status' in child development, affording children opportunities to discover and learn to understand that mental and internal reality is distinct from – though related to – external reality. This is a developmental achievement that is crucial for mature, full-blown mentalizing capacities (Fonagy & Target, 1996a, 2000; see also Chapter 2), as expressed in the ability to 'play with reality' or to 'treat ideas as ideas' (Fonagy & Target, 1996a, 1996b).

In children who have experienced complex trauma, early traumatic circumstances have often interfered with the healthy development of play and, more broadly, representational and symbolising capacities (such as playing, drawing, and telling a story to verbalise experiences) (see also Chapter 2). The most severely disturbed of these children cannot play at all: they are unable to engage in any playful mutual interaction. In other traumatised children, play is inhibited or shows the particular overwhelming characteristics of 'traumatic play' (Chazan et al., 2016). With these children, play often remains empty or repetitive or is restricted to preparatory play activities: the doll house gets tidied up and cleaned, the scene is set, but the real play never begins. By shutting down processes of expressing and symbolising aspects of their inner world, these children protect themselves from psychic pain and anxiety.

In recent years, neuroscientific trauma literature has offered empirical support for play as vital for a process of change and healing (Gaskill & Perry, 2014). It points to three key elements of play which pave the way for effective therapeutic interventions for traumatised children. Play approximates a purposeful behaviour, fostering the child's perceived sense of control. Play is voluntary, pleasurable and has no immediate or obvious 'purpose' and can thus be experienced as rewarding by the child. Play takes place in a non-threatening, low-stress context and thus constitutes

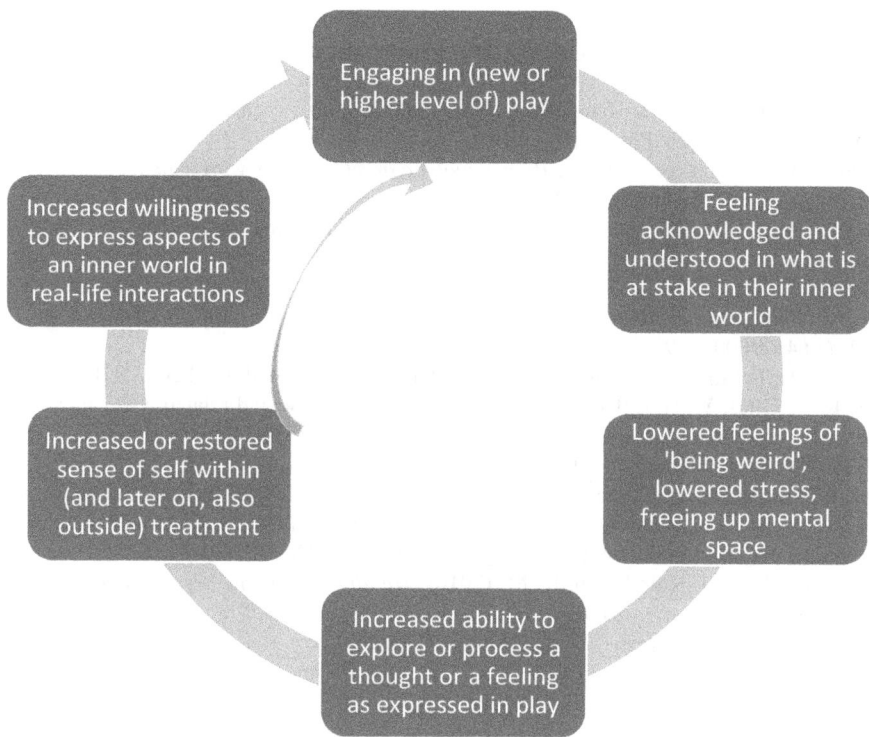

Figure 1.4 A broaden-and-build model of the child's growing capacity for playing with as well as in reality.

a manageable level of stress for the child. As such, play is an effective therapeutic agent when it provides a developmentally appropriate means to regulate, communicate, practise and master. It is important for growth and development, and the capacity to play is central to mental flexibility. Moreover, as trauma impairs the capacity to frame and reframe experiences (Luyten & Bateman, in press), helping a child to be able to enter a playful state and engage in playful interactions is of major importance to make experiences accessible for framing and reframing. As such, fostering the (re-)emergence of imaginative (pretend) play capacities as the core of developmental recovery – often first discernible in treatment but ideally, eventually transferring to real life – is at the centre of a contemporary psychodynamic treatment approach to children who have experienced complex trauma (see Figure 1.4).

These four basic assumptions, i.e., the importance of a developmental perspective, of mentalizing relationships, of balancing process and content and of play and playfulness, underpin the treatment approach set out in Part II of this book. How these assumptions have been operationalised into core features and basic principles of this three-track approach will be addressed in Chapter 4.

References

Allen, J. G. (2013). *Mentalizing in the development and treatment of attachment trauma.* Karnac.

Allen, J. G., Fonagy, P., & Bateman, A. W. (2008). *Mentalizing in mental health practice.* American Psychiatric Publishing.

Alvarez, A. (1992). *Live company. Psychoanalytic psychotherapy with autistic, borderline, deprived and abused children.* Routledge.

Alvarez, A. (2012). *The thinking heart: Three levels of psychoanalytic therapy with disturbed children.* Routledge.

Alvarez, A., & Phillips, A. (1998). The importance of play: A child psychotherapist's view. *Child Psychology and Psychiatry Review, 3*(3), 99–103. https://doi.org/10.1017/s1360641798001579

Anda, R. F., Felitti, V. J., Bremner, J. D., Walker, J. D., Whitfield, C., Perry, B. D., Dube, S. R., & Giles, W. H. (2006). The enduring effects of abuse and related adverse experiences in childhood. *European Archives of Psychiatry and Clinical Neuroscience, 256*(3), 174–186. https://doi.org/10.1007/s00406-005-0624-4

Bervoets, E., Meurs, P., Luyten, P., Tang, E., & Vliegen, N. (2021). Walking the tightrope: Ego support and exploration with a child with complex trauma. *Journal of Child Psychotherapy, 47*(3), 415–432. https://doi.org/10.1080/0075417X.2021.2014935

Blaustein, M. E., & Kinniburgh, K. M. (2010). *Treating traumatic stress in children and adolescents: How to foster resilience through attachment, self-regulation, and competency.* The Guilford Press.

Boston, M., & Szur, R. (Eds.). (1983). *Psychotherapy with severely deprived children.* Routledge & Kegan Paul.

Briggs, A. (2012). *Waiting to be found: Papers on children in care.* Karnac.

Briggs, A. (Ed.). (2015). *Towards belonging: Negotiating new relationships for adopted children and those in care.* Karnac.

Camoirano, A. (2017). Mentalizing makes parenting work: A review about parental reflective functioning and clinical interventions to improve it. *Frontiers in Psychology, 8,* 14. https://doi.org/10.3389/fpsyg.2017.00014

Caspi, A., Houts, R. M., Belsky, D. W., Harrington, H., Hogan, S., Ramrakha, S., Poulton, R., & Moffitt, T. E. (2016). Childhood forecasting of a small segment of the population with large economic burden. *Nature Human Behaviour, 1*(1), Article 0005. https://doi.org/10.1038/s41562-016-0005

Chazan, S., Kuchirko, Y., Beebe, B., & Sossin, K. M. (2016). A longitudinal study of traumatic play activity using the Children's Developmental Play Instrument (CDPI). *Journal of Infant, Child, and Adolescent Psychotherapy, 15*(1), 1–25.

Cicchetti, D., & Banny, A. (2014). A developmental psychopathology perspective on child maltreatment. In M. Lewis & K. D. Rudolph (Eds.), *Handbook of developmental psychopathology* (pp. 723–741). Springer. https://doi.org/10.1007/978-1-4614-9608-3_37

Cicchetti, D., & Toth, S. L. (2009). The past achievements and future promises of developmental psychopathology: The coming of age of a discipline. *Journal of Child Psychology and Psychiatry, 50*(1–2), 16–25. https://doi.org/10.1111/j.1469-7610.2008.01979.x

Davis, D. E., DeBlaere, C., Owen, J., Hook, J. N., Rivera, D. P., Choe, E., Van Tongeren, D. R., Worthington, E. L., & Placeres, V. (2018). The multicultural orientation framework: A narrative review. *Psychotherapy, 55*(1), 89–100. https://doi.org/10.1037/pst0000160

DeJong, M. (2010). Some reflections on the use of psychiatric diagnosis in the looked after or "in care" child population. *Clinical Child Psychology and Psychiatry, 15*(4), 589–599. https://doi.org/10.1177/1359104510377705

Emanuel, L. (2002). Deprivation x 3. *Journal of Child Psychotherapy, 28*(2), 163–179. https://doi.org/10.1080/00754170210143771

Esposito, E. A., & Gunnar, M. R. (2014). Early deprivation and developmental psychopathology. In M. Lewis & K. D. Rudolph (Eds.), *Handbook of developmental psychopathology* (pp. 371–388). Springer. https://doi.org/10.1007/978-1-4614-9608-3_19

Fonagy, P., Gergely, G., Jurist, E., & Target, M. (2002). *Affect regulation, mentalization, and the development of the self.* Other Press.

Fonagy, P., Luyten, P., & Allison, E. (2015). Epistemic petrification and the restoration of epistemic trust: A new conceptualization of borderline personality disorder and its psychosocial treatment. *Journal of Personality Disorders, 29*(5), 575–609. https://doi.org/10.1521/pedi.2015.29.5.575

Fonagy, P., & Target, M. (1996a). Playing with reality: I. Theory of mind and the normal development of psychic reality. *International Journal of Psycho-Analysis, 77,* 217–233.

Fonagy, P., & Target, M. (1996b). Playing with reality: II. The development of psychic reality from a theoretical perspective. *International Journal of Psycho-Analysis, 77,* 459–479.

Fonagy, P., & Target, M. (2000). Playing with reality: III. The persistence of dual psychic reality in borderline patients. *International Journal of Psycho-Analysis, 81*(5), 853–873.

Fonagy, P., Target, M., & Gergely, G. (2006). Psychoanalytic perspectives on developmental psychopathology. In D. Cicchetti & D. J. Cohen (Eds.), *Developmental psychopathology: Vol. 1. Theory and method* (2nd ed., pp. 701–749). John Wiley & Sons, Inc.

Freud, A. (1973). *The writings of Anna Freud, Vol. III: Infants without families. Reports on the Hampstead Nurseries (1939–1945).* International Universities Press.

Gaskill, R., & Perry, B. (2014). The neurobiological power of play. Using the neurosequential model of therapeutics to guide play in the healing process. In C. A. Malchiodi & D. A. Crenshaw (Eds.), *Creative arts and play therapy for attachment problems* (pp. 178–194). The Guilford Press.

Hindle, D., & Shulman, G. (Eds.). (2008). *The emotional experience of adoption: A psychoanalytic perspective.* Routledge.

Juffer, F., Palacios, J., Le Mare, L., Sonuga-Barke, E. J. S., Tieman, W., Bakermans-Kranenburg, M. J., Vorria, P., van IJzendoorn, M. H., & Verhulst, F. C. (2011). II. Development of adopted children with histories of early adversity. *Monographs of the Society for Research in Child Development, 76*(4), 31–61. https://doi.org/10.1111/j.1540-5834.2011.00627.x

Kenrick, J., Lindsey, C., & Tollemache, L. (Eds.). (2006). *Creating new families: Therapeutic approaches to fostering, adoption, and kinship care.* Karnac.

Kim, S. (2015). The mind in the making: Developmental and neurobiological origins of mentalizing. *Personality Disorders: Theory, Research, and Treatment, 6*(4), 356–365. https://doi.org/10.1037/per0000102

Koss, K. J., & Gunnar, M. R. (2018). Annual research review: Early adversity, the hypothalamic-pituitary-adrenocortical axis, and child psychopathology. *Journal of Child Psychology and Psychiatry, 59*(4), 327–346. https://doi.org/10.1111/jcpp.12784

Lanyado, M. (2004). *The presence of the therapist: Treating childhood trauma.* Brunner-Routledge.

Lanyado, M. (2018). *Transforming despair to hope: Reflections on the psychotherapeutic process with severely neglected and traumatised children.* Routledge.

Leve, L. D., Harold, G. T., Chamberlain, P., Landsverk, J. A., Fisher, P. A., & Vostanis, P. (2012). Practitioner review: Children in foster care – vulnerabilities and evidence-based interventions that promote resilience processes. *Journal of Child Psychology and Psychiatry*, *53*(12), 1197–1211. https://doi.org/10.1111/j.1469-7610.2012.02594.x

Levy, T. M., & Orlans, M. (2003). Creating and repairing attachments in biological, adoptive, and foster families. In S. M. Johnson & V. E. Whiffen (Eds.), *Attachment processes in couple and family therapy* (pp. 165–190). The Guilford Press.

Lieberman, A. F., & Van Horn, P. (2005). *Don't hit my mommy!: A manual for child-parent psychotherapy with young witnesses of family violence*. Zero To Three.

Luyten, P., & Bateman, A. (in press). In A. Bateman, P. Fonagy, C. Campbell, M. Debbané, & P. Luyten (Eds.), *The Cambridge guide to mentalization-based treatment*. Cambridge University Press.

Luyten, P., Mayes, L. C., Blatt, S. J., Target, M., & Fonagy, P. (2015). Theoretical and empirical foundations of contemporary psychodynamic approaches. In P. Luyten, L. C. Mayes, P. Fonagy, M. Target, & S. J. Blatt (Eds.), *Handbook of psychodynamic approaches to psychopathology* (pp. 3–26). The Guilford Press.

Luyten, P., Nijssens, L., Fonagy, P., & Mayes, L. C. (2017). Parental reflective functioning: Theory, research, and clinical applications. *The Psychoanalytic Study of the Child*, *70*(1), 174–199. https://doi.org/10.1080/00797308.2016.1277901

Luyten, P., Vliegen, N., Van Houdenhove, B., & Blatt, S. J. (2008). Equifinality, multifinality, and the rediscovery of the importance of early experiences. *The Psychoanalytic Study of the Child*, *63*(1), 27–60. https://doi.org/10.1080/00797308.2008.11800798

Lyons-Ruth, K., & Jacobvitz, D. (2008). Attachment disorganization: Genetic factors, parenting contexts, and developmental transformation from infancy to adulthood. In J. Cassidy & P. R. Shaver (Eds.), *Handbook of attachment: Theory, research, and clinical applications* (2nd ed., pp. 666–697). The Guilford Press.

Mahler, M. S., Pine, F., & Bergman, A. (1975). *The psychological birth of the human infant: symbiosis and individuation*. Basic Books.

McCrory, E. J., Gerin, M. I., & Viding, E. (2017). Annual research review: Childhood maltreatment, latent vulnerability and the shift to preventative psychiatry – The contribution of functional brain imaging. *Journal of Child Psychology and Psychiatry*, *58*(4), 338–357. https://doi.org/10.1111/jcpp.12713

Midgley, N. (2011). Test of time: Anna Freud's normality and pathology in childhood (1965). *Clinical Child Psychology and Psychiatry*, *16*(3), 475–482.

Midgley, N., Ensink, K., Lindqvist, K., Malberg, N., & Muller, N. (2017a). The development of mentalizing. In *Mentalization-based treatment for children. A time-limited approach* (pp. 15–37). American Psychological Association.

Midgley, N., Ensink, K., Lindqvist, K., Malberg, N., & Muller, N. (2017b). *Mentalization-based treatment for children. A time-limited approach*. American Psychological Association.

Midgley, N., Ensink, K., Lindqvist, K., Malberg, N., & Muller, N. (2017c). When the capacity for mentalizing is underdeveloped or breaks down. In *Mentalization-based treatment for children. A time-limited approach* (pp. 39–60). American Psychological Association.

Music, G. (2019). *Nurturing children. From trauma to growth using attachment theory, psychoanalysis and neurobiology*. Routledge.

Nathanson, A., Music, G., & Sternberg, J. (Eds.). (2022). *From trauma to harming others. Therapeutic work with delinquent, violent and sexually harmful children and young people*. Routledge.

National Scientific Council on the Developing Child. (2004). *Young children develop in an environment of relationships: Working Paper No. 1*. Retrieved from https://developing-child.harvard.edu/wp-content/uploads/2004/04/Young-Children-Develop-in-an-Environ-ment-of-Relationships.pdf

Pace, C. S., Cavanna, D., Velotti, P., & Cesare Zavattini, G. (2014). Attachment representations in late-adopted children: The use of narrative in the assessment of disorganisation, mentalising and coherence of mind. *Adoption & Fostering, 38*(3), 255–270. https://doi.org/10.1177/0308575914543235

Pace, C. S., Zavattini, G. C., & D'Alessio, M. (2012). Continuity and discontinuity of attachment patterns: A short-term longitudinal pilot study using a sample of late-adopted children and their adoptive mothers. *Attachment & Human Development, 14*(1), 45–61. https://doi.org/10.1080/14616734.2012.636658

Palacios, J., & Brodzinsky, D. M. (2010). Review: Adoption research: Trends, topics, outcomes. *International Journal of Behavioral Development, 34*(3), 270–284. https://doi.org/10.1177/0165025410362837

Perry, B. D. (2009). Examining child maltreatment through a neurodevelopmental lens: Clinical applications of the neurosequential model of therapeutics. *Journal of Loss and Trauma, 14*(4), 240–255. https://doi.org/10.1080/15325020903004350

Rustin, M. (1999). Multiple families in mind. *Clinical Child Psychology and Psychiatry, 4*(1), 51–62. https://doi.org/10.1177/1359104599004001005

Schechter, D. S., & Willheim, E. (2009). When parenting becomes unthinkable: Intervening with traumatized parents and their toddlers. *Journal of the American Academy of Child and Adolescent Psychiatry, 48*(3), 249–253. https://doi.org/10.1097/CHI.0b013e3181948ff1

Schofield, G., & Beek, M. (2005). Providing a secure base: Parenting children in long-term foster family care. *Attachment & Human Development, 7*(1), 3–26. https://doi.org/10.1080/14616730500049019

Schore, A. (2009). Attachment trauma and the developing right brain: Origins of pathological dissociation. In P. Dell & J. O'Neil (Eds.), *Dissociation and the dissociative disorders. DSM-V and beyond* (pp. 107–141). Routledge.

Sharp, C., Fonagy, P., & Goodyer, I. M. (2006). Imagining your child's mind: Psychosocial adjustment and mothers' ability to predict their children's attributional response styles. *British Journal of Developmental Psychology, 24*(1), 197–214. https://doi.org/10.1348/026151005x82569

Slade, A. (1994). Making meaning and making believe: Their role in the clinical process. In A. Slade & D. P. Wolf (Eds.), *Children at play: Clinical and developmental approaches to meaning and representation* (pp. 81–107). Oxford University Press.

Slade, A. (2005). Parental reflective functioning: An introduction. *Attachment & Human Development, 7*(3), 269–281. https://doi.org/10.1080/14616730500245906

Steele, M., Hodges, J., Kaniuk, J., & Steele, H. (2009). Mental representation and change: Developing attachment relationships in an adoption context. *Psychoanalytic Inquiry, 30*(1), 25–40. https://doi.org/10.1080/07351690903200135

Tarren-Sweeney, M. (2013). The Brief Assessment Checklists (BAC-C, BAC-A): Mental health screening measures for school-aged children and adolescents in foster, kinship, residential and adoptive care. *Children and Youth Services Review, 35*(5), 771–779. https://doi.org/10.1016/j.childyouth.2013.01.025

Tessier, V. P., Normandin, L., Ensink, K., & Fonagy, P. (2016). Fact or fiction? A longitudinal study of play and the development of reflective functioning. *Bulletin of the Menninger Clinic, 80*(1), 60–79. https://doi.org/10.1521/bumc.2016.80.1.60

van der Kolk, B. A., Pynoos, R. S., Cicchetti, D., Cloitre, M., D'Andrea, W., Ford, J. D., Lieberman, A. F., Putnam, F. W., Saxe, G., Spinazzola, J., Stolbach, B. C., & Teicher, M. (2009). *Proposal to include a developmental trauma disorder diagnosis for children and adolescents in DSM-V.* Retrieved from https://complextrauma.org/wp-content/uploads/2019/03/Complex-Trauma-Resource-3-Joseph-Spinazzola.pdf

Vliegen, N., Tang, E., & Meurs, P. (2023). *Children recovering from complex trauma: From wound to scar.* Routledge.

Welsh, J. A., Viana, A. G., Petrill, S. A., & Mathias, M. D. (2007). Interventions for internationally adopted children and families: A review of the literature. *Child and Adolescent Social Work Journal, 24*(3), 285–311. https://doi.org/10.1007/s10560-007-0085-x

Winnicott, D. W. (1971). *Playing and reality.* Tavistock Publications.

Chapter 2

Complex trauma and profound disruptions in four domains of child development

In normal development, emotional and relational capacities emerge in the context of early caregiving relationships. Infants are hardwired to engage in social interaction from birth onwards. In good-enough circumstances, the process of developing intrapsychic and interpersonal capacities is part and parcel of ordinary parent-child interactions. As such, day-to-day good-enough interactive experiences with primary caregivers not only result in secure mental representations of self and other in the child but also provide the child with ample opportunity to learn about the links between mental states and behaviours that scaffold the development of mentalizing capacities (Allen et al., 2008; Fonagy & Allison, 2012; Midgley et al., 2017a). However, in the context of complex trauma, early adverse experiences interfere with the development of intrapsychic and interpersonal capacities that are critically needed for adaptive development later in life. In this regard, contemporary neuroscientific findings have informed us how trauma-induced vulnerability in the neurobiological circuitry implicated in stress and affect regulation may lead to considerable regulation problems, which, in turn, may set in motion a cascade of social-emotional and behavioural difficulties (for recent reviews, see e.g., Koss & Gunnar, 2018; McCrory et al., 2017). As such, early adverse experiences have been found to disrupt normal patterns and processes of development in four important domains: representational capacities, affective development and affect regulation strategies, attachment development and relational capacities and sense of self and identity.

In this chapter, we elaborate on the theoretical underpinning of each of these domains. For ease of presentation, we discuss each of these domains and how these are impacted by complex traumatic experiences separately, but as will become apparent, in reality, these developmental domains are of course interwoven. In Part II of this treatment guide, we will outline how the knowledge about the impact of complex trauma on these four developmental domains runs as the main common thread throughout the treatment model. Moreover, we will outline how the therapist may address problems in each of these four domains through direct work with the child, work with the parents/carers and work with the broader network caring for the child.

DOI: 10.4324/9781003044918-4

Representational capacities as expressed in play and narrative

As discussed in Chapter 1, playing, drawing and talking about their inner world helps children to process experiences, feelings and thoughts. Play is the child's primary way of dealing with experience by creating model situations and of mastering reality by experiment and planning (Erikson, 1940). As such, play has been argued to be the primary vehicle for enhancing mentalizing processes in children (Midgley et al., 2017b; Tessier et al., 2016). The capacity to represent inner experiences in an imaginative way in some form of play or narrative develops in the context of caregiving relationships (see Table 2.1). Early on in life, there is no awareness of mental states as underlying goal-directed behaviour. In this so-called teleological mode, there is only (motor) action leading to an immediate result.

Table 2.1 Definition and expressions of pre-/non-mentalizing modes

Pre-mentalizing mode	Definition	Expression in normal development	Expression in pathological development
Teleological mode	Mental states are expressed in goal-directed actions	Infant expecting an immediate solution when experiencing something negative (e.g., hunger, cold, boredom)	Child expecting the carer/therapist to solve a problem or a negative affect immediately, is demanding and controlling and becomes angry and frustrated when the other doesn't solve the negativity here and now
Psychic equivalence mode	Reality is equated with mental states	Infant or toddler convinced they have bad parents, because they experience something negative (e.g., shouting 'bad Mum' when having to wait, feeling pain, being told 'no')	Child convinced the carer/therapist is a bad person and only has bad intentions when the other does something that elicits a negative feeling (e.g., setting a boundary, ending a treatment session); overwhelmingly negative and destructive play
Pretend mode	Mental states are decoupled from reality	A toddler or pre-schooler engaging in play, without being aware of the flexible link between the play content and aspects of external reality	Child losing themselves in play, rigidly holding on to staying in the 'play' and not being able to make use of play to process aspects of reality (play as an escape from reality)

For example, the infant experiences that a problem is resolved on the spot: 'when I cry, Mum picks me up'. Later on, an awareness of mental states emerges, but these 'are not felt to be representations but, rather, direct replicas of reality, and consequently always true' (Fonagy et al., 2002, p. 259); the young child is said to function in a 'psychic equivalence mode'. For example, the infant is imagined to be thinking 'When Mummy puts me to bed leaving me all alone, she is awful wholly and truly'.

As a result of cognitive and emotional development in a scaffolding and playful environment, a new, more representational way of experiencing psychic reality develops, i.e., the 'pretend mode' emerges, in the second and third year of life. The child is aware of inner experiences and mental states and is fully engaging with these in make-believe play and stories, i.e., 'pretend play'. However, in this mode of functioning, the toddler is not yet able to link their pretend play world to features of external reality. For example, playing doctor and wanting Dad to pretend crying in anxious anticipation of the vaccine shot does not help the child yet to reflect on their own anxiety or to be less anxious about the next time they need to be vaccinated. The absence of a flexible link between 'pretend' and 'real' in this pretend mode of functioning becomes clearly visible when an adult, observing the child's play, comments on it from external reality (e.g., 'Oh, was this what you felt when we were at the doctor's?'). Then, often, the child's play will break down, as the 'suspension of disbelief' has been broken.

Around the age of four, facilitated by and embedded in language and narrative development, the 'integrative mode' develops. At this level of psychic functioning, the child is conscious of mental states *as mental states*: they understand that elements of their inner world map onto – yet do not coincide with – features of external reality and vice versa. This enables the child to flexibly alternate between pretend play and real life. Consequently, pretend play can serve to fulfil wishes ('I'm building a round house, so Mum can't make me stand in a corner to punish me'), to express thoughts and feelings ('I'm a big girl now, but I can pretend I'm still a baby that needs to be taken care of'), to practise with gender and other life roles ('Today, I am a boy, a doctor, a teacher') and to learn to consider thoughts as thoughts ('I feel like hitting my annoying little sister, but I won't, otherwise I'll get in trouble'). As such, pretend play not only offers a window into the child's mind but constitutes a prerequisite for mental processing. In pretend play, toys or persons can be used as if they were something or someone else and be part of imaginary stories which help to master and process experiences. Moreover, in the integrative mode, the child becomes able to give words to experiences: they can talk about what happened in external reality but also about how that affected them internally (e.g., 'We went to Aunt Maggie, and I was afraid of the dog, but Granny took my hand and said the dog really loves children. So, I petted the dog. He really is a sweet dog, you have to see him!'). As such, these early years of life in good-enough circumstances offer ample opportunity for the child to develop representational capacities as crucially important precursors of later mentalizing capacities.

Children who have experienced complex trauma are often compromised in these abilities to use play, visual symbols and language to make sense of their emotional experiences. As stated by Slade (1994, p. 89) 'living in a chaotic emotional universe [that], by virtue of its very disorganization, precludes disguise because it precludes symbolization'. For severely disturbed children, playing, drawing and talking about inner experiences, affects and states 'can make them seem more real than they already are' (Slade, 1994, p. 89), comparable to how infants experience the world in a psychic equivalent mode. In case of complex trauma, language does not aid in containing and processing difficult feelings 'but instead amplifies the sense of lack of control that results from the failure to separate language from action and actuality' (Slade, 1994, p. 89). As such, the inability to play is considered as a mental processing impairment, requiring intervention to bring to life unutilised and inhibited mental processes (Fonagy et al., 1993).

As introduced in Chapter 1, impaired play in traumatised children can take various forms. Some children are unable to play at all, unable to be in the presence of someone else in a playful way. Such children haven't developed the mental openness, the peace or the trust in the other, to participate in playful interactions. Other children's play is considered 'traumatic play' (Chazan et al., 2016), characterised by tediously repetitive feelings and/or narratives. The traumatised child's play activity appears constricted, mechanistic and inhibited to an extreme extent, or it results in disorganisation (Chazan et al., 2016). In such traumatic play, aggressive and even sadistic themes occur alongside themes of rescue or reparation. This kind of play often proves ineffective in processing difficult experiences, as it stands in the way of a truly constructive resolution.

Several processes involved in complex trauma underlie the inability to play freely, coherently or meaningfully: (a) a profound lack of experiences of being treated as a mental agent; (b) being overwhelmed by negative experiences, which may be unthinkable and unplayable for the child and (c) trauma triggers entering play activity, which render play unsafe and anxiety-provoking.

A profound lack of experiences of being treated as a mental agent

Lisa nearly died as a baby due to parental neglect, and only after several kinship foster placement breakdowns has she been placed with her current (non-kinship) foster family. In a court-ordered visit with her biological mother, supervised by a child psychotherapist, Mother has brought her baby brother along. When the therapist says hello to her baby brother and asks how he is doing, this is met by Lisa's puzzled look and uneasy giggles, as she says in a high-pitched voice: 'What are you doing? He doesn't understand what you're saying, he's too small, right?'

A precondition for the development of representational abilities lies in the earliest experiences of being addressed by primary caregivers as an individual with one's own inner world and mental life. Growing up in the context of essentially positive and mentalizing relationships engages the infant in myriad processes that scaffold early representational capacities via ordinary family discourse (e.g., 'You must have felt very angry') and playful interactions (e.g., 'Are you so upset because you have to go to bed? Shall we play horsey on the way up to your bedroom?'). Long before a child can talk or play about how external experiences and events impact upon their inner world and vice versa, they are addressed as a feeling, thinking and knowing individual. Within such a mentalizing environment, early notions of what bodily sensations, such as warmth, cold or hunger, mean can emerge, as well as first gestures to express a need or longing (e.g., for a cookie or being carried) and first words to verbalise an intention (e.g., 'go walk', 'no'). For nine-year-old Lisa, however, it is a new and surprising experience to witness someone treating her baby brother as having his own inner world that is worthwhile to try to address. This is puzzling in a curious but somewhat uncomfortable way for Lisa because growing up with her biological parents she rarely experienced being treated as a mental agent by them.

In social environments characterised by early adversity (e.g., abuse or neglect), caregivers less often engage their children in emotional discussions; they are impaired in their capacity to understand their children's expression of affect and consequently are less accurate in their reflections of the child's mental states (Edwards et al., 2005; Ensink et al., 2015; Shipman & Zeman, 2001). Hence, the child grows up without having experienced the benefits of an adult reflecting accurately and thoughtfully on their inner world, impeding the development of skills to represent, express and mentalize feelings and thoughts. Early adversity and early trauma can thus be argued to be incompatible with mentalizing the child's experience and to compromise the development of mentalizing (Allen, 2013; Ensink et al., 2015). As such, in the presence of undifferentiated or unpredictable parents, the child is unable to identify and represent what is at stake in their own world and to find ways to express themselves in a genuine and appropriate way in play, drawing or narratives. Due to the discontinuities in their early caregiving relationships, children who have experienced complex trauma usually have had less consistent scaffolding opportunities regarding representational capacities as a basis for later mentalizing (Fonagy, 2000; Fonagy & Luyten, 2009; Midgley et al., 2017c).

Being left behind with what is unthinkable and unplayable

During the assessment, the therapist gets to know Mei-Lan as a child who exhibits extremely disruptive behaviour in situations that make her anxious and who is overwhelmed by nightmares night after night. When the therapist invites Mei-Lan to make a drawing, she answers forcefully: 'But you don't understand, I can't draw! I can only copy, because I don't have any imagination. Can you give me something I can copy?'

From early on in life, the continuous stream of internal and external stimuli of everyday life confronts infants with arousal and affective states which they cannot make sense of themselves (yet). For mental representations and meaning-making to emerge, infants are in need of primary caregivers' ability for what Bion (2002) has called 'containment'. Containment refers to the caregivers' willingness and capacity to receive, bear and give meaning to the unbearable mental content, which can then be returned to the child in a more manageable form (Bott Spillius et al., 2011).

Having been subjected to neglect of basic needs and/or maltreatment interferes with the acquisition of representational skills in several ways. First, early adverse experiences that are not acknowledged or named become stored in pre-verbal, procedural memory. This leaves the child literally without words to process these experiences. Consequently, the child falls victim to the inner terror of unprocessed experiences. In an attempt to lock out experiences, feelings and thoughts that are too hard to bear, the psychological capacities of thinking, imagining, dreaming and phantasising then get shut down. As such, a child's inability to mentalize may in fact include an active (though often unconscious) avoidance to mentalize: 'a form of decoupling, inhibition, or even a phobic reaction to mentalizing' (Fonagy & Allison, 2012, p. 17). This often manifests as rigid mental functioning, as expressed in Fish-Murray et al.'s (1987) finding that 'the inflexibility of organized schemata's and structures in all domains' (p. 101) was the strongest effect of abuse on children's thinking. In the earlier vignette, Mei-Lan's anxious reaction to the therapist's invitation to draw whatever comes to mind can be understood as an incapability as well as an active attempt to avoid being potentially overwhelmed by the unbearable contents that have settled in her mind as a result of having been repeatedly subjected to parental neglect in childhood. Third, children who have experienced complex trauma have often been confronted with a 'reflective discourse' that is not congruent with their feelings, such as a parent describing them as 'naughty' when actually they may be frightened or confused. Children who were involved in violent or sexually charged interactions with their primary caregiver(s) have been subjected at a far too early age to an intensification of complex feelings of aggression or sexual arousal that at the same time were mirrored inadequately or even intentionally named wrongly. Abusive caregivers may even have used language to actively deny what is happening or 'to attack and disorganize rather than to facilitate emotional communication, language then functions to increase conflict and further disrupt relations' (Slade, 1994, p. 90).

As such, continuous misattunement to or inadequate reading or mirroring of the child's affective states reduces the child's ability to understand and mentalize verbal explanations of their own and other people's actions. Such children are likely to struggle to accurately identify mental states underlying actions. What remains in the child's inner world are experiences of being overwhelmed and left alone, a sense of being aroused beyond bearable limits and thresholds, threatening the child's emergent sense of self and basic trust in relationships. Such undigested traumatic experiences stored as memory traces may subsequently act as trauma triggers, which can be acted out in behaviour barely comprehensible to the child or well-intentioned, new caregivers around the child (see later).

From this perspective, it makes perfectly good sense that children like Mei-Lan hold off the images in their mind and revert to copying an image that is much less threatening. In this sense, 'inhibitions of play' form part of an inhibition of the exploration of thoughts and feelings, and play remains restricted to empty or repetitive play or to preparatory play activities in order to protect oneself from psychic pain and anxiety. However adaptive to the original early adverse circumstances, these self-protective measures are often to no avail: they seldom prove effective in the long run and become maladaptive when the caregiving environment has changed for the better, for instance, in foster or adoptive care.

Trauma triggers rendering play unsafe and anxiety-provoking

 Once Mei-Lan is engaged in drawing, copying an image of a banana from a card she and her therapist found in the therapy room, she starts talking about why drawing is so difficult for her. She says: 'When I start to draw and to imagine, nightmare-like images come to my mind, like my dad changing into a zombie, or me playing tennis with a guinea pig. . . . It really scares me a lot, when I don't know what I have to draw'.

Beyond the anxiously guarded rigidity, nightmare-like terror often lurks around the corner for children who have experienced complex trauma. When the child's vigilance eases and they dare to engage in play, drawing or talking, often painful, terrorising and traumatising experiences forcefully penetrate their psychic shield. The child may suddenly find themselves reliving or even re-enacting aspects of an adverse experience. When play is possible, it is often characterised by high levels of disorganisation and destruction. Excessive arousal leads to inhibition, regression and catastrophic play (Desmarais, 2006).

This kind of play is disturbing to the child because it is accompanied by feelings of anxiety, distress and pain but also to the carers witnessing this play. In a qualitative study of how parents of late-adopted children perceived parent-child play (Desmarais, 2006), one of the emerging themes was 'play as frustration: a field of parental avoidance': parents admitted to feelings of discomfort and distress when observing the level of destructiveness in their children's play. It is hard for parents and other caregivers to empathically witness the disorganised form and the destructive content of these children's play. Moreover, they do not feel eager to engage in play with their child and often feel unsure about how to react. Sometimes they unwittingly attempt to forbid the child to handle the dolls so rudely or ignore the child's destruction of a drawing that was originally created with so much attention and pleasure. However understandable such reactions from parents, children whose early caregiving environment was unsuccessful in treating them as mental agents direly need an adult who is able and willing to mentalize their difficult affects and experiences. As long as traumatic memories and experiences – and the accompanying difficult affects – remain tucked away in procedural memory, they will fail to connect or transfer to 'processable' memories or thoughts that can be represented in words or play (Modell, 1996, 2008). And these traumatic memory traces will have no other way out than to be compulsively repeated as if they are occurring in the present. It is only when children who have experienced complex trauma can be helped to process their traumatic memories at a symbolised and mentalized level that more adaptive functioning and development can emerge. The fact that Mei-Lan, in the previous vignette, can begin to reflect on what happens to her when she starts to draw is itself a hopeful sign of this process starting to take place.

Taken together, the specific vulnerabilities and the fluctuations in capacities and levels of play and other forms of representation that characterise traumatised children require specific attention in psychotherapy. These children are in need of a therapeutic space in which their play can become the scene for connecting to inner experience 'in order to master it or omnipotently reinvent it, or, more hopefully, to procure a renewed experience in which the failure situation will be able to be unfrozen and re-experienced' (Desmarais, 2006, p. 351). In this context, parents/carers and other caregiving adults will need to be helped to understand (e.g., through trauma-informed psycho-education) as well as to bear – often for a long time – these children's impairments in the capacity to represent and communicate in constructive ways about what is at stake in their inner world.

Affective development and regulation strategies

Although negative and potentially overwhelming experiences are part and parcel of every young child's development, good-enough parents quickly learn to know their baby by meticulous observation of small signs and signals expressing the child's state of arousal and affect and to use this knowledge to co-regulate: 'When she gets upset, she loves to be wrapped up in her blanket. That calms her down', 'When he is screaming that intensely, you better wait to give him his bottle, otherwise he will just throw up'. Regulation evolves from a substantial contribution of the primary caregivers monitoring and responding to the child's needs, states and emotions, with the child participating to the best of their ability, to increasing self-regulatory abilities in the child. Helpful processes in this gradual development of self-regulatory capacities are the parents' capacities to provide a containing response in an accurate and timely manner, thereby fostering the development of the child's representation of affect, the child's sense of agency and mastery and the child's ability to express affective experiences in words and to process difficult feelings and anxieties (Fonagy et al., 2002).

Children who have experienced complex trauma are often compromised in their development of affect regulation strategies and defence mechanisms. Regulation strategies and defence mechanisms refer to psychological strategies that a person has developed to protect themselves from anxiety that arises from difficult or unacceptable thoughts or feelings (Lingiardi & Bornstein, 2017). In case of children who have experienced complex trauma, these strategies have remained of a rather primary level in an attempt to adapt to their early adverse environment. Yet, these primary affect regulation strategies (fight-flight-freeze) make them vulnerable to intense, often lifelong regulation problems: their inner world often feels like an emotional rollercoaster, with their emotional life's temperature switching rapidly back and forth between freezing and boiling point. 'Following a history of early deprivation, even mild stress later in life can elicit severe reactivity and dysfunction' (Cook et al., 2003, p. 10). These once adaptive strategies become maladaptive in the context of a good-enough environment provided by the new foster or adoptive family. This renders such children not only unpredictable to themselves but also to their caregiving environment, meaning that they can be hard to manage and to raise in a way that feels rewarding. Yet, it is these children who are in high need of co-regulating parents and other caregivers who are willing and available to take over regulation for a much longer period than is necessary in normal development.

Several processes in complex trauma underpin these impairments in affective development, regulation strategies and defence mechanisms: (a) a lack of opportunities to develop mature coping and defence mechanisms; (b) unmentalized intense arousal triggering primary fight, flight and freeze mechanisms and dissociative processes in a desperate attempt to evacuate difficult affects and (c) the meaning that has been ascribed to some signals of stress, affect and emotions during these early years interfere with adaptive development.

A lack of opportunities to develop mature coping and defence mechanisms

For a long time, Youri, aged eight, uses the word 'annoying' for everything that he experiences as negative. He is able to recognise that when he is feeling 'annoyed' his foster family members get angry. However, understanding why he finds something 'annoying' or knowing whether 'annoyed' relates to feeling angry, sad or lonely remains a mystery to Youri for a long time.

Similarly, Lisa (nine years) struggles for a long time to give words to that undefined 'annoying' feeling inside her, which she seems only to be able to get rid of by evacuating it in a massively bodily way: toys are thrown through the therapy room, furniture gets knocked over, Lisa crawls across the floor and laughs uncontrollably. At home, when upset, she circles around the house on her bike and absolutely needs to be left alone until she is exhausted and comes back in on her own.

As discussed previously, early life is much about regulation and being regulated (Stern, 1985), with primary caregivers having a full-time job regulating the infant's inner states. Children whose early caregiving environment has been characterised by the absence of available and predictable co-regulating caregivers are often compromised in their abilities to recognise and identify physical sensations and perceptions (e.g., being hungry, cold or in need of stimulation). Such lack of awareness of basic physical experiences precludes sensations from obtaining meaning in the child's inner world. And where there is no psychological space or psychic organisation to feel or think, experiences and emotions cannot be modulated or processed, conferring vulnerability in managing day-to-day emotional and social problems and processing emotion-laden life events. Children like Youri and Lisa, in the earlier vignettes, have lacked opportunities in their early caregiving environment to practise with identifying, labelling and modulating physical sensations and affective states. Consequently, these children continue to struggle to understand and regulate their affective experiences, and sometimes there is no other way out than resorting to an intense and imperative discharge in physical and motor activity, like in Lisa's case.

Unmentalized intense arousal triggering primary defensive strategies

In early life, Lisa has been exposed to parental neglect, and based on child protective services reports, probably also to physical as well as sexual abuse. During the assessment sessions, she generally presents as a talkative and likable girl. Yet, the therapist quickly notices that Lisa seems 'hypersensitive', noticing every single sound – however faintly audible – outside of the therapy room. At times like these, Lisa's facial expression quickly 'flattens', she stops talking in the middle of her sentence and her gaze goes blank. When the therapist gently calls out her name, Lisa is able to re-engage with the therapist yet does not seem to be able to recollect what just transpired. Lisa's foster carers report similar incidents at home whenever unexpected company rings at the door.

For some children, early life has not only been characterised by deprivation of necessary support and regulation but also by being subjected to intrusive experiences of maltreatment and violence. When confusing and overwhelming experiences have not been regulated by caregiving others but, to the contrary, have been caused by the very people a young child normally turns towards in times of anxiety and dysregulation, the development of healthy ways of modulating and processing intense arousal, such as in aggression and sexuality, can get severely disturbed. A child's neurophysiological system may adapt in different ways. The child's stress system may become hypersensitive, making them vulnerable for persisting hyperarousal-related symptoms, such as physiological hyperarousal and hyperactivity, eating and sleep disturbances, affect regulation problems or generalised anxiety (Perry, 2001). Children who were subjected excessively to violence, physically and/or sexually, will be left with feelings of aggression or sexuality that are easily triggered, even in 'normal' situations. Growing up in unpredictable circumstances, children like Lisa may become hypervigilant: always prepared for an attack, eyes and ears constantly scanning the environment for signs of danger 'that may come down from the sky or from over land' as phrased by Jemal when playing with knights in a castle during his first therapy session. Such persistent physiological hyperarousal, anxiety and/or aggression activates primary defensive strategies, such as fight, flight and freeze mechanisms and dissociative processes, in a desperate attempt to evacuate all these complex and difficult feeling states. Yet, these strategies become maladaptive in the good-enough environment of a new family and, due to their relatively persistent nature, confer vulnerability to psychopathology later in life.

The specific meaning ascribed to particular signals of stress, affect and emotion

In a peaceful and cosy family moment, Youri starts to annoy his brother, spoiling the moment of being together and exasperating and antagonising his brother. Subsequently, both boys start annoying one another, resulting in their foster mother getting angry because the atmosphere of a family moment has gotten spoiled.

Arousal, affect and emotions are about what experienced sensations, perceptions, states and feelings have come to mean to a child. For instance, why does a child get so enraged at the very hint of a hunger sensation (arousal)? Can an experience of disappointment (emotion; 'My teacher forgot it was my birthday this weekend') initiate a reflective process about people making mistakes and about how to reconnect in a relationship after a difficult incident, or rather, does it immediately mean 'I'm furious, and will never trust the teacher again because she doesn't care about me'? Does a moment of boredom (affect) initiate a creative impulse, or does it instead make the child panicky, counter-reactively leading to overly excited or risk-seeking behaviour? For some children, like Youri, peaceful quietness has acquired the meaning of unbearable boredom and emptiness, and quarrelling and fighting has become a way of actively avoiding these feelings of boredom and emptiness by drawing others into turbulent interactions. In children who have experienced complex trauma, bodily experiences such as hunger and cold and feelings such as boredom or even cosiness may have acquired a very specific meaning, which threatens the child's affective equilibrium and induces dysregulated behaviour. The same applies to children who have been subjected to violence or to sexualised arousal and/or behaviour when they were too young to understand the seriousness and wrongness of what was being done to them or of what they were observing: a well-intended appropriate touch may quickly though inappropriately elicit an aggressive or sexualised reaction in the child. This, in turn, interferes with adaptive development and taxes relationships.

In sum, the often underdeveloped and disturbed processes of regulation in traumatised children require particular – and as a rule of thumb, prompt – attention in direct work with the child as well as in working with parents and other carers, as dysregulation is a major stressor in the life of all involved. Being able to regain a basic level of regulation, again and again, is a prerequisite for a mental(izing) space in which any other emotional and relational learning can take place: 'regulate, then relate, then reason', as Perry (2016) has taught us. Only when the child is helped to recognise, experience, contain and regulate their difficult affective world over and over again can more constructive relationships between the child and their caregiving environment grow, and the child can move beyond self-representations of being 'mad' or 'bad'. This is a learning process for child and parents or carers alike, which ideally takes place in all important relationships and which receives particular attention both in the direct work with the child and in the work with parents and network. Carers need support to come to terms with and manage the fact that the child's urgent needs for co-regulation interfere with other duties and plans and will so probably for a long time and with 'predictable unpredictability'. In this regard, helping carers to remain patient as well as to observe small steps forward in the child's self-regulatory capacities is key, as development of adaptive and mature regulation capacities is a slow process. In this domain, progress comes about through seemingly endless repetition and in small steps rather than by swift and deep insight inciting one great leap forward. In this regard, child dysregulated behaviour requires a benevolent, developmentally informed as well as a trauma-informed perspective and approach (Lieberman et al., 2015).

Attachment development and relational capacities

Physical characteristics inherent to a new-born – an endearing, soft and sweet-smelling creature – as well as the inborn capacities to cry when upset and smile when content enable the baby to keep caregivers close. Based on numerous early caregiving experiences, a child builds inner representations of caregiving others as expectations that generalise to new relationships. In circumstances of loving care provided by good-enough parents, the child can be relatively carefree – free of intense hunger, pain or anxiety – and develops a 'secure base' (securus in Latin means 'without worries'). As development proceeds, a child gradually learns to be more autonomous with regard to regulation of arousal and affect and exploration of the world, and the parental secure base comes to also function as a 'safe haven', a place to come home to, to calm down and refuel emotionally (salvus in Latin means 'unharmed'). Developing a secure attachment is thus not only about close-ness and proximity but equally about being supported in becoming autonomous and in exploring as a self-evident part of growing up. As such, the development of attachment representations in the context of early caregiving relationships is to be considered part of a lifelong process of growth and maturation (Allen, 2013). A mature, adaptive personality is characterised by autonomy-within-relatedness, i.e., a relative and flexible balance between a capacity to establish and maintain relatedness to others, on the one hand and a capacity to explore the world autono-mously and curiously, on the other.

Early adverse experiences disorganise the attachment system (Cicchetti & Valentino, 2006) and cause the development of secure attachment representations and adaptive relational capacities to go awry. Several processes underpin relational impairments: (a) children who have experienced complex trauma draw – as it were – a map of their first relational territory as a barren, rough or hostile area; (b) without a secure base a safe haven for emotional refuelling cannot develop and (c) learning from others becomes impaired. (d) Going through life with this kind of relational map is at best not very helpful and at worst counter-productive in new safe caregiving circumstances.

A map of a barren, rough or hostile area

 Lisa comes into a therapy session around Christmas time raging that her foster carers are going to the Christmas fair without her. She is absolutely convinced that they purposefully chose the time of her therapy session to visit the fair, so as to cruelly deprive her of the opportunity to join in.

When a child is subjected to unpredictable early caregiving experiences, they are robbed of the opportunity to develop a secure base. Instead, such children develop inner representations of caregiving others as rejecting/abandoning, unpredictable and/or harsh and punitive. They draw an inner map of social circumstances and social traffic characterised by emptiness or deep sadness, intense unpredictability or continuous hostility and conflict, where remaining hypervigilant for 'booby-traps' or being ready to fight to 'fend for yourself' are ways to survive mentally. For children such as Lisa, as shown in the previous vignette, the world is often interpreted in hostile ways, confirming their inner belief that those who are supposed to care for them are in fact rejecting and nasty.

Without a secure base a safe haven for emotional refuelling cannot develop

 On the way to the therapy room, Lisa tells her therapist nervously that her class teacher will be visiting school tomorrow with her new-born baby. Lisa recalls that she herself was never breastfed, because she was born prematurely and her mum didn't have enough milk for her. While Lisa is telling this to the therapist, her agitation grows tangibly. Suddenly, Lisa pulls up her shirt and shows the therapist a nasty scratch on her tummy. She says that the physical education class was in another room at school today, but she wasn't sure where exactly, so she started to run around frantically looking for the right room; she ran through some bushes while crossing the playground to another school building and that's how her tummy got scratched. As Lisa normally presents as a very talkative and articulate girl, the therapist feels herself being baffled by Lisa's complete lack of awareness that she might rely on any familiar adult at school to find her way to the right classroom.

A lack of a secure base impairs the child from feeling comfortable and agentic in exploring the world around them. If the infant could put their experience into words, it would be as if they are saying: 'when I cry because I long for Mummy's familiar face and smell, a stranger appears above my cot, and distress and anxiety only grow' or 'Nobody notices that I'm scared to death when I hear that meowing sound so near to me'. These kinds of experiences result in the child believing that grown-ups are non-available passers-by without any particular bond or even that they are to be avoided because they are scary or cause even more stress. Or a certain caregiving act brings the child to a state of alarm, announcing that something bad is going to happen. In such circumstances, a child becomes preoccupied with relationship issues. This preoccupation can take different shapes depending on the prevalent early caregiving relationship patterns. Some children will frantically 'explore' the outside world in a conscious attempt not to appeal to the caregiver's proximity too much, like Lisa in the previous vignette. These 'avoidantly attached' children have learnt not to rely on others for nurturance or consolation. Other children will frantically attempt to keep the caregiver close, to the detriment of developing autonomy and agency. These 'anxious-ambivalently attached' children have learnt that they need to keep the caregiver close for fear that they will otherwise retreat. Finally, highly inconsistent caregiving may lead to more 'disorganised' attachment representations and behaviours, because the child has no clue which attachment strategy will work at any particular time.

Without a secure base learning from others becomes impaired

Early relationship patterns form the basis of the ability to learn from others, as conceptualised in the concept of 'epistemic trust' (Fonagy et al., 2017; Luyten et al., 2020). Epistemic trust refers to the capacity to open up one's mind to new learning experiences within a relationship with an adult whom the child can trust. It allows a child to learn from parents, teachers and other supportive figures such as mental health professionals. In normal development, an infant's innate epistemic vigilance quickly makes place for epistemic trust in the context of secure attachment relationships with its primary caregivers. By contrast, growing up in an environment lacking predictable and reliable sources, the development of social learning may become impaired in two different ways. Some children show epistemic hypervigilance or epistemic mistrust. They are unable to rely on others for help and information and react with suspicion and anxiety towards others and the new experiences/thoughts/information they have to offer. Such epistemic hypervigilance gravely impedes children from learning and growing through relationships. Other children exhibit 'epistemic credulity' (Fonagy et al., 2019), characterised by a profound lack of epistemic vigilance. Epistemic credulity puts a child at high risk of being misinformed, for example, by adults with well-intentioned but unprofessional rescue phantasies or of being retraumatised by people with bad intentions.

Relying on 'old' relational maps taxes new caregiving relationships

 When her foster carers come to fetch Lisa after her therapy session, she sarcastically enquires whether they had a good time at the Christmas fair without her, making sure to emphasise the latter. She continues raging about the unfairness of the whole situation. Her foster carers' baffled response is that, as they already explained to her on the way to the therapy centre, they were intending to take her along after her session. Lisa suddenly stops raging, as if it is the first time that she hears about these plans.

Due to the relative stability of mental representations, it is insecure or disorganised mental representations of self and other that traumatised children bring with them into their new foster or adoptive family (Hodges et al., 2005). Profound distrust is often central to how this presents itself. These representations act as expectations about how one will be treated by others (e.g., 'Obviously, I will not get those new shoes, whereas my brother gets all he wants') and lenses through which children look at how they are treated by others (e.g., 'I saw it in Mum's eyes, in the way she looked at me, she didn't like to give me that sandwich'). These lenses filter what a traumatised child hears and sees, what catches their attention, and how perceptions are interpreted and given meaning. In turn, these perceptions confirm what the child expects and often fears, rendering mental representations as self-fulfilling prophecies. If a child expects to be abandoned, any experience of being unattended to, any time someone looks away for a moment or any experience of being left alone for a moment is interpreted as evidence confirming an 'old' expectation: 'See, I knew it! You are abandoning me again!' Parental structuring of and limit-setting to 'odd' behaviour may be experienced as neglectful: 'They always say no, I never receive what I want'. Experiences concordant with 'old' but persistent mental representations of self and other are readily accepted, whereas discordant experiences are much less easily held on to or are actively rejected as impossible, as if unimaginable that others are trustworthy and/or one is worthy of care, as illustrated in the previous vignette. As such, children who have experienced complex trauma risk re-enacting mental representations of self and other built up from past caregiving relationships in present good-enough relationships. This can tax the solidity of these relationships and risks 'double deprivation' (Henry, 1974; see also Chapter 3), where the child who is already deprived now deprives themselves further of what they need by the way they relate to others. Or, as so aptly phrased by Patrick Casement (2002, p. 110), 'a sure way of getting lost, is to rely on a familiar map in unfamiliar territory'.

Precisely because of the relative tenacity of such 'old' mental representations in the mind of the traumatised child, it will take a tremendous amount of good-enough experiences for them to even attempt to try out new relational patterns. The context of a safe and predictable therapeutic relationship may then provide the child with a 'practising field' before trying out new relational patterns with significant others in real life, such as foster carers or teachers and coaches. For the most severely disturbed children, we might hope and work towards

> a new template of emotional relating . . . one that would never completely re-place the old one, but might steadily take root alongside it, hopefully becoming [the child's] 'go-to' neuronal pathway through which [the child] might filter more future experiences.
>
> (Music, 2019, p. 44)

As discussed, the traumatised child's impairments in attachment development and relational capacities severely and often chronically tax the relationships with the adults who care for them in everyday life. This requires the therapist in working with the parents/carers and with the network to pay particular attention to support them to tolerate and manage constructively being 'treated badly' by the child, as if they were neglectful or abusive. Often, this work also involves helping carers to come to terms with the fact that the traumatised child will never fully become 'securely attached', that under pressure, they will often revert back to an insecure or disorganised relational style, while at the same time supporting carers to keep providing good-enough care to the child as well as remaining hopeful that they can help the child to benefit (more) from that care.

Sense of self and identity

Creating one's own version of one's life story is an essential part of identity development. The quest for knowledge about one's birth and heritage is a central and universal aspect of this process of identity construction (McAdams, 2020; Sharp & Wall, 2021; Wright, 2009). However, this quest is often deeply compromised in children who have experienced complex trauma. To children in foster or adoptive care, parts of their life story often remain unknown or sometimes are even kept secret. The latter sometimes originates in the 'good intention' to protect the child; in other cases, the intention may be less benign. Regardless, not knowing (parts of) one's history makes it harder to develop a sense of self characterised by continuity and coherence. Moreover, often the experiences children with complex trauma went through were so traumatising and hurtful that these are impossible to be thought about and remembered without the child becoming dysregulated (see earlier).

At the most profound level of disturbance, children who have experienced complex trauma lack feelings of being alive and vital. They struggle with experiences of not knowing who they are, what they feel, what is important to them, what is vital and vitalising. At times, they may be barely aware of basic physical sensations and perceptions, such as a runny nose, let alone be able to ascribe meaning to these sensations and perceptions and have a mental space where thoughts can be thought about and feelings can be felt. Several processes involved in complex trauma underlie these impairments in the development of a sense of self and identity, including: (a) a lack of support to explore who the child is and what they want, (b) adapting to negative circumstances and (c) profound experiences of discontinuity and loss that are difficult to integrate.

A lack of support to explore who the child is and what they want

> During an intake session, ten-year-old Jemal seems rather flat in affect: he plays joylessly and absent-mindedly. At the end of the intake, when the therapist suggests he chooses a game, Jemal chooses to play a board game with his adoptive father. When he's ahead, a faint smile appears around his lips; when he falls behind, Jemal's facial expression tenses. The therapist, noticing these minor changes in his expression, enquires whether he enjoys playing board games. Jemal nods barely noticeably. His adoptive father adds that at home they don't play board games that often anymore, since Jemal prefers to play outside. When the therapist asks what games he likes to play outside, Jemal responds in a rather flat and soft tone of voice that he likes to shoot hoops, and in a somewhat stronger tone of voice and with some more facial expression, he adds that he plays football. When the therapist enquires whether he thinks he's any good at football, Jemal turns to his adoptive father, gently asking 'Is there anything I'm good at?' His adoptive father, resting his hand on Jemal's shoulder, replies: 'I wish you could believe that'.

Growing up amidst traumatising circumstances often means that caregivers lacked interest in the child as a developing individual, with their own talents, interests and so on. Is the child passionate about moving about? About discovering new, unfamiliar things by observing? Is the child talkative or rather receptive to sounds and words? Caregivers who are preoccupied with their own worries or who are responsible for the care of too many children may well be providing adequate nutrition, hygiene and sleep routine for the child yet often lack the time and mental space to help the child discover who they are, what touches them, what interests them and so on. It is in such circumstances, characterised by a consistent lack of genuine curiosity and interest in all facets of the developing child's being, that the child lacks the mirroring back of their emerging sense of who they are and wish to become. In that sense, such children risk dying a psychic death unless caregiving adults pick up on and foster any sign of the child's 'vital spark' (Winnicott, 1971), like Jemal's therapist and adoptive father attempted to do in the previous vignette.

Adapting to negative circumstances

 In an assessment session, Mei-Lan is looking at the play materials with flat affect. When the therapist enquires what she would prefer to play with, she shrugs and looks helpless and sad. 'It can be hard to know what you would like to do', the therapist comments. Mei-Lan nods, with a sigh of recognition and relief. 'Maybe we can start with something, and see how it feels? What about . . . the marble run or . . . maybe the colouring stencils?' the therapist wonders aloud. Mei-Lan whispers, 'The marble run' and hesitantly starts to explore the pieces.

 The therapist accompanies Youri, who essentially lacked parental care as a baby, to the playroom for the first time. On the way there, Youri complains about being thirsty. As the therapist shows him to the water fountain, Youri grasps a cup and holds it against his body with a protecting gesture as if someone is going to take it away from him. Once in the playroom, spotting a candy that someone has dropped on the floor, he shoves the candy in his mouth before the therapist realises what's happening.

Exposure to adverse experiences in early life can thus lead to a state of devitalisation and a lack of self-agency. This is often accompanied by a lack of feelings of curiosity, interest, enthusiasm and passion but instead feelings of futility and anhedonia, engendering a suffocating sense of emptiness and senselessness. This may be expressed in statements such as 'There is no point to my life' or 'I might as well not be alive'. In an attempt to adapt to early adverse circumstances, the child loses a sense of self, rendering their living a mere reacting rather than a thriving, with the child expending massive amounts of energy in reacting to (perceived) threats instead of having the peace of mind to discover and develop their own sphere of interest. In this regard, mechanisms of 'numbing' difficult feelings, such as fear and sadness, may underpin a lack of connectedness to one's own body and one's core sense of self (van der Kolk, 2014). When feelings are too difficult to bear for the child's developing psyche, the child may forcefully attempt to evacuate or shut out those feelings or discard them in any way possible. For instance, in play we might see a child who has experienced complex trauma struggling to begin to play, like Mei-Lan or suddenly put all the play characters to sleep or break off the play altogether. The problem with such numbing mechanisms is that it is impossible to shut out only part of one's feelings without getting out of touch with one's inner world in its entirety. It is like attempting to remove the dark colours from a painting: as soon as you remove one colour, the entire palette of the painting changes. Hence, children who numb feelings that are too difficult to bear often do not experience any other kind of affects either, making them feel 'dead' inside (van der Kolk, 2014). Other traumatised children like Youri have often learnt to proactively 'take what they need' and protect it at any cost based on the hard-wired expectation that no one will offer it to them but instead might try to rob them. As a result, a sense of self as 'not needing other people', like expressed in Jemal's 'anti-dependent' or even 'arrogant' stance, may emerge. Children exposed to violence or sexualised behaviour may counter-reactively assimilate these overly aggressive or sexualised parts into their identity to the extent of experiencing the whole of the self as an aggressive or sexual being.

Profound experiences of discontinuity and loss that are difficult to integrate

Jemal enters the playroom with an excited though somewhat tense look on his face. When the therapist notices and gently enquires about this, Jemal responds: 'Huh? . . . Yeah. . . . Did you know it was my birthday this weekend?' The therapist responds affirmatively, congratulates Jemal on this birthday and then enquires further: 'Is that what's on your mind and makes you look a bit excited but also nervous maybe?' Jemal talks about having a surprise birthday party his adoptive parents organised at an Ethiopian restaurant. 'I didn't know what was going to happen . . . they wanted to surprise me . . . but I don't like surprises! At all!! So, I was kind of mad, at least at first. . . . But once we were seated . . . it was a nice place, and the people were friendly, so. . . . Then . . . the food came . . . all of these brightly coloured plates with food on! And the smells! It was . . . it was . . . kind of . . . nice . . . like I remember them, you know . . . but I don't remember anything about Ethiopian food, you know, I didn't know what the food on the plates was, but the smells. . . .' Jemal looks really puzzled.

For children who have been placed in adoptive or foster care in particular, the development of a coherent and continuous sense of self and identity is compounded by the experience of loss in continuity in their sensory and cultural world of birth. Being placed in a substitute family indeed not only entails the loss of (the relationship with) the primary caregivers but actually a breach with all aspects of the familiar surroundings: smells, flavours, colours and sounds but also habits, values and norms belonging to the subculture of origin. The subsequent placement into another (sub-)culture requires the child to successfully negotiate the integration of – sometimes vastly – different aspects of the 'old' and the 'new' self. This constitutes a doubly challenging task for children who feel little mirrored in their new surroundings (e.g., a dark-skinned internationally adopted child among mostly Caucasian adults and peers). Or like Jemal who has got used to the food of his European Caucasian adoptive family but for whom the smells of food from his birth country elicit a deep layer of his earliest (bodily) memories. For some children, the challenge also lies in – rightly so or otherwise – experiencing little acknowledgement for their identity struggles (e.g., by adoptive parents who may unwittingly 'really not believe' that their child is being subjected to racial micro-aggressions).

Taken together, for many children who have experienced complex trauma, a profoundly scanty, incoherent or negative sense of self and identity constitutes an almost insurmountable roadblock on the way to a happy and fulfilling life. Yet, similar to the seeds in Death Valley National Park in the US that may lay dormant for years on end until the rain sets in motion a super-bloom of wildflowers, seeds of vitality may lay dormant in traumatised children who may appear deadened. It takes an extremely observant caregiving adult – a new parent, teacher or child psychotherapist like Mei-Lan's therapist in the previous vignette – to patiently water these vital seeds in order to foster the child's development of an essentially positive and eventually more coherent sense of self. In this regard, it is of paramount importance to cherish for the traumatised child each and every vital spark that can be discerned. This is true for the therapist working with the child in the playroom but even more so for the caregiving adults who surround the traumatised child on a day-to-day basis. The latter requires the therapist working with these adults, in parent work as well as in the work with the network, to help carers become aware of their vital and vitalising role and to scaffold their abilities to foster the child's sense of self. Moreover, with internationally adopted children and children placed in foster care in particular, a specific sensitivity and active approach to themes regarding (sub-) cultural differences and the child's difficult – often lifelong – task in integrating these into a coherent and essentially positive sense of self is warranted in all three tracks of intervention.

References

Allen, J. G. (2013). *Mentalizing in the development and treatment of attachment trauma.* Karnac.

Allen, J. G., Fonagy, P., & Bateman, A. W. (2008). *Mentalizing in mental health practice.* American Psychiatric Publishing.

Bion, W. R. (2002). A theory of thinking. In J. Raphael-Leff (Ed.), *Parent-infant psychodynamics: Wild things, mirrors and ghosts.* Routledge.

Bott Spillius, E., Milton, J., Garvey, P., Couve, C., & Steiner, D. (2011). *The new dictionary of Kleinian thought.* Routledge.

Casement, P. J. (2002). *Learning from our mistakes. Beyond dogma in psychoanalysis and psychotherapy.* The Guilford Press.

Chazan, S., Kuchirko, Y., Beebe, B., & Sossin, K. M. (2016). A longitudinal study of traumatic play activity using the Children's Developmental Play Instrument (CDPI). *Journal of Infant, Child, and Adolescent Psychotherapy, 15*(1), 1–25.

Cicchetti, D., & Valentino, K. (2006). An ecological-transactional perspective on child maltreatment: Failure of the average expectable environment and its influence on child development. In D. Cicchetti & D. J. Cohen (Eds.), *Developmental psychopathology: Risk, disorder, and adaptation* (Vol. 3, pp. 129–201). John Wiley & Sons.

Cook, A., Blaustein, M. E., Spinazzola, J., & van der Kolk, B. A. (2003). *Complex trauma in children and adolescents: White paper from the National Child Traumatic Stress Network Complex Trauma Task Force.* National Center for Child Traumatic Stress

Desmarais, S. (2006). 'A space to float with someone': Recovering play as a field of repair in work with parents of late-adopted children. *Journal of Child Psychotherapy, 32*(3), 349–364. https://doi.org/10.1080/00754170600996879

Edwards, A., Shipman, K., & Brown, A. (2005). The socialization of emotional understanding: A comparison of neglectful and nonneglectful mothers and their children. *Child Maltreatment, 10*(3), 293–304. https://doi.org/10.1177/1077559505278452

Ensink, K., Normandin, L., Target, M., Fonagy, P., Sabourin, S., & Berthelot, N. (2015). Mentalization in children and mothers in the context of trauma: An initial study of the validity of the Child Reflective Functioning Scale. *British Journal of Developmental Psychology, 33*(2), 203–217. https://doi.org/10.1111/bjdp.12074

Erikson, E. H. (1940). Studies in the interpretation of play: Clinical observation of play disruption in young children. *Genetic Psychology Monographs, 22*, 557–671.

Fish-Murray, C. C., Koby, E. V., & van der Kolk, B. A. (1987). Evolving ideas: The effect of abuse on children's thought. In B. A. van der Kolk (Ed.), *Psychological trauma* (pp. 89–110). American Psychiatric Publishing.

Fonagy, P. (2000). Attachment and borderline personality disorder. *Journal of the American Psychoanalytic Association, 48*(4), 1129–1146.

Fonagy, P., & Allison, E. (2012). What is mentalization? The concepts and its foundations in developmental research. In N. Midgley & I. Vrouva (Eds.), *Minding the child: Mentalization-based interventions with children, young people and their families* (pp. 11–34). Routledge.

Fonagy, P., Gergely, G., Jurist, E., & Target, M. (2002). *Affect regulation, mentalization, and the development of the self*. Other Press.

Fonagy, P., & Luyten, P. (2009). A developmental, mentalization-based approach to the understanding and treatment of borderline personality disorder. *Development and Psychopathology, 21*(4), 1355–1381. https://doi.org/10.1017/S0954579409990198

Fonagy, P., Luyten, P., Allison, E., & Campbell, C. (2017). What we have changed our minds about: Part 2. Borderline personality disorder, epistemic trust and the developmental significance of social communication. *Borderline Personality Disorder and Emotion Dysregulation, 4*(1), 1–13. https://doi.org/10.1186/s40479-017-0062-8

Fonagy, P., Luyten, P., Allison, E., & Campbell, C. (2019). Mentalizing, epistemic trust and the phenomenology of psychotherapy. *Psychopathology, 52*, 94–103. https://doi.org/10.1159/000501526

Fonagy, P., Moran, G. S., Edgcumbe, R., Kennedy, H., & Target, M. (1993). The roles of mental representations and mental processes in therapeutic action. *The Psychoanalytic Study of the Child, 48*(1), 9–48. https://doi.org/10.1080/00797308.1993.11822377

Henry, G. (1974). Doubly deprived. *Journal of Child Psychotherapy, 3*(4), 15–28. https://doi.org/10.1080/00754179708257300

Hodges, J., Steele, M., Hillman, S., Henderson, K., & Kaniuk, J. (2005). Change and continuity in mental representations of attachment after adoption. In D. M. Brodzinsky & J. Palacios (Eds.), *Psychological issues in adoption* (pp. 93–116). Praeger Publishers.

Koss, K. J., & Gunnar, M. R. (2018). Annual research review: Early adversity, the hypothalamic-pituitary-adrenocortical axis, and child psychopathology. *Journal of Child Psychology and Psychiatry, 59*(4), 327–346. https://doi.org/10.1111/jcpp.12784

Lieberman, A. F., Ghosh Ippen, C., & Van Horn, P. (2015). *Don't hit my mommy!: A manual for child-parent psychotherapy with young children exposed to violence and other trauma* (2nd ed.). Zero To Three.

Lingiardi, V., & Bornstein, R. F. (2017). Profile of mental functioning – M axis. In V. Lingiardi & N. McWilliams (Eds.), *Psychodynamic diagnostic manual: PDM-2* (pp. 75–133). The Guilford Press.

Luyten, P., Campbell, C., Allison, E., & Fonagy, P. (2020). The mentalizing approach to psychopathology: State of the art and future directions. *Annual Review of Clinical Psychology, 16*, 297–325. https://doi.org/10.1146/annurev-clinpsy-071919-015355

McAdams, D. P. (2020). Psychopathology and the self: Human actors, agents, and authors. *Journal of Personality, 88*(1), 146–155. https://doi.org/10.1111/jopy.12496

McCrory, E. J., Gerin, M. I., & Viding, E. (2017). Annual research review: Childhood maltreatment, latent vulnerability and the shift to preventative psychiatry – The contribution of functional brain imaging. *Journal of Child Psychology and Psychiatry, 58*(4), 338–357. https://doi.org/10.1111/jcpp.12713

Midgley, N., Ensink, K., Lindqvist, K., Malberg, N., & Muller, N. (2017a). The development of mentalizing. In *Mentalization-based treatment for children. A time-limited approach* (pp. 15–37). American Psychological Association.

Midgley, N., Ensink, K., Lindqvist, K., Malberg, N., & Muller, N. (2017b). *Mentalization-based treatment for children. A time-limited approach*. American Psychological Association.

Midgley, N., Ensink, K., Lindqvist, K., Malberg, N., & Muller, N. (2017c). When the capacity for mentalizing is underdeveloped or breaks down. In *Mentalization-based treatment for children. A time-limited approach* (pp. 39–60). American Psychological Association.

Modell, A. H. (1996). Trauma, memory, and the therapeutic setting. In L. E. Lifson (Ed.), *Understanding therapeutic action: Psychodynamic concepts of cure* (pp. 41–50). Analytic Press.

Modell, A. H. (2008). Implicit or unconscious?: Commentary on paper by the Boston Change Process Study Group. *Psychoanalytic Dialogues, 18*(2), 162–167. https://doi.org/10.1080/10481880801909534

Music, G. (2019). Attachment and jumpy untrusting kids. In *Nurturing children. From trauma to growth using attachment theory, psychoanalysis and neurobiology* (pp. 39–53). Routledge.

Perry, B. D. (2001). The neurodevelopmental impact of violence in childhood. In D. Schetky & E. P. Benedek (Eds.), *Textbook of child and adolescent forensic psychiatry* (pp. 221–238). American Psychiatric Press.

Perry, B. D. (2016). *In The trauma therapist project podcast Episode 94: Bruce Perry, MD, PhD*. G. Macpherson. Retrieved from www.thetraumatherapistproject.com/podcast/bruce-perry-md-phd/

Sharp, C., & Wall, K. (2021). DSM-5 level of personality functioning: Refocusing personality disorder on what it means to be human. *Annual Review of Clinical Psychology, 17*, 313–337. https://doi.org/10.1146/annurev-clinpsy-081219-105402

Shipman, K. L., & Zeman, J. (2001). Socialization of children's emotion regulation in mother – child dyads: A developmental psychopathology perspective. *Development and Psychopathology, 13*(2), 317–336. https://doi.org/10.1017/s0954579401002073

Slade, A. (1994). Making meaning and making believe: Their role in the clinical process. In A. Slade & D. P. Wolf (Eds.), *Children at play: Clinical and developmental approaches to meaning and representation* (pp. 81–107). Oxford University Press.

Stern, D. N. (1985). *The interpersonal world of the infant. A view from psychoanalysis and developmental psychology*. Basic Books.

Tessier, V. P., Normandin, L., Ensink, K., & Fonagy, P. (2016). Fact or fiction? A longitudinal study of play and the development of reflective functioning. *Bulletin of the Menninger Clinic, 80*(1), 60–79. https://doi.org/10.1521/bumc.2016.80.1.60

van der Kolk, B. A. (2014). *The body keeps the score: Brain, mind, and body in the healing of trauma*. Viking Penguin and The Penguin Group.

Winnicott, D. W. (1971). *Therapeutic consultations in child psychiatry*. The Hogarth Press and the Institute of Psychoanalysis.

Wright, J. L. (2009). The princess has to die: Representing rupture and grief in the narrative of adoption. *The Psychoanalytic Study of the Child, 64*(1), 75–91. https://doi.org/10.1080/00797308.2009.11800815

Complex trauma and the challenge to mentalizing capacities in parents and the network

Parenting and caring for a typically developing child is hard work and can be challenging at times. Parenting and caring for a traumatised child, as introduced in Chapter 1, constitutes a huge challenge to carers' caregiving skills in general and their mentalizing capacities in particular. Even well-intentioned new caregivers, such as foster carers or adoptive parents or well-trained professionals, such as most teachers, are likely to be challenged to a much greater extent and for much more extended periods of time than those caring for a child who has not experienced complex trauma. Different caregivers deal with these intense challenges very differently, ranging between two extremes. Some carers go to extraordinary lengths to continue to invest energy and care in a child who does not seem able and/or willing to benefit from such engagement, up to the point of exhaustion or harm to their own or other family members' well-being. Other carers find themselves on the verge of complete and utter disengagement from and rejection of the child, often in a desperate attempt to get away from the 'bad' – the unbearable feelings stirred up by the child's behaviours and dynamics.

In this chapter, we first discuss how traumatised children's development and functioning that is so fundamentally different from that of 'normal' children strain carers' resources in different ways. We then explain what these particular strains mean to caregivers' mentalizing capacities in raising and caring for a child suffering from complex trauma. In conclusion, we set out the need for a mentalization-informed approach to working with parents/carers and the network around the child, the aim of which is to scaffold an environment as conducive as possible to the child's developmental recovery. What such a mentalization-informed approach to the work with a traumatised child's primary caregivers and with the network may look like in practice will subsequently be addressed in Chapters 7 and 8, respectively.

The strains of caring for a traumatised child

Caring for children who have experienced complex trauma is inherently different from caring for normally developing children. The additional strains of caring for such children lie in the particular combination of their being harder to read and their impaired capacities to benefit from social, emotional and cognitive experiences

DOI: 10.4324/9781003044918-5

(Perry, 2001), while at the same time, their need for interactions and relationships that foster growth and development is so much greater.

A child that is hard to read, a challenge to caregivers' mentalizing

 Rebecca, Jemal's adoptive mum, talks to the parent worker about an incident earlier this week. Jemal was playing basketball by himself on the driveway. Rebecca could see him through the living room window. She let him play by himself for a while, only occasionally throwing a glance, knowing that Jemal doesn't like her to 'pry'. After half an hour or so, seeing him huffing and puffing, Rebecca decides to ask whether Jemal would like some lemonade. 'He started yelling and screaming, that I should leave him alone, in a way that really. . . . I was really flabbergasted!'

In 'normal' development, parents learn from the child's birth onwards to meticulously read their infant's behavioural signals as to what affective states underlies their behaviour and what then the infant needs from the parent in terms of response. For example, when an infant becomes 'fussy' in a particular way, the parent may infer that it's nursing time or the baby needs a change in type or level of stimulation. This process of trying to make sense of behavioural signals in terms of mental states and subsequent attuned responding is what has been termed 'parental mentalizing' (Midgley et al., 2017a), involving processes of 'keeping mind in mind' (Allen & Fonagy, 2006, p. xix) and 'seeing oneself from the outside and others from the inside' (Midgley et al., 2017a, p. 15). Features of good-enough parental mentalizing have been described by Midgley et al. (2017a, p. 24) to include the following:

- a benign interest in the mind of the child and emotional availability to help the child make sense of their own reactions and those of others;
- a capacity to look past the child's behaviour to determine what it communicates about their experience, feelings and difficulties;
- a capacity to play, joke and imagine with the child;
- a motivation to consider the meaning and sense of a child's thoughts and feelings, even if one cannot be exactly sure what is in the child's mind;
- availability to help to put feelings into words and elaborate autobiographically meaningful narratives;
- a motivation to see the child's perspective and awareness that the child's experience may be very different from one's own;
- an ability to have a sense of one's own thoughts and feelings when interacting with the child and modulate one's own aggression; and/or
- an appreciation that one's own feelings and moods will affect – and have an impact on – one's children.

As parents learn to know their infant, these mentalizing processes become more automatic or implicit, that is, they require less conscious effort on the part of the parent to tease out what the infant needs (Luyten et al., 2012; Midgley et al., 2017a). Parents often infer their child's mental state via rapid processing of facial and behavioural information and have the experience they 'know' their child and 'just see' when they are happy, frightened, nervous or angry. More explicit mentalizing comes to the fore when something happens that the parent needs to reflect on more explicitly (e.g., when the child reacts to something in a way that seems 'out of character'). Parental mentalizing is thus about what parents do in daily life; it fluctuates between background (implicit) when everything is continuing smoothly and foreground (explicit). In sum, in normal family life, implicit mentalizing is common, and explicit mentalizing comes to the fore only when parents are faced with situations that require more conscious and thoughtful understanding and management. As such, mentalizing in ordinary life is subject to difficulties under circumstances of stress, ranging from small daily moments of stress or sorrow (e.g., having to prepare a meal when tired and running out of time) eliciting minor difficulties in mentalizing which a parent can recover from easily, to moments of greater stress (e.g., having a child run away after a huge conflict) resulting in breakdowns in mentalizing. 'There is no doubt that family life and being a parent' – even under normal circumstances – 'place huge strains on our capacity to mentalize' (Midgley et al., 2017b, p. 41), with 'no context more likely to induce a loss of mentalizing than family interactions' (Fonagy & Allison, 2012, p. 24).

In parenting and caring for a child who has experienced complex trauma, explicit mentalizing and mentalizing breakdowns are much more common (see the section 'Mentalizing in the context of complex trauma'). Traumatised children's underdeveloped capacities to know and to show who they are and what they feel and their difficulties in regulating and modulating affect, emotion and behaviour (see Chapter 2) often result in their everyday behaviour being more difficult to understand and to manage. For example, Jemal's adoptive mother struggles to understand how an innocent question on her part about whether Jemal would like some lemonade could trigger such a massively aggressive reaction from him. She had left him playing on his own during half an hour, knowing well this is what he often prefers. His disproportional reaction easily arouses thoughts about him 'being rude' and finding him 'difficult to interact with'. Similarly, traumatised children's difficulties in basic functions (e.g., sleeping or eating), behavioural regulation, relationships with family members and friends, engaging in education and school functioning, result in caregivers being much less able to resort to usual types of implicit/automatic mentalizing which we do all the time, by implicitly reading others' behaviour in terms of intentional states. In order to foster developmental recovery in children like Jemal, it is of major importance that caregivers continue to respond in a constructive and mentalizing way to rather 'unusual' or 'incomprehensible' behaviour. Consequently, sorting out feelings, helping to identify what the child feels, wants or means, is part of a caregiver's activity for a much more extended period of time than with a 'normally' developing child.

A child less equipped to benefit from positive experiences: the risk of 'double deprivation' and getting caught in a 'biopsychosocial trap'

 Youri is little in touch with his bodily sensations. He often looks scruffy, doesn't seem to feel when his hands or face are dirty. His classmates find him to be 'weird'. He also seems out of touch with his impulses and his longings. When he sees other children playing, he abruptly joins in without asking and ends up disrupting their play and reaping annoyance. Having been neglected early in life, he runs the risk of being rejected in his school environment once again.

 Jemal is extremely sensitive to stressful events and reacts with an avoidant, almost unreachable attitude when he gets anxious. His adoptive parents know that he will warm up again as soon as he relaxes and that he can accept their help or comfort after he regains some calm. At school, the new teacher is a warm but temperamental man who easily raises his voice. Consequently, Jemal feels uncomfortable and becomes hypervigilant. Towards his teacher, he becomes ever more untouchable and unreachable and is unable to accept his help. The teacher, in turn, feels uneasy, finds Jemal distant and at times even arrogant. Being anxious of stressful and negative relationships, with his 'arrogant' behaviour, Jemal runs the risk of evoking negative and even dismissive reactions from caregiving adults such as his teacher.

The multiple and complex developmental impairments in children who have experienced complex trauma, as described in Chapter 2, render these children less able to benefit from growth-promoting experiences in the cognitive, emotional and social realm. For example, the continuous state of hyperarousal and overarching anxiety, leading to frequent yet unpredictable emotional outbursts or else the mechanisms of numbing or avoidance (Lieberman & Van Horn, 2004) undermine the child's capacities to learn in class (Perry, 2006). This makes perfect sense considering the fact that a certain amount of inner safety and peace of mind is required to be able to learn anything. So, as long as all energy is absorbed in scanning for and surviving perceived threat and danger, little mental space and attentional focus is left for maths, science or history. To no surprise, academic 'underperformance' or otherwise 'inexplicable' attentional or learning difficulties are often reasons for referring traumatised children to mental health services.

Moreover, trauma mechanisms interfere with the ability to rely on the help of others as a way of restoring a sense of safety (Shalev, 2000). In a state of hypervigilance, the child is always ready to defend themselves, sometimes by aggressively and violently attacking what they perceive to be an unsafe, scary and threatening environment. Consequently, children who have experienced complex trauma are often perceived by those around them as over-reacting (fighting, running away, making a big deal out of 'nothing') and easily over-generalising (e.g., 'I knew you were going to say no, you always say no when I ask to do/get something'). Age-inappropriate and disproportional tantrums and externalising behaviour problems are therefore a common reason for referral. Other children, like Jemal, withdraw into an 'anti-dependent' or 'arrogant' stance in an attempt to defensively disavow the importance of relatedness to or relationships with others.

The excessive aggression or profound mistrust some of these children bring into close relationships can severely tax these relationships. It is hard to maintain a positive relationship with a child with whom one can have a reasonable and agreeable conversation at one moment but who starts kicking and punching the next moment, triggered by a small comment or a minimal frustration. When even a seemingly neutral event is experienced as threatening, evoking fight or flight responses, when an otherwise adequately structuring 'no' is experienced as neglectful or an instruction or correction is interpreted as a harsh intrusion, a caregiver may feel treated as a source of constant potential threat. Or when the child's hyperalert, scanning, distrustful attitude makes one feel constantly watched and controlled, it requires hard work to keep mentalizing 'online' and to not get drawn into negative or unpredictable communication. With other children, like Youri, it is their profoundly devitalised state or their 'lack of social skills' that makes it so hard to find relating to them rewarding. In this regard, Henry (1974) has drawn attention to the risk of 'double deprivation' for traumatised children. While manipulating or controlling caregivers or peers to protect themselves against the painfulness of a dependent relationship or by their 'off-putting' demeanour, children like Jemal and Youri are at major risk of being deprived a second time around (Boston & Szur, 1983). In addition to 'the early deprivation inflicted by external circumstances, they deprive themselves by their crippling defences' (Boston & Szur, 1983, p. 3) that make them so hard to read and to reach. As aptly explained by Boston and Szur (1983), 'the essence of this double deprivation, observed to some degree in all children in out-of-home care, is the identification with an unfeeling, cruel, abandoning parental figure' (p. 3). This figure in the child's representational world is perceived in other people. The child might experience caregivers (parents, teachers, therapists) as cold, unfeeling, cruel, because this fits with the 'old' mental representations of caregivers that they carry with them. It makes a great deal more sense of much of the seemingly unreasonable behaviour of many traumatised children, 'if one bears in mind that they are often doing unto others what they experience as being done to them, both externally and internally' (Boston & Szur, 1983, p. 3). However understandable from a trauma-informed perspective, it is also one 'of the greatest tragedies of human interaction . . . when an individual misinterprets or is cut off from the language of mind and hence cannot fully grasp the many meanings of gestures of love, friendship, or hostility' (Mayes, 2012, p. xi).

Reaping negative reactions and comments from others also taxes the child's developing sense of self and identity. Many traumatised children struggle with feelings of being 'mad' or 'bad', often accompanied by overwhelming feelings of shame and guilt, which only add to the child's inner dysregulation. Feelings of intense shame and guilt also make it more difficult for the child to further invest in building and maintaining relationships with others.

Finally, traumatised children's pervasive developmental impairments also make growing-up so much harder in the longer run. 'Successfully' negotiating the developmental tasks of maintaining friendships and learning new skills during elementary school age or developing a coherent and essentially positive sense of identity as an adolescent becomes that much more difficult for these children.

Taken together, traumatised children's neurobiological reprogramming, which occurred as an adaptation to early adverse life circumstances, may initiate a cascade of problems in the domain of psychological and social development – the so-called 'biopsychosocial trap' (Shalev, 2000). Traumatised children run a higher risk of getting caught in this complex entanglement of problems that severely compromises their chances of getting back on a more adaptive developmental track.

The imperative need for growth-promoting interactions

Youri doesn't talk much about his daily experiences and activities. It is one of the things that really frustrates his foster mother. She is doing her utmost to be an interested and sensitive parent by asking every day how Youri's day at school was, but all he does is shrug his shoulders and respond with a sparing 'fine'. Youri's foster mother also vents her frustration to the parent worker about all the 'useless stuff' Youri always brings home in his pockets and school bag: pebbles and twigs from his walk home from school, scraps of paper with doodles and scribbles from a game on the playground, a candy wrapper from a schoolmate's birthday treat . . . 'My other kids also come home with stuff, but with Youri . . . it's e-ve-ry-thing! And he gets so so angry, and sad, whenever he even thinks that something is missing from his "collection"!' Mum exclaims. The parent worker helps Youri's foster mother to see how Youri may be using all these 'things' as a first step in building a narrative about himself: gathering things helps him to 'tell' his 'story of the day'. This helps Youri's foster mother to feel less frustrated about Youri's 'hoarding' and to show interest in all these little things. To the parent worker, she talks about feeling less frustrated in her daily interactions with Youri as well as how these 'things' have become the starting point of sharing the story of Youri's day with her. It takes Youri's foster mother a lot of time and energy, as she also has other children in need of her, but she's really glad to feel more 'connected' to Youri. This after-school 'ritual' of emptying Youri's bag and pockets together and sharing the stories of the day has become a cherished part of their relationship.

Children who have experienced complex trauma are in dire need of a therapeutic environment that immerses them in the positive experiences that growth-promoting interactions are. Ideally, they need more than good-enough give-and-take with mentalizing caregivers, which provides experiences that are tailored to their unique developmental profile and personality style. In that way, the child can really benefit from relationships that build on their own interests, capabilities and initiative and that stimulate the growth of their heart and mind (National Scientific Council on the Developing Child, 2004). For traumatised children, such interactions often require low adult-to-child ratios (often 1:1) and may involve activities frequently associated with children of a much younger age. Parents often bring to the fore situations in which their child persistently shows behaviour that feels inadequate, too young for their age, such as asking for or even claiming help which children of this age usually no longer need. This might include an eight-, nine-, or ten-year-old child asking to be dressed or to have their hair combed by a parent every morning or only being able to fall sleep with a parent beside them and falling prey to extreme anxieties when the parent does not meet this need.

We are not advocating for 'corrective' experiences, in the sense of contending that developmental milestones that have been missed can be accomplished this time round. However, contemporary neuroscientific knowledge does indicate that for children who have experienced complex trauma, many foundational experiences (neural networks) have been missed or are incomplete (Ludy-Dobson & Perry, 2010; Perry, 2006, 2009). Furthermore, neuroscientific findings suggest that 'the number of interactions required to change ingrained low-brain patterns call for extensive commitment from parents, teachers, therapists, and extended family, as the time required exceeds the capabilities of a single individual' (Gaskill & Perry, 2014, p. 186). It may help parents and carers to understand that the child is not 'just acting small or immature' but rather that the child's behaviour stems from an almost ingrained need, and this, in turn, may help the parent or carer to feel less antagonised and to engage with the child's need in a more thoughtful way, as Youri's foster mother did.

Mentalizing in the context of complex trauma

Beyond the normal fluctuations, mentalizing is 'fragile, liable to break down at least temporarily, especially when we are under stress or in a state of emotional arousal' (Midgley et al., 2017b, pp. 40–41). As discussed earlier (see the section 'A child that is hard to read, a challenge to caregivers' mentalizing'), in caring for a child who has experienced complex trauma, caregivers are faced with extremely difficult time- and energy-consuming situations, requiring more than ordinary mentalizing skills.

Complex trauma requires a much higher degree of explicit mentalizing

Jemal's adoptive parents talk about the moment he decided that he no longer wanted drawings on the wall in his room and removed all the stuffed animals from his bed, claiming to be 'too old for such childish stuff' (see introductory chapter). When they describe him as 'hard to reach', the therapist can feel their desperation about him pushing away every well-intentioned parental gesture on their part, making it almost impossible for them to think about what may lie beneath their adoptive son's 'anti-dependent' attitude. The therapist consciously spends a large part of the remainder of the session thoughtfully wondering aloud and inviting the parents to explore possible reasons for Jemal's 'anti-dependent'

stance. This helps the parents to start seeing Jemal somewhat differently, as a child who does have dependency needs, but who may be scared to express them. Soon after this session, the therapist learns from Jemal's adoptive parents that he has re-adopted his teddy bears and other stuffed animals and that he asked Mother to sit by him on his bed until he falls asleep. The latter continues for months, until Jemal's sleeping difficulties gradually subside. The parents were not aware that they had done anything massively different in how they related to him, but they were aware that they saw him differently. Aside from Jemal's adoptive parents being able to enjoy this more 'dependent' side of their son, it also helped them realise that his 'counter-dependent' behaviour was not so much a rejection of their parental care as it was his defence against a previously disavowed profound need for parental care and nurture.

In parenting a child who has experienced complex trauma, explicit mentalizing may need to be at the foreground more frequently and during larger episodes of family life. For example, Jemal's way of relating and behaving is confusing: it might be read as him not needing anyone to rely on, while there are indications that this 'anti-dependent' stance functions as a defence against conflicts around autonomy and relatedness. Carers may need to make much greater use of explicit/controlled mentalizing – a process that requires more conscious and explicit reflection on the child's intentions, thoughts and emotions (Midgley et al., 2017a). In Jemal's story, his adoptive parents needed first to bear being pushed away and subsequently to engage in fulfilling deep regressive needs for parental love and availability.

The same holds true for people caring for the child in other contexts, such as at school (teachers) or in leisure contexts (e.g., sports coaches). In such contexts, additional strain on caregivers' mentalizing abilities also stems from other processes.

Jemal is sporty and started to play football at a young age. After a violent fight though, he got kicked off the team. His adoptive parents found a new team, where they hoped Jemal would have a better chance to find his way. The new team is headed by coach Michael, a seasoned coach with a big heart for 'kids with temperament' as he calls them. Coach Michael describes Jemal as an enthusiastic player, a welcome asset to his team: 'You know, I've known him for a while now, and he can be a real team player, but when frustration runs high he loses it. I've learnt what works and what doesn't at such moments. Sometimes, when I notice him getting upset, it's enough that I make a calming gesture with my hands. It's amazing how he will always look at me at those moments and notice my gesture. Now and then, that isn't enough, and I will get him off the field for a while, to calm down on the bench. I never spend much words on what happened. It rarely gets so bad that Jemal can't get back on the field. What really works as a red rag to a bull is when I lose my patience and get angry, so I try to keep my cool'.

For the group of professional caregivers, like coach Michael or Jemal's teacher (see earlier), having a child in the group whose developmental needs are larger, more complex and more difficult to understand compounds the task of balancing the need to address this child's needs while also being responsible for meeting the needs of the other children in the group. Unsurprisingly, the traumatised child, who may require a lot of individual attention and support at the most unpredictable and 'inconvenient' moments, can be experienced as making life harder for the teacher or coach as well as for the peer group. So, although these professionally trained network partners may have plenty of knowledge and skills with regard to children's developmental needs, the presence of a child such as Jemal in the group confronts them with the difficult task of being able to access and apply this knowledge and these skills in highly challenging circumstances. Michael, who was already a very experienced coach, was willing to make an extra effort to get to know Jemal and to learn to manage his particular way of functioning, in close collaboration with Jemal's adoptive parents.

For Mei-Lan, doing homework after an already intense school day seems an insurmountable task. School materials have been thrown across the table more than once, and help offered by one of her adoptive parents only seems to make things worse. In talking about these difficulties in parent work sessions, the idea of asking Mei-Lan's cousin William for help emerges. The family of Uncle Thomas, who is a child psychiatrist, is of major importance to Mei-Lan and her family. Cousin William, who is a medical student, approaches Mei-Lan warmly and patiently. His presence and support seems to help Mei-Lan to stay calm most days after school. The first time Mei-Lan falls prey to a tantrum while doing homework with William, he is shocked. Fortunately, Mei-Lan's adoptive mother was close by. William tells her: 'I know you told me it could get "too hot", but I really wouldn't have known how to react if I would have been all alone with Mei-Lan! I never imagined she could rage like that!'

For the caregivers in the informal network, like William, the challenge in interacting with a child such as Mei-Lan lies elsewhere. The important and supportive personal relationship which they offer the child, while hopefully characterised by patience, time and goodwill, can become strained in the face of a lack of professional knowledge and skills about how to understand and respond to the very particular developmental needs of a traumatised child. Consequently, these informal caregivers sometimes tend to withdraw or disengage from the child when the child becomes 'too difficult to handle'. This may happen when facing interactions that are unexpectedly intense (as in the vignette earlier), feeling 'manipulated' by the child or when getting entangled in difficult interactions, for example, when unwittingly colluding with the child in stories about receiving bad care at home, based on 'old' representations rather than on actual reality.

Complex trauma inevitably evokes mentalizing breakdowns

Consequently, breakdowns in mentalizing – however normal in all families – are more likely to occur in parents and networks caring for a child suffering from complex trauma. In parents or carers, expressions of one or several non-mentalizing modes may then become apparent (see Table 3.1).

Table 3.1 Definition and expressions of non-mentalizing modes in parents or carers

Non-mentalizing mode	Definition	Possible expressions
Teleological mode	Mental states are expressed in goal-directed actions	• Acting demanding towards the therapeutic team, expecting problems to be solved immediately by concrete actions ('quick fix') and becoming angry when problems persist • Putting the child to the fore as the problem, focusing solely on the child's problems and behaviour, and expecting these to be 'eradicated', without attention to mental states or inner experience
Psychic equivalence mode	Reality is equated with mental states	• Seeing the child's behaviour as the whole and only truth about the child, and trying to control the child's behaviour through authoritarian styles of parenting/caregiving • Excessive blaming or fault-finding towards the child, trying to convince the therapeutic team of 'what a difficult child it really is' and other unmentalized ideas and feelings about the child • Demonstrating negative distortions and attributions to the child (e.g., asserting that the child is behaving like this 'because they're out to ruin the atmosphere for everyone, because they have a sadistic pleasure in harassing everyone') • Exhibiting unmodulated mental states, without awareness of the impact these may have on the child
Pretend mode	Mental states are decoupled from reality	• Elaborating the child's inner world in a way that is 'decoupled' from the child's personal reality and doesn't lead to an attuned and growth-promoting relationship (e.g., talking about the interesting drawings the child made about monsters and demons, without awareness of the affective charge encompassed in the content and what the child may then need from them as parents/carers)

Such difficulties to mentalize the child may increase the risk of parents or carers disengaging from or rejecting the child. Aside from problems in mentalizing about the child, parents or carers may also struggle to (keep) mentalizing about themselves as caregivers. It is not uncommon for parents or carers, for instance, to be able to remain empathic and caring towards the traumatised child at length, going to extraordinary lengths to continue to invest energy and care in a child who does not seem able and/or willing to benefit from such engagement, to the detriment of their own well-being (e.g., becoming exhausted or 'burnt out').

Such mentalizing breakdowns in carers increase the risk of negative and even retraumatising interactive cycles (see Figure 1.1, Chapter 1). Hence, a traumatised child's process of recovery needs to be embedded in a network that is united in holding dear 'going on reflecting' and restoring breakdowns in mentalizing. In mentalization-based work with parents and network, restoring parents' and other caregivers' mentalizing capacities is thus at the heart of treatment. What this may look like will be the topic in Chapters 7 and 8, respectively. At this point, it seems important to tease out what processes may be involved in these mentalizing breakdowns.

Particular vicissitudes of caregivers' mentalizing skills in the context of complex trauma

Being confronted with threatened levels of energy and unexpected strong negative feelings

Mei-Lan shows intense behaviour problems at home: frequent anger outbursts, temper tantrums and her never-ending message to her adoptive parents that she hates them. When asked about their perspective on their adoptive child's problems, the therapist is somewhat taken aback by the parents' almost opposite perspectives. Mother, who is an engineer, has not been able to work for almost a year due to exhaustion and medically unexplained somatic symptoms. The therapist feels Mother's deep compassion with Mei-Lan, spurring almost endless attempts to understand the difficulties underlying her adoptive daughter's negative behaviour. Father, who is a physician, seemingly speaks in a more detached way, with covert hostility seeping through. He talks about his adoptive daughter as 'a disturbed child with a psychiatric problem, unable to engage in positive relations' as if speaking about a patient rather than about a daughter. Nevertheless, the therapist is able to discern father's loving stance towards Mei-Lan in the caring and available way he acts towards her in day-to-day interactions.

Maïté is a young teacher, substituting for Lisa's class teacher who is on maternity leave for some months. She is new to having a child with complex trauma in class. During the first few months of the school year, she exerts huge efforts to keep Lisa on track, supported by a strong

> special educational needs team at school. After an incident in which Lisa could make her believe that her foster carers gave her unhealthy and mouldy bread for lunch (see also Chapters 7 and 8), Maïté feels how she tends to keep her distance from Lisa.

As children who have experienced complex trauma require much more of their caregivers and over much longer periods, the child's needs may interfere with the needs and the life rhythm of their caregivers, often leading to reduced levels of energy. Feelings of weariness, loneliness and exhaustion are commonplace. In some families, moments of serenity and peacefulness are rare. In others, space for activities that give the parents energy, or time for the parents as a couple, like a weekend getaway, is lacking, to the extent of being 'unimaginable'. Some parents, like Mei-Lan's adoptive mother, struggle with symptoms of burnout and depression.

Moreover, caring for a child who has experienced complex trauma may evoke myriad strong negative feelings, which one might not have expected and at least would prefer to avoid, compounding the inevitable breakdowns in mentalizing. Intense feelings of love, compassion and empathy may get entangled with unexpected feelings of anger, exhaustion and anxiety, sadness and guilt, harm and even trauma. Rage, hate and sadism may also come to the fore. These disturbing feelings may induce the risk of withdrawal or disengagement from the child, as discernible in the way Mei-Lan's adoptive father talks about her or even rejection of the child.

The aforementioned scenario does not only hold for the traumatised child's immediate carers (e.g., adoptive parents or foster carers) but also for members of the informal and professional network around the family. The more involved the teacher or coach, the more they may become intensely engaged in trying to keep these children on track, like Lisa's teacher did, potentially increasing the risk of crossing their personal boundaries. Others tend to disengage when challenged by difficult behaviour, experiencing the child as interfering with their 'core tasks'. For example, in teaching a class group a new mathematical concept or coaching a group to acquire new sports skills, or in helping the child to complete their homework after school while the parents are still at work, the child's disruptive and disturbing behaviour interferes with the task at hand and makes one's job more difficult. Then, it is only natural *not* to wonder about the reasons behind it or to experience the behaviour as intentional, as meant to disturb and make things harder. This, in turn, may easily evoke disengagement or alienation from the child or even rejection of the child.

Staying with the child at the hard place

> Mei-Lan struggles intensely with being separated from her adoptive mother. On school days, getting out of bed and leaving for school is often extremely difficult and stressful. Mei-Lan wants to get dressed by Mum, needs to make a drawing for her mother while having breakfast, can't leave the house without all her colouring pencils sorted in a particular order, and keeps wanting to give the cat 'just one more hug'.

> Every morning tends to end up in a struggle. Mother has learnt – the hard way – that trying to put a stop to Mei-Lan's 'rituals' is to no avail; on the contrary, it only makes the process of getting ready for school that much more of a struggle. At the same time, arriving late at school almost daily violently clashes with Mother's aspirations for her adoptive daughter (see later).
>
> At school, a comparable but milder dynamic can be observed. When having to leave the familiar classroom to go to the gym class, Mei-Lan insists on checking her gym bag several times: 'Do I really have everything? My gym clothes, my gym shoes, my drink and biscuit for after gym class?' After having reacted impatiently several times, the teacher has learnt that this only makes things worse. In talking about it at a network meeting, the idea emerges to assign a peer to help Mei-Lan. Doris, one of the few classmates Mei-Lan regularly plays with on the playground and seems close to, comes to mind. For every gym class, Doris stays by Mei-Lan while she reassures herself. Once calm and convinced that everything is okay, Mei-Lan and Doris run to the gym class and arrive in a light-hearted mood.

Caregivers dealing with children who have experienced complex trauma are often faced with situations in which the child's behaviour is difficult to understand, 'weird', provoking or challenging – situations that require them to continuously function as containers for the child's difficult emotional life, often without a clear understanding of what precisely is going on. This evokes stress and may cause caregivers' ability to think and respond calmly and adequately to break down. When even experienced therapists find it challenging to understand the signs and expressions of complex developmental difficulties, it is extremely taxing and overwhelming for ordinary parents and other caregivers to understand and to thoughtfully respond to. In the previous vignette, both Mei-Lan's adoptive mother and her teacher have found ways not to let situations escalate too much, by affording Mei-Lan control over her 'rituals', but this doesn't mean that the continual tolerance for and thoughtful responses to such situations don't tax resources or that the mornings aren't still stressing Mother out and exhausting her.

Torn between hope and despair, feelings of loss and mourning

> Mei-Lan's adoptive parents talk about their concerns: In Kindergarten, Mei-Lan was unable to accept her adoptive mother departing before she was in her classroom, but even now – at elementary school age – this has hardly improved. Mei-Lan seems to remain a needy and demanding toddler-like child. Her adoptive parents see little growth, despite their best efforts, making them profoundly anxious about Mei-Lan's future. When the therapist invites them to imagine their daughter in the future, they talk about seeing a woman who will never be able to take care of herself, a kind of an 'invisibly disabled child'.

Caregiving in the context of complex trauma not only requires an ability to bear and contain the child's anxiety and anger, pain and suffering, in the moment but often also involves coming to terms with feelings of loss and mourning accompanying the realisation of the long-lasting scars and vulnerabilities the child has to live with. Because of traumatised children's often complex and pervasive needs, good-enough care often proves *not* enough. When caregiving efforts feel like an endless task, the risk of disengagement becomes greater: 'Whatever we do for her, it doesn't make any difference'. Moreover, treatment of complex trauma seldom succeeds in 'curing' the child quickly or completely. Change often comes in small steps, and enduring vulnerability turns new developmental steps into difficult challenges for the child and family. Indeed, for the most vulnerable children, new phases in development may put old injuries under pressure anew, leading to difficulties and challenges for the child and caregivers all over again. In this context, feelings of despair often (re-)surface, incapacitating parents in continuing to do what is in the child's best interest and to treat the child in a nurturing, kind and supportive way. This may also apply to members of the child's informal or formal network. The aunt/uncle or grandparent, or the foster care worker or teacher at school, who invests emotionally in a relationship with the child across several years, will also face the challenge of mourning the loss of a normal development for the child. Some network members run the risk of exhausting themselves; others tend to disengage, for example, by expelling the child from school. In this regard, it is important to remember that every new developmental phase also brings with it a new opportunity to work through old problems at a more advanced level. Developmental change in traumatised children concerns a slow unfolding of difficult inner dynamics and a repeated working-through of the same dynamic at a more advanced level. For instance, when distrusting others has been part of who a child is throughout childhood, having to trust in adolescence brings old anxieties to bear in new romantic relationships – even if the child has already managed to learn to trust parents and teachers in an earlier developmental phase.

In light of this, parents of children who have experienced complex trauma will inevitably – and often repeatedly – go through an episode of mourning. For instance, when realising their child will remain dependent on their parental presence much longer or is not able to make use of their cognitive capabilities due to extreme sensitivity to stress. Or because of the realisation that they will have to include other safe adults in the child's care, which may be experienced as parental failure. Paradoxically, (realistic) hope is the fuel that keeps parental engagement and mentalizing going. Yet, often it is not until the more advanced phases of the work with parents that they can come to terms with the fact that although children suffering from complex trauma mostly remain scarred for life, a scar is a much more human and liveable perspective than having to live with the raw wounds from which it originates (Vliegen et al., 2023). A different kind of confidence has to develop, in which caregivers can accept the persistent vulnerability as a basis for change, often without really being able to envision the profundity of the child's wounds or the scope of their scars. As difficult as it is to foretell any child's exact developmental trajectory, this is even more true for children who have experienced complex trauma, making it even harder for their carers to negotiate being continually torn between despair and hope.

Actively scaffolding coherence and integration

Jemal's adoptive parents enter the consulting room in high arousal. The parent worker learns that Jemal was involved in a heavy conflict after football training. He ended up damaging a teammate's (Bruce) bike. Jemal's adoptive parents are angry about what happened, and worried about what this means for Jemal's future development seeing him 'becoming a thug'. They tried to talk to Jemal – for the umpteenth time – that a dispute is best solved in a non-violent way. They wanted Jemal to apologise and to pay for the bike to be repaired. Jemal agreed to pay for the reparation from the pocket money he saved but adamantly refused to apologise, which made his adoptive parents worry even more.

In listening to and thinking about this incident, the parent worker shares the parents' surprise at Jemal's level of aggression in reacting. Having become rather sensitive to racial micro-aggressions in working with children of colour, she wonders aloud whether Jemal could possibly have a good reason to not want to apologise and whether racism could play a part in that. Jemal's adoptive parents react with surprise. They are convinced that no one can ever have a good reason to destroy someone else's belongings. While the therapist acknowledges the grain of truth in this idea, she also sticks to the possibility that a person can feel so deeply hurt that they don't feel they have to apologise for reacting so angrily. The parents admit that they hadn't thought of racial issues being involved at any moment and are willing to talk to Jemal about that.

In the next session, the parents talk about how Jemal felt deeply hurt and became extremely angry again when they tried to talk to him again about the incident with Bruce's bike. They did, however, manage to get a clearer picture of what exactly happened: Bruce was angry about Jemal not passing him the ball during the football match and started calling Jemal names – names, with a clear racial undertone, that Jemal didn't even want to repeat to his adoptive parents. Together with Jemal, they decided to ask coach Michael, the team's seasoned and skilled coach, to mediate between Bruce and Jemal.

As discussed in Chapter 1, adopted and foster and children are inherently 'children of two (or more) (sub-)cultures'. In this regard, they not only face the loss of continuity in their primary caregiving relationships and (sub-)culture of origin, but they often embody characteristics and expectations, as well as values and norms belonging to another (sub-)culture than the one their new carers (adoptive parents or foster carers) belong to. Moreover, the developmental consequences of having gone through complex traumatic experiences, such as having learning difficulties or lacking emotional and behavioural control, often make these children 'stand out' even more, adding to them feeling very different to the people in their new surroundings. Consequently, adoptive parents and foster carers, as well as others belonging to the child's caregiving network, are faced, to a much greater extent than with biological children, with the challenge of helping the child in their attempts at integrating aspects of 'different worlds' into a sense of self-continuity and self-coherence. This task may be especially challenging when carers' (sub-)culture of origin is profoundly different from the child's. For example, when Caucasian adoptive parents or foster carers had no prior first-hand experience with racial micro-aggressions, as was the case with Jemal's adoptive parents.

Aside from the more obvious cultural differences, such as skin colour, there are the differences in subculture between the child's family of origin and their new adoptive or foster family. Most obviously, this pertains to the issue of contact with the biological parents, how this challenges the child in reconciling these two worlds and the new carers in supporting the child therein. With foster children who still have a legally recognised bond with (one of) their biological parents, this means that foster carers have to take into account the biological parents' perspective in everyday (e.g., haircut) as well as major decisions (e.g., school) with regard to their foster child. But even in situations in which there is no real relationship to maintain with the child's biological parents (e.g., if they are deceased or no longer have contact with the child), child and adoptive parents or foster carers are faced with the task of reconciling the phantasised biological parents' and family members' intentions and wishes for the child with their own wishes and values and norms stemming from their own subculture of origin. The emotional upheaval this may bring about often proves to be much more difficult than anticipated, as it relates to the (phantasised) biological parents/family as well as their own dynamics, sensitivities and anxieties regarding issues of family belonging.

Mei-Lan, who is of average intelligence, doesn't seem to be able to make optimal use of all the chances she receives. Despite all Mother's efforts to help her to make progress at school, Mei-Lan seems to fall back after short periods of progression and seems to develop severe learning difficulties. Mother often feels helpless, frustrated and angry. 'How is it possible that a child who receives so much support and so many chances does not grasp all these chances to the fullest?' she wonders aloud.

Mei Lan's adoptive mother grew up in a hard-working working-class family. Her warm and loving parents worked hard to give their children every chance in life, but it was up to them to really grasp and capitalise on these chances. For example, she and her brothers were allowed to pursue a higher education in their discipline of choice, but in Mother's experience, her parents did not have the skills to support their children when they struggled with academic work. Mother looks back on her

> youth with gratitude but also with feelings of loneliness. There was
> this continuous threat that she could fall behind. She became an en-
> gineer and is committed as a mother to support her children in their
> development.

Differences in subculture and possible difficulties in integrating these may also
stem from carers' vulnerabilities related to specific aspects of their personal history and upbringing. Internalised values and norms may play out as strengths and
resources, which caregivers may fall back on in their own caring for the next gen-
eration, but these may also function as vulnerable spots when put under pressure
by the child's functioning or dynamics. For example, in the case of Mei-Lan's
adoptive mother, her internalisation of the importance of academic performance
is something that has successfully supported her in her own academic and professional aspirations, as well as in her dedication to her children's academic achievements. Yet, confronted with Mei-Lan's more vulnerable academic functioning, she
struggles to understand and to come to terms with the fact that the same academic
'standard' may not apply to Mei-Lan. The carers' task of actively scaffolding processes of trying to find coherence and integration becomes all the more challenging
when the child's dynamics trigger unresolved vulnerabilities in new carers, this is,
when carers 'get hit where it hurts' as it were.

Vulnerabilities in carers may range from rather 'minor' and thus easier to disentangle from the child trigger, as was the case with Mei-Lan's adoptive mother, to
more severe in nature, with the risk of impinging on the carer's relationship with the
child and subsequently on the child's development. In this regard, psychodynamic
writings as early as the 1970s have taught us valuable concepts such as 'ghosts in
the nursery' (Fraiberg et al., 1975) to better understand the dynamics underpinning
the intergenerational transmission of psychopathological vulnerability in general –
and of trauma in particular – from parent to child. Clinical and personal experience
attest to the fact that parents are at their most vulnerable when their own issues are
triggered or re-activated by their children's behaviour. Whereas this is true for all
parents and children, adoptive parents and foster carers often bring specific aspects
from their own history into their parenting. Sometimes issues around 'being a real
parent or not' can be triggered, for instance, when infertility issues have played a
role to come into adoptive parenthood or fostering in the first place. Grappling with
infertility issues in and of itself constitutes a process centred around multiple losses
and identity transformation – themes that may be re-activated when adoptive or
foster parenthood proves to be more challenging than perhaps anticipated.

Children who have experienced complex trauma thus tend to put greater strain
not only on parental skills but also on parental vulnerabilities. At the most extreme,
for parents struggling with their own vulnerabilities due to difficult or traumatising experiences in their own childhood or in becoming a parent, the risk of getting
entangled in negative and even retraumatising interactive cycles with the child is
even greater. Although work with parents of traumatised children is never meant to
replace individual psychotherapy, the parents' own vulnerabilities and issues will

inevitably enter the parent worker's consultation room. These issues should thus be a topic in therapeutic work with parents as far as they relate to this parent's care of and relationship with this child. How the therapist may address these topics in the present treatment approach will be discussed in Chapter 7.

'It takes a village . . .': complex trauma and the need for mentalizing partnerships around the child

Mei-Lan has a strong tendency to run away from any conflict, whether at home or during family outings. This has led to episodes of huge panic in her adoptive parents and crises requiring police intervention. In parent work, Mei-Lan's adoptive parents have been helped to re-frame her fugitive behaviour as a pervasive defence mechanism which their daughter is really struggling with and which will not be solved by parental or police force. In thinking together about what might be helpful, Mei-Lan's parents become able to talk about this with family, in attempting to create a network of people whom Mei-Lan could turn to. Father's brother, 'Uncle Thomas' – who is a child psychiatrist – and his family are immediately willing to be involved. Mei-Lan has a good bond with her cousins there, especially with William who helps her with homework (see earlier vignette), and feels helped when 'running away from difficulties' can be reframed as 'running to William, or to the uncle Thomas' family, a safe place to calm down'. As soon as this construction is agreed on, moments of crisis diminish.

In the context of complex trauma, it is crucial to not only involve the parents/carers and the family but to create a social care system surrounding the child, in order to establish a growth-facilitating context. The rationale for this need for mentalizing partnerships is twofold. First, sometimes the child's needs exceed what a single family can offer, as in Mei-Lan's case. In such situations, loving and mentalizing parents are in need of an understanding network that is capable of supporting them in specific, sometimes crisis-like situations – people who remain reflective when parents feel their mentalizing skills collapsing or who offer places where child or parent may turn to when family relationships have become overly tense. As described in Chapter 2 and illustrated in the vignette about Mei-Lan earlier, traumatised children's tendency to fall back on fight or flight mechanisms in moments of distress results in them and their parents being in need of safe places to turn to.

Moreover, the problems which traumatised children are struggling with are often not limited to the family relationships but also occur in other contexts, such as school, friendships or extracurricular activities. Meeting with teachers or special educational needs services may be needed to get a child back on track. Furthermore, difficulties may have been challenging to the extent that intensive involvement from foster care or child protection services has been required. It is important to keep these relevant partners involved, attempting to create a shared representation of the child's internal experience when seen from a range of perspectives (Zevalkink et al., 2012). This shared understanding can be used in the service of fostering the child's adaptive functioning in as many domains of daily life as possible.

In most cases, it is possible to mobilise such a safe, trauma-informed and mentalizing network surrounding the traumatised child and their family. Yet, sometimes, this may prove less straightforward than anticipated because of several additional challenges. Often, the caregiving system around these children has necessarily become large. Paradoxically, the large number of stakeholders often complicates the mentalizing collaborative efforts towards a shared understanding. Each network partner adheres to different priorities, goals and premises, often resulting in different perspectives on the child and their functioning. Thinking and talking together and agreeing and deciding on a shared plan of action may prove a difficult task, leading to moments of disintegration or even splitting (see later) in a network (Bevington et al., 2017). Large and complex networks 'naturally do *not* work, their resting state is to be disintegrated' (Bevington, 2019, March 29). Constructive communication and collaboration without falling prey to mutual frustration about, for example, 'the other not doing a satisfactory job' understandably but almost inevitably proves to be a major challenge to the networks surrounding traumatised children.

Children who have experienced complex trauma further compound this disintegrated state of their networks by their propensity towards inducing splitting mechanisms. Such children, in a desperate attempt to manage anxieties, often resort to primary defence mechanisms in which they attempt to keep good and bad experiences and representations split off from each other by projecting these on to different people. In this way, traumatised children are often – although unintentionally or at least unconsciously – at the source of tense relationships among the people responsible for their care who have been designated 'good' and 'bad' carers. At any one moment, the parents might be all good and the social worker all bad, or Dad may be Mr Perfect, and Mum is Mrs Monster. Especially for those who are seen as the 'good' figure, it can be hard to see that is part of the challenge in caring for the child, rather than starting to believe that they are actually the 'right' one, and others have got it wrong. (When Mr Perfect suddenly turns into Mr Monster, the reversal can be quite a shock and may lead to anger and rejection.) At the same time, it is these same children who cannot stand the slightest sign of tension in or among the caregiving adults surrounding them. Relational tension or splitting mechanisms in the caregiving adults can really drive these children 'insane' and further make them lose balance and control. Network partners are faced with the difficult task to withstand such child-induced splitting mechanisms to not get drawn into 'triple deprivation' (Emanuel, 2002), i.e., dynamics and interactions which deprive the traumatised child for the third time from the care they so direly need. This requires each of these stakeholders to almost continuously be wary of such splitting mechanisms or the risk thereof, as well as to almost continuously mentalize about network dynamics. It follows that the creation and sustenance of 'one consistent, positive, thinking and caregiving network' (Boston & Szur, 1983, p. 5) around the child who has experienced complex trauma, in order to provide the child as well as the parents with the growth-promoting relationships they need, should be a major issue of concern to the network partners, including psychotherapists, involved in caring for traumatised children.

References

Allen, J. G., & Fonagy, P. (2006). Preface. In J. G. Allen & P. Fonagy (Eds.), *Handbook of mentalization-based treatment* (pp. xix–xxi). John Wiley & Sons.

Bevington, D. (2019, March 29). *AMBIT in practice: Working across complex and disintegrated professional networks* Vlaamse Vereniging voor Psychoanalytische Therapie [Dutch-speaking Association for Psychoanalytic Therapy] 2019 conference: A day of teaching with . . . Dickon Bevington, Kortenberg, Belgium.

Bevington, D., Fuggle, P., Cracknell, L., & Fonagy, P. (2017). *Adaptive mentalization-based integrative treatment: A guide for teams to develop systems of care*. Oxford University Press.

Boston, M., & Szur, R. (Eds.). (1983). *Psychotherapy with severely deprived children*. Routledge & Kegan Paul.

Emanuel, L. (2002). Deprivation x 3. *Journal of Child Psychotherapy, 28*(2), 163–179. https://doi.org/10.1080/00754170210143771

Fonagy, P., & Allison, E. (2012). What is mentalization? The concepts and its foundations in developmental research. In N. Midgley & I. Vrouva (Eds.), *Minding the child: Mentalization-based interventions with children, young people and their families* (pp. 11–34). Routledge.

Fraiberg, S., Adelson, E., & Shapiro, V. (1975). Ghosts in the nursery. *Journal of the American Academy of Child Psychiatry, 14*(3), 387–421. https://doi.org/10.1016/s0002-7138(09)61442-4

Gaskill, R., & Perry, B. (2014). The neurobiological power of play. Using the neurosequential model of therapeutics to guide play in the healing process. In C. A. Malchiodi & D. A. Crenshaw (Eds.), *Creative arts and play therapy for attachment problems* (pp. 178–194). The Guilford Press.

Henry, G. (1974). Doubly deprived. *Journal of Child Psychotherapy, 3*(4), 15–28. https://doi.org/10.1080/00754179708257300

Lieberman, A. F., & Van Horn, P. (2004). Assessment and treatment of young children exposed to traumatic events. In J. D. Osofsky (Ed.), *Young children and trauma: Intervention and treatment* (pp. 111–138). Guilford Press.

Ludy-Dobson, C. R., & Perry, B. D. (2010). The role of healthy relational interactions in buffering the impact of childhood trauma. In E. Gil (Ed.), *Working with children to heal interpersonal trauma: The power of play* (pp. 26–43). The Guilford Press.

Luyten, P., Fonagy, P., Lowyck, B., & Vermote, R. (2012). Assessment of mentalization. In A. W. Bateman & P. Fonagy (Eds.), *Handbook of mentalizing in mental health practice* (pp. 43–65). American Psychiatric Publishing.

Mayes, L. C. (2012). Foreword. In N. Midgley & I. Vrouva (Eds.), *Minding the child: Mentalization-based interventions with children, young people and their families* (pp. xi–xii). Routledge.

Midgley, N., Ensink, K., Lindqvist, K., Malberg, N., & Muller, N. (2017a). The development of mentalizing. In *Mentalization-based treatment for children. A time-limited approach* (pp. 15–37). American Psychological Association.

Midgley, N., Ensink, K., Lindqvist, K., Malberg, N., & Muller, N. (2017b). When the capacity for mentalizing is underdeveloped or breaks down. In *Mentalization-based treatment for children. A time-limited approach* (pp. 39–60). American Psychological Association.

National Scientific Council on the Developing Child. (2004). *Young children develop in an environment of relationships: Working Paper No. 1*. Retrieved from https://developingchild.harvard.edu/wp-content/uploads/2004/04/Young-Children-Develop-in-an-Environment-of-Relationships.pdf

Perry, B. D. (2001). The neurodevelopmental impact of violence in childhood. In D. Schetky & E. P. Benedek (Eds.), *Textbook of child and adolescent forensic psychiatry* (pp. 221–238). American Psychiatric Press.

Perry, B. D. (2006). Applying principles of neurodevelopment to clinical work with maltreated and traumatized children: The neurosequential model of therapeutics. In N. B. Webb (Ed.), *Social work practice with children and families. Working with traumatized youth in child welfare* (pp. 27–52). The Guilford Press.

Perry, B. D. (2009). Examining child maltreatment through a neurodevelopmental lens: Clinical applications of the neurosequential model of therapeutics. *Journal of Loss and Trauma, 14*(4), 240–255. https://doi.org/10.1080/15325020903004350

Shalev, A. Y. (2000). Post-traumatic stress disorder: Diagnosis, history and life course. In D. Nutt, J. R. T. Davidson, & J. Zohar (Eds.), *Post-traumatic stress disorder: Diagnosis, management and treatment* (pp. 1–15). Martin Dunitz.

Vliegen, N., Tang, E., & Meurs, P. (2023). *Children recovering from complex trauma: From wound to scar*. Routledge.

Zevalkink, J., Verheugt-Pleiter, A., & Fonagy, P. (2012). Mentalization-informed child psychoanalytic psychotherapy. In A. W. Bateman & P. Fonagy (Eds.), *Handbook of mentalizing in mental health practice* (pp. 129–158). American Psychiatric Publishing.

Part II

The three-track treatment approach

> As every captain knows: a ship has to change its course by only a few degrees to end up in another port.
>
> van Dis, 2007, September 18

In the second part of this treatment guide, we outline a contemporary psychodynamic psychotherapeutic approach for children who have experienced complex trauma. At this point, we wish to remind the reader that the treatment model set out in this book has primarily evolved in the context of an outpatient mental health centre servicing children in adoptive or long-term foster care placements, rather than children on the edge of care (e.g., children at risk of being removed from their biological parents or children in short-term foster care) or children in other living arrangements than a family environment (e.g., children in group homes). This implies that the work conducted with the child's primary caregivers, which we will refer to as 'Track 2', primarily relates to adoptive parents and foster carers (caring for a child in long-term foster care). Therefore, for reasons of parsimony and readability, in the next chapters, we will refer to the child's adoptive parents or foster carers (i.e., the primary caregivers who take care of the child on a day-to-day basis) as 'parents'. When it is important to differentiate between biological parents on the one hand and adoptive parents or foster carers on the other hand or between adoptive parents and foster carers, we have attempted to do so. Although this model was primarily developed for children who have experienced complex trauma living in stable family relationships offering them a relatively long-term perspective, it is our hope and objective that the model set out in this book might inspire and be useful for working with a broader group of traumatised children and the caregiving adults surrounding them.

Second, this book is primarily aimed at (child) psychotherapists who have a core knowledge about psychodynamic concepts and have core competencies in psychodynamic treatment models. However, as we also hope to inspire a broader group of professionals surrounding traumatised children and their families, we

DOI: 10.4324/9781003044918-6

have attempted to articulate relevant psychodynamic concepts and processes in accessible and jargon-free language as much as possible. For further reading, we refer to primers on psychodynamic child psychotherapy (e.g., Blake, 2011; Dowling, 2019; Grünbaum & Vibeke Mortensen, 2017).

In integrating the theoretical and clinical frameworks described in Part I, the importance of treating traumatised children while also offering support to those around the child, both within and outside the family, was emphasised. This has formed the very foundation of the present three-track treatment approach, encompassing direct work with the child, work with the parents, and work with the network. In Part II of this book, we set out each of the components of this three-track treatment approach, including a consideration of when all three tracks need to be offered side-by-side or when it may be better to start with one or two tracks (e.g., working with the parents and network before starting direct work with the child).

In Chapter 4, we introduce the core features of this way of working, by outlining each of the three tracks and by describing the basic principles and attitudes that inform the work done across these three components and across the phases of treatment. In later chapters, we discuss how these general principles play out in the work with the child, their parents and the network in the different phases of treatment.

In Chapter 5, we describe the aims and the structure of the assessment phase at all three levels of intervention (child, parents and network). Getting to know the child within their context and thoroughly assessing their developmental vulnerabilities and strengths helps lay the groundwork for a coherent case formulation to guide further treatment. Moreover, getting to know the parents and their strengths and vulnerabilities helps to form a much-needed working alliance. As clinicians, we must understand the support parents will need to keep being good-enough parents to their child. Finally, relevant partners in the network around the child and their family are included from the very beginning of the therapeutic trajectory.

In Chapters 6, 7 and 8, we discuss the direct work with the child, the work with parents and with the network, respectively. These tracks, when followed side-by-side, aim at facilitating developmental recovery in the child, recovery of mentalizing capacities in parents and other caregiving adults, as well as more positive relationships among child, parents and significant others in their life. The overall aim is to promote a more balanced way of living and being with one another.

In Chapter 9, we outline how the therapists can work towards ending in the three tracks of this treatment approach. Work in the ending phase aims at consolidating the developmental progress that has been achieved throughout the therapeutic process. In addition, working through a separation experience in a non-traumatising and growth-promoting way is of crucial importance for children with a history of discontinuity and breakdowns in care relationships. Finally, the fact that children who have experienced complex trauma may remain vulnerable to new or re-activated difficulties in subsequent developmental phases is specifically considered in the way the ending phase has been shaped in the present treatment approach.

References

Blake, P. (2011). *Child and adolescent psychotherapy*. Karnac.

Dowling, D. (2019). *An independent practitioner's introduction to child and adolescent psychotherapy: Playing with ideas*. Routledge.

Grünbaum, L., & Vibeke Mortensen, K. (2017). *Psychodynamic child and adolescent psychotherapy: Theories and methods*. Karnac Books.

van Dis, A. (2007, September 18). *Knack*.

Chapter 4

The three-track treatment approach: core features and basic principles

As argued in Part I, complex trauma is not only a problem of the individual child but deeply affects parents and the broader network. The treatment approach set out in this book aims to foster developmental recovery in the child as well as recovery of parents' and other caregiving adults' mentalizing abilities. The latter is geared towards creating a 'facilitating environment' (Winnicott, 1971) around the child in which growth-promoting interactions can be fostered as much as possible and positive and rewarding adult-child interactions can emerge. Such embeddedness in mentalizing relationships forms the crucial backdrop against which any developmental recovery and progress can emerge. Following Howe (2005), we strongly believe that 'If relationships are where things developmental[ly] can go wrong, then relationships are where they are most likely to be put right' (p. 278). Hence, the present treatment approach has been conceptualised as a three-track trajectory in which the different aspects are taken into account: the child's particular developmental injuries and problems, the parents struggling to keep mentalizing their child, and network partners facing hard-to-understand behaviour in the child and unexpected responses in themselves (see Figure 4.1).

In this chapter, we first outline the three tracks of the present treatment approach and discuss how therapists can assess the appropriateness of this treatment approach at the level of a particular child, their parents and the network. In doing so, we pay particular attention to the need for a therapeutic couple embedded within a mentalizing team, in order to be able to keep in mind the many minds involved with a traumatised child. We then outline the basic principles and attitudes of this approach, which form the common threads throughout the treatment.

A three-track trajectory of intervention

Given traumatised children's developmental difficulties (see Chapter 2) and the impact of these difficulties on carers' well-being (see Chapter 3), it is clear that merely treating the child individually or only working with parents or with the network will often prove to be 'too little'. Similarly, it will often not be enough to merely keep parents informed without a full engagement in real parent work, or, referring parents to a 'trauma-sensitive' parenting programme may be helpful but

DOI: 10.4324/9781003044918-7

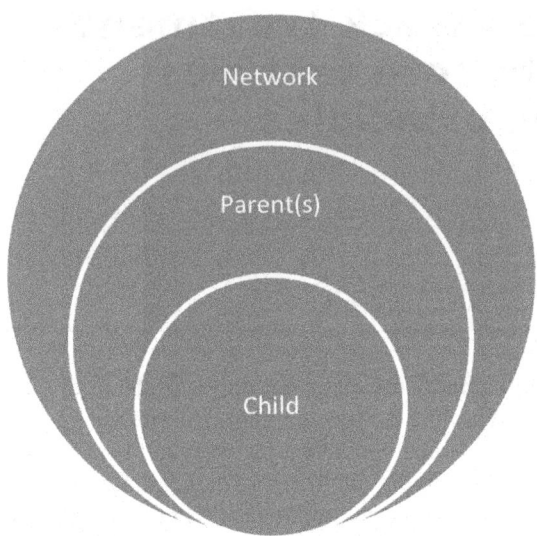

Figure 4.1 A three-track treatment approach, with the direct work with the child embedded within the work with the parent(s), in turn, embedded within the work with the network.

in some cases may be insufficient to really support them in tackling their child's specific problems.

Yet, what may sometimes be less straightforward is the timing and pacing of the three tracks. Given that intense suffering and disruptive and disturbing behaviour is common in traumatised children, it is natural to assume that the child must be helped directly and that individual therapy is thus a good place to begin (Track 1). However, it is important to consider that direct work with a traumatised child can only fulfil its potential when it is fundamentally embedded in the work that can be done with parents (Track 2) and the network (Track 3). The additional value of direct work with the child in fostering developmental recovery is thus dependent upon the extent to which the child's family and network can be supported to form a positive and growth-promoting everyday environment around the child. This implies that in circumstances in which the safety and stability of the child's caregiving environment are at stake, we advocate careful consideration of starting up direct work with the child. Some traumatised children are referred for treatment not knowing what family they will be living with next month (e.g., because foster placement has not yet been secured). Others are living in families in which they are chronically confronted with being misunderstood or with their caregivers' overwhelming suffering. Such circumstances entail that the child cannot rely on their parents' or carers' mentalizing capacities when distressed. As such, it would be very difficult, if not impossible, for the child to find the mental space to engage in a therapeutic process that would surely strain their capacities and abilities. When

Table 4.1 Basic features of the three-track treatment approach

Track 1: Direct work with the child	Track 2: Work with the parents	Track 3: Work with the network
• Once-weekly sessions	• Every three to four weeks • In-between-sessions availability as appropriate	• Network meetings once a term • In-between meetings with one or more network partners as appropriate
• Time-limited, namely period spanning about 40–60 sessions with child • Two therapists • Mentalizing team		

the setting is too unstable or unsupportive, in a first phase, work with network partners may be offered to clarify what the current concerns are and what the child needs first and foremost (which is usually not psychotherapy). Prematurely starting up direct work with a traumatised child when the setting is very unsettled may increase the risk of premature endings, which will leave the child with a potentially retraumatising experience of yet another relationship breakdown.

In the following sections, we outline each of the three tracks of intervention (see Table 4.1) and introduce specific interventional principles associated with each of these tracks that are further discussed in subsequent chapters. In doing so, we aim to provide the reader with specific guidelines as to the timing and pacing of a focus on each of these tracks and their interrelationships.

Track 1: direct work with the child

Track 1 concerns direct work with the child, preferably in once-weekly sessions, in order to provide the child with a much-needed transitional space to experiment and practise with more adaptive ways of tackling the problems they are struggling with, in the safety of the therapist's presence. As discussed in Chapter 2, traumatised children's problems are complex and pervasive and are often related to several of the four developmental domains which have been found to be compromised by complex traumatic experiences. Therefore, a time-limited long-term treatment trajectory is indicated. The time-limited nature is meant to create momentum: it helps to keep everyone involved (child, parents and other adult carers, including the therapists) focused on the task at hand (i.e., the therapeutic goals agreed upon: see Chapter 5, also Chapter 9). A duration of about 40 sessions (corresponding to a school year) is usually considered as essential but minimal to provide the child optimal opportunity to form a firm enough bond with the therapist in order for therapeutic progress to ensue. An extended trajectory (to about 60 sessions) can help to bridge the transition to the next school year, which provides the caregiving network more opportunities to evaluate whether therapeutic gains have transferred to real-life relationships. This may be more important, for example, if therapeutic change takes place more slowly and/or the child faces particular challenges in real life that weigh on therapeutic progress.

In this context, two issues are worth considering. From a traumatised child's perspective, entrusting oneself to yet another unknown adult who, at least based on most of their prior experiences, might not be all that trustworthy or reliable, is a huge thing to ask. This requires from the child's parents to have a fair level of emotional and mental balance to enable them to support and encourage the child in the risky venture of entrusting themselves to the therapist.

Second, many traumatised children suffer from a range of problems, some of which having been labelled with one or more psychiatric diagnoses. For instance, some children struggle with learning difficulties, a language delay or other cognitive impairments. Others show ADHD-like hyperactive behaviour or struggle to hold or switch attention. Still others present with an autism-like relational pattern, characterised by social withdrawal and a lack of imagination, or even dissociative or psychotic moments. For clinicians and therapists working with such children, it is often impossible to disentangle whether these problems are part of the clinical presentation of complex trauma or rather have to be considered as 'comorbid' conditions relatively distinct from the impact of complex traumatic experiences. Regardless of this chicken-or-egg question, such multiple problems require therapists to be very mindful of the child's particular profile of vulnerabilities and to adapt the treatment approach accordingly. Moreover, some children may benefit from a psychopharmacological add-on or from an additional intervention at school or at home aside from psychotherapy. In other words, the three-track model presented in this book doesn't mean that the child shouldn't receive any other intervention. As we will discuss in Chapter 5, one outcome of the assessment phase may be to assess what else, aside from the three tracks, the child might need in terms of additional intervention to address some of the difficulties. The process and any outcomes of such 'service needs assessment' will need to be discussed and agreed upon with the child's parents in Track 2 as well as with the network in Track 3. And ideally, the service provider of the additional intervention will be included as a network partner in Track 3. In sum, most traumatised children with additional mental health needs can benefit from the present treatment approach if the treatment implications of their particular needs are fully integrated and implemented in all three tracks.

Track 2: work with the parents

The second track involves work with the child's primary caregivers, starting prior to and running parallel with the direct work with the child. As the work conducted in this track is primarily aimed at containing parents' worries and suffering and supporting them in keeping their mentalizing abilities online, sessions with parents are scheduled every three to four weeks, depending on the phase in treatment and the urgency of the child's problems. For some families, this may need to be complemented with additional availability of the therapist or the service in cases of crisis and emergency.

As indicated in Chapter 3, detecting, containing and understanding why mentalizing abilities in parents will inevitably break down in everyday life and how to recover from such breakdowns is a major focus in parent work. Parents' mentalizing abilities are the basic prerequisite to foster growth and development in their child as well as to facilitate a more balanced family life. Mentalizing helps parents to better understand their child in terms of their particular inner world and dynamics underlying any 'intractable' behaviour, as well as to better understand themselves and their responses as being part and parcel of living with a traumatised child. Ultimately, mentalizing aims at fostering parents' skills to manage day-to-day difficult moments and conflicts with their child and to help encourage and build on experiences where parent and child 'connect'.

In the context of starting up this track of work with the child's parents, therapists may consider two issues. The first one concerns the child's as well as the family's safety. Safety – including physical, educational and emotional safety (Struik, 2019) – is always paramount. This means that the therapist, while listening to parents, needs to assess whether this family is in a safe space for every family member. Physical and emotional safety refer to the parents' ability to safeguard family members from harming each other physically or emotionally, or to at least be aware of and willing to talk about what happened to find a way out of destructive interactions. Educational safety refers to the parents' ability to provide a structured environment to the child on a day-to-day basis – with daily rhythms and patterns – and to meet the child's basic attachment needs. Only in the context of a basic level of safety and predictability in the family environment can the child fully benefit from child psychotherapy (Novick & Novick, 2011). Consequently, if the child's family relationships are assessed as posing a risk to any family member's physical and/or mental integrity, work with the parents or network may take place as part of putting a safety plan into place, in accordance with national or regional professional ethical and legal guidelines on child protection and safety. In such cases, the direct work with the child only comes into view when basic safety has been secured.

Second, in normal circumstances but even more so in caring for a child who has experienced complex trauma, parents' mentalizing capacities are subject to periods of stress and vulnerability. This makes the clinician's task of assessing parents' 'basic level' of mentalizing – and whether this level will sustain an intensive and challenging treatment process – a difficult one. This becomes even harder when confronted with caregivers whose parenting skills and/or mentalizing abilities seem to be severely and persistently impaired. For instance, severe mental impairment or chronic psychiatric problems (e.g., severe personality disorder, psychosis, severe chronic depression) in parents may interfere with their ability to offer a good-enough relationship to a child. Such instances require therapists to further scrutinise, assess and, if needed, take appropriate measures prior to considering the present three-track approach as a treatment option for this family. For instance, if the clinician assesses that parental issues interfere with good-enough parenting and/or basic parental mentalizing but that this interference is temporary, a 'parental module' to foster the re-emergence of good-enough parenting skills and/or parental mentalizing may be useful as a starting point for further therapeutic work.

Describing these considerations one by one may give the impression that we can deal with these considerations in a stepwise manner, as if first we assess the child's and family's safety and take appropriate action, then we assess and tackle the parents' mentalizing abilities, and 'all will be well' for the remainder of the treatment trajectory. In reality, as noted, both issues are closely interwoven and resemble iterative rather than linear processes. For instance, parents often only dare to talk freely about incidents of 'losing it' and acting aggressively towards their child or about phantasies of giving up this child when they start to feel safe in the emerging working alliance with the therapist. This means that no such reports by parents at referral are not to be considered as an absolute 'green light' to start treatment. Nor is the emergence of such reports by parents to be interpreted as a sign that the therapist did not do a good job. Rather, such 'shifting' windows into parenting practices is often part and parcel of the parents' therapeutic process. Similarly, parents' mentalizing abilities may appear largely absent at referral, only to start recovering in the context of being mentalized by the therapist during the early phase of treatment. Hence, the issues we have discussed with regard to the work with the child's parents are to be considered less as absolute contra-indications but rather as concerns to be considered and adequately responded to by the therapist in an ongoing process. How this can be done will be the focus of Chapter 7.

Track 3: work with the network

As discussed in Chapter 3, parents of a traumatised child depend on a supportive network to be able to provide a sufficiently safe and predictable environment to their child. Informal caregivers (e.g., family members and friends) as well as professionals (e.g., the child's teacher or foster care worker) can support the child in their particular developmental challenges and the parents in their parenting and mentalizing efforts. Track 3 therefore involves working with these network partners in order to create a much-needed facilitating environment. To this end, meetings in which – ideally – all the network partners participate are organised, complemented by one-to-one or smaller group meetings, in-between video or phone calls and/or crisis meetings.

Network meetings are among the most constructive means to build and maintain partnerships and to get every partner moving in the same direction. They form the prime stage for the work with the network and require agreements about the overall aims and frequency of the network meetings as well as about how to keep communication lines open in between meetings. A workable rhythm is to convene once a term, three to four times a year, irrespective of whether there are pressing problems at that moment or not. These meetings are indispensable in creating a shared understanding of the child's functioning. Based on this, a shared plan of action/care can be agreed upon as a necessary – but insufficient – condition for the child's development as well as their relationships to recover. Meeting each other and learning to know each partner's mandate and perspective and discussing ways of managing difficult situations at more quiet times is important in order to be able to act united when crisis situations do emerge. Aside from these formally organised network meetings, important work with members of the network is conducted in smaller or one-to-one meetings, depending on what is needed to provide good support to this child or family. Really sustaining and capitalising on these growing partnerships 'in smaller company' will foster the much-needed facilitating environment.

Despite the importance of creating and maintaining such a facilitating environment around the child and the family, one of the greatest challenges of this work is that it evokes strong feelings, including annoyance, fear, anger, disengagement, distrust and aversion. It challenges us to recognise and allow such feelings in the work, while remaining benign in our approach towards the people we are working with. In this regard, it is important to consider that working with a large(r) network is inherently complicated, as partners may enter the collaboration with different explicit and implicit ideas about the child's main issues, about what actions would be in the child's best interest and/or who should be responsible to take these actions (Bevington et al., 2017). In case of complex trauma, this 'usual' divergence in perspectives may be compounded by two processes. First, the traumatised child's level of behavioural difficulties or emotional suffering often leads to a sense of urgency which strains the mentalizing space in and among network partners. This may lead to premature or misguided actions, for instance, expelling the child from school because of disruptive behaviour without taking into consideration all the implications or exploring other viable options. Second, these children often 'disperse' their problems in their social environment, leading to different parties experiencing different aspects of the child's functioning. For instance, behaviour problems may be especially perceptible at home, while the same child conducts themselves as rather easy-going at school or vice versa, leading to meetings in which adults from different contexts can hardly imagine that they are talking about the same child. In some instances, the child may even be able to conduct themselves as well-behaved and lovable in one situation or relationship, while acting out their controlling, manipulative or destructive parts in another. These dynamics can easily trigger splitting mechanisms among network partners if these remain undetected or managed inappropriately. For instance, these may elicit phantasies of the 'good' child needing to be rescued from their 'bad' parents. In this regard, network partners may need to be supported to realise that one perspective on the child is not necessarily more 'true' than another but rather that the child's complex trauma history spurs such 'fragmented' functioning and dynamics. How this can be done will be discussed in Chapter 8.

In sum, in working with network partners, it may prove hard work to translate 'good intentions' into mentalizing and collaborative interventions. With mentalizing breakdowns almost inevitable and splitting processes lurking around the corner, network partners, including therapists, need to be aware of as well as prepared to manage these potential threats to their collaborative efforts. In some cases, considerable time and effort needs to be invested in reaching a shared understanding among network partners prior to or parallel with the work in Tracks 1 and 2.

Two therapists: two mentalizing and interacting minds, embedded in a mentalizing team

As discussed, children who have experienced complex trauma bring intense feelings of anxiety, sadness, anger and 'madness' into all close relationships. In doing so, they bring about unexpected, sometimes inappropriate and even retraumatising, reactions in the adults who care for them, including mental health professionals such as psychotherapists. As a result, therapeutic work with such children and their carers may be fraught with high levels of arousal, negative or even explosive affects and an almost continual risk of misunderstandings and relationship breakdowns. Being able to keep oneself regulated enough to be able to keep in mind not only the child's mind but also the parents' mind as well as the mind of the teacher, the foster care worker, the sports coach etc. is far from straightforward. This is why we have found it so important to advocate in this treatment approach the intense collaboration between two therapists embedded within a mentalizing team. Although we are aware of how services may struggle with shortages of staff, it is our experience and conviction that these children and the adults involved in their care require more than 'one thinking mind', due to the complexity of the cases, the impact on the therapist's resources and the threat of splitting mechanisms.

In our experience, having two therapists working together as two mentalizing and interacting minds around a traumatised child and their carers is anything but a luxury. With one therapist being able to focus on doing the direct work with the child and the other on working with the child's parents and with the network around the child, we aim to provide an environment which can hold and contain the strong dynamics which are often at play in such cases. Mental health services may already be struggling with shortages of staff and heavy caseloads, and even if working in pairs is a viable option, it often proves to be anything but pragmatic. Yet, this choice has been based on considerations regarding the inherent fragility of the capacity to mentalize in all of us in circumstances of heightened stress, which is compounded by the particular dynamics that traumatised children tend to set in motion. This also means that the idea of two therapists is not about two people working side-by-side, like two cyclists racing separately. Instead, the therapists need to work hard to align their 'racing strategy', with regard to direction but also with regard to pace. Moreover, rather than imagining the treatment approach as two separate tracks (one determined by the child psychotherapist and the other by the parent/network worker), we have often found it more helpful to think about it as part of one 'racing strategy', with at times one therapist 'riding point' and at other times the other, depending on what is needed 'to travel the distance'. In order for such a 'two-headed cycling team' to run smoothly – or as smoothly as possible – the two therapists need not only to work on the same case and exchange information but to commit to genuine communication and collaboration with one another. For instance, there is a risk of over-identifying with one of the parties involved and under-identifying with another. This mostly takes the shape of the child therapist over-identifying with the child and finding it hard not to think about the parents in terms of 'bad parents' and the parent worker over-identifying with the parents and finding it hard not to think about the child in terms of 'a bad' or 'a mad child'. As discussed earlier, a traumatised child's relational dynamics may elicit non-mentalizing splitting mechanisms in the adults around them. In our experience, the force of two genuinely collaborative minds is needed to counter this potent pull towards fragmentation and disintegration.

Moreover, both therapists being embedded in a mentalizing team can offer a setting to detect and uncover how frictions between the child psychotherapist and parent worker may reflect processes of over- and under-identification among those involved with a particular child and family. For instance, the child psychotherapist sighing in a team meeting that 'things would change faster for [the child] if only the parents would be a little more reflective' may bring about a reaction in the parent worker about how these parents have been doing their utmost for this child. Or, the parent worker may be empathising so much with the child's parents in their suffering that they react with marked disbelief when the child therapist talks about the feelings of profound sadness and loss which the child expresses in therapy. In such instances, a mentalizing team may provide the therapist pair with the much-needed mentalizing space to take a step back from the affect-laden dynamics in which they have become entangled and, in doing so, help them see their 'blind spot' and regain a more mindful stance.

Basic principles and attitudes

Across all three tracks of intervention and across the phases of treatment of the present model, certain basic principles and corresponding attitudes inform the work conducted (see Table 4.2). In the following sections, we aim to outline these guiding principles as well as give the reader a sense of how these principles may be particularly challenged in working with children who have experienced complex trauma. In later chapters, we will address in detail how we try to deal with and respond to these challenges in growth-promoting ways.

A solid but flexible therapeutic frame: developing a mentalizing structure around child, family and network

A first basic principle is the therapist's commitment to establishing and maintaining a solid therapeutic frame and to handling this frame with adequate flexibility. Psychodynamic approaches attach great value to a solid, enduring and reliable therapeutic frame. As traumatised children and their families and surrounding networks

Table 4.2 Basic principles and attitudes of the three-track treatment approach

- A solid but flexible therapeutic frame, as a structure conducive to (regain) mentalizing
- A continuous focus on supporting relatedness
- Keeping a mentalizing stance front and centre
- Looking through a trauma- and developmentally informed lens

often face intense and even dysregulating and crisis-like situations, they are in need of a stable framework to avoid drowning in negativity and to keep or restore mentalizing capabilities 'online'. When the time, rhythm and space of the therapeutic encounter starts to be experienced as predictable and reliable, a basic sense of 'feeling safe' can emerge, often meaning 'feeling safe enough to experience and communicate about feelings of unsafety, distrust, fears of being judged'. It is the safety of the external frame that makes it possible for a strong, understanding and essentially positive working alliance with child, parents and network partners alike to develop. Within such a frame, the benign and collaborative intent of interpersonal interactions in the therapeutic encounter can be conveyed, and therapeutic processes and change can ensue (see also 'epistemic trust'; Fonagy et al., 2019).

However, there is no straight line from 'offering a firm frame' via 'feeling safe' to 'therapeutic change'. The task of establishing and maintaining such a therapeutic frame goes hand-in-hand with feelings of friction, perhaps even anger or distrust, thus requiring a lot of reflectivity and flexibility. At the level of all three treatment tracks, specific dynamics may set in motion that adjustments to the therapeutic frame need to be considered. How this may play out and how the therapist can respond to such challenges to the therapeutic frame will be addressed in Chapters 6, 7 and 8, respectively.

A continuous focus on supporting relatedness

Parallel to the therapeutic frame constituting the therapist's external frame, a core element of the therapist's inner frame is their attempts to support relatedness. Scaffolding the child's relationships with significant others and supporting a sense of belonging and relatedness – which is a basic principle of any psychodynamic child psychotherapeutic work (Novick & Novick, 2011) – is often more complicated in working with children who have experienced complex trauma. These children can bring about a variety of difficulties in their close relationships by approaching new relationships with 'old' and often burdening relationship patterns. Precisely because of this and because mentalizing breakdowns in these children's parents and other caregiving adults are common, therapists need to keep these multi-layered and complex relational dynamics in mind. The cocktail of a hard-to-care-for child and almost inevitable mentalizing breakdowns in carers needs to be at the core of the therapist's attention, sometimes explicitly in the foreground, at other times more in the background. In this context of 'high stakes' and low mentalizing, keeping others in mind as well as helping others to keep each other in mind is a central part of the psychotherapeutic work that has to be done within all three tracks. How the therapist can go about this will be addressed in Chapters 6, 7 and 8, respectively.

Keeping a mentalizing stance front and centre

The idea that human behaviour – no matter how weird or difficult – is meaningful forms the basis of a 'mentalizing stance' and is at the core of contemporary psychodynamic treatment approaches. To keep this idea on the fore is a real challenge when working with children who have experienced complex trauma and the caregiving adults surrounding them. Having to live with the given that you frequently behave in ways that are incomprehensible to yourself evokes feelings of being weird or even mad. Having to face 'incomprehensible' and challenging behaviour on a daily basis makes parents and other caregiving adults struggle with uneasy feelings of not being able to understand why the child does what they do. To break the vicious non-mentalizing cycle of difficult behaviour resulting in misunderstandings and negative reactions, a genuine commitment to almost continuously attempting to restore reflection about the possible meanings of what seems to be weird and incomprehensible is essential. A therapist who is capable of 'stubbornly' remaining mindful and who is committed to helping child, parents and network partners make 'weird' behaviour comprehensible again and again functions like an antidote against being overwhelmed by fear and anger and against un-mindful reactions to trauma triggered arousal. This requires the therapist to continuously construct and reconstruct the child and their family in their mind (Fonagy et al., 2014), rooted in profound knowledge about and understanding of trauma dynamics.

Looking through a trauma- and developmentally informed lens

In psychotherapeutic work with traumatised children and their carers, maintaining a mentalizing stance or recovering from mentalizing breakdowns swiftly enough is a mission impossible without developmental and trauma-informed knowledge. A traumatised child's 'difficult' behaviour and what this evokes in parents and other caregiving adults often remains incomprehensible unless one can consider it in light of developmental adaptations and trauma dynamics (e.g., fight, flight or freeze reactions to trauma triggers; expressions of a hypervigilant stress response system or manifestations of 'old' relational expectations). Moreover, general knowledge about trauma and its impact on development is of little use when not embedded in a genuine commitment to attempt to 'know' (i.e., to keep mentalizing) this particular child in this family and these circumstances. Part of this coming to 'know' this child and their family also entails helping both child and carers come to terms with aspects that will remain unknowable, such as parts of the child's early childhood history (e.g., in case of international adoption) or the child's exact future developmental trajectory. Sometimes clients come to psychotherapy expecting the therapist to be able to see into people's minds and predict how they will fare in the future or to 'fix' the child so that they will be able to attain whatever aspirations or dreams their parents have for them. The therapist will then need to support both child and adults to mourn the loss of unrealistic expectations, aspirations and dreams and, at the same time, to hold on to a (realistically) hopeful perspective. This requires the therapist to have profound knowledge of the impact of complex traumatic experiences on the child's subsequent development as well as on the well-being of those involved in caring for and raising them. How the assessment work with a particular child and their carers can be conducted will be the focus of Chapter 5. The focus of the subsequent therapeutic work then hinges on the therapist's ability to use such a developmental and trauma-informed perspective to inform the treatment approach at the level of all three tracks. How this can be done will be addressed in Chapters 6, 7 and 8, respectively.

References

Bevington, D., Fuggle, P., Cracknell, L., & Fonagy, P. (2017). *Adaptive mentalization-based integrative treatment: A guide for teams to develop systems of care*. Oxford University Press.

Fonagy, P., Luyten, P., Allison, E., & Campbell, C. (2019). Mentalizing, epistemic trust and the phenomenology of psychotherapy. *Psychopathology, 52*, 94–103. https://doi.org/10.1159/000501526

Fonagy, P., Rossouw, T., Sharp, C., Bateman, A., Allison, L., & Farrar, C. (2014). Mentalization-based treatment for adolescents with borderline traits. In C. Sharp & J. Tackett (Eds.), *Handbook of borderline personality disorders in children and adolescents* (pp. 313–332). Springer.

Howe, D. (2005). *Child abuse and neglect: Attachment, development and intervention*. Bloomsbury Publishing PLC.

Novick, K. K., & Novick, J. (2011). *Working with parents makes therapy work*. Jason Aronson.

Struik, A. (2019). *Treating chronically traumatized children: The Sleeping Dogs method* (2nd ed.). Routledge.

Winnicott, D. W. (1971). *Therapeutic consultations in child psychiatry*. The Hogarth Press and the Institute of Psychoanalysis.

Chapter 5

Assessment of 'child within family' development

Understanding the child's development is essential if we want to find out what may be helpful for a particular child and their family, as 'adopting a developmental perspective fosters compassionate understanding' (Allen, 2013, p. 1). This includes understanding early environmental factors that may be shaping the child's development, as well as the interactions between development and the child's current environment. The assessment phase is, in the first place, essential to *get to know the child*, their inner world and the way they experience the outer world of relationships and events and to understand the child's strengths and vulnerabilities in different developmental domains. Furthermore, we aim to *get to know and understand the parents*, their concerns regarding the child and their abilities to mentalize their child and themselves. By organising and phrasing the information gathered during the assessment in a transparent and recognisable case formulation, we aim to *help the parents to understand* their child's difficulties in terms of what is happening in the child's inner world and how these problems are challenging their parental skills and resources. A shared understanding about the particular problems the child is struggling with, as well as the underlying dynamics that lie at the heart of these problems, fosters parental mentalizing abilities and helps the family to engage in an – often demanding – therapeutic process based on a shared agreement about the kind of help that is required (Cregeen et al., 2017). Finally, the assessment phase *helps the child to begin to understand* the connection between their behaviour – often experienced or even named as weird, crazy or bad – and what is going on in their mind. We aim to foster the child's engagement in the therapeutic process by getting them involved from the very beginning. As such, throughout the assessment, the therapist attempts to hold the balance among information gathering, reflection on internal experience and creating working alliances with all involved (Cregeen et al., 2017).

The four basic principles, as outlined in Chapter 4, run as central threads throughout the work conducted from the outset. As understanding what is at stake in the child's and the parents' minds forms the crux of the assessment phase, a mentalizing stance is required from the first moments of encountering the family members. Therefore, a clear – but flexible – assessment frame is set out, offering the therapist the opportunity to enter into a reflective dialogue with child and family – a

DOI: 10.4324/9781003044918-8

process that contributes towards a deeper understanding of the child's as well as the parents' thoughts and feelings. The emphasis on relational embeddedness and the trauma- and developmentally informed lens are inherently part of the way the assessment phase is shaped: the assessment work is meant to understand how this child's development has been shaped by traumatising early circumstances and may recover (in part) through current mentalizing relationships.

In this chapter, we first frame the work to be done when parents consult or are referred, prior to the 'actual' assessment sessions. We then outline the structure of the assessment process as conceptualised in the present treatment approach. Next, using the composite case of Jemal and his adoptive family, we describe the aims and the content of each of the assessment stages and sessions and formulate guidelines on specific topics in these sessions. At this point, we wish to remind the reader that this principle-based treatment guide is not so much meant to be used as an exhaustive checklist but rather as a source of inspiration to guide the therapist's thinking and observing.

Prior to getting started: paving the way, identifying the obstacles

Julian and Rebecca are the adoptive parents of Jemal, aged ten, who was born in Ethiopia and came to live with them when he was three years old. As soon as Jemal started elementary school, his adoptive parents witnessed him struggling with severe behavioural and educational problems. They transferred Jemal to a special educational needs school. After two years, when he was able to return to his previous elementary school, his adoptive parents dared to be hopeful again. They expected Jemal to develop better due to the intense help he had received at the special educational needs school, and they had always experienced the first school as helpful. Some months into the new school year, their hope gets dashed as Jemal seems to relapse into bad behaviour. Jemal's adoptive parents decide to contact the special educational needs school to talk about their worries. The psychologist, who supported the family during Jemal's two years at the school, refers them for psychotherapeutic treatment.

Sometimes, parents are referred for psychotherapeutic treatment by services or colleagues who are well-informed about what to expect. As in Jemal's case, parents/carers may have already received some support in parenting their adopted or foster child, for instance, from the adoption or the foster care service; other carers may have followed a 'trauma-informed parenting' programme and are seeking more intensive treatment. Such parents have already advanced through part of the process: they have experienced how it can help to reflect on the interactions between parents and child; they have learnt how to remain loving, secure and mentalizing parents across difficult situations; and/or they have realistic expectations of how psychotherapy may be of additional help and how intensely we will have to cooperate to sometimes only move small steps forward. In such cases, referrers and parents have a fairly good idea, i.e., relatively accurate expectations, about what therapeutic help can mean for their family and are, in that sense, 'ready' for a psychotherapeutic trajectory to be started up.

However, in other situations, families are referred for psychotherapy in the midst of a crisis because of difficulties with their child, with merely the hope that difficulties can stop and things will get better, with only little notion about how their parenting behaviour can influence their child's behaviour and sometimes with unrealistic expectations that psychotherapy will simply 'fix' their child's problems without them having to get involved. In such circumstances, some work needs to be done to translate the parents' and/or referrer's concerns into more realistic expectations about treatment. In other situations, a referral is made and parents consult, yet reluctantly, because they feel pressured. For example, when the teacher is alarmed by the child's behavioural problems at school but the parents, observing how the child is only just starting to calm down and settle in their new family, are hesitant to put additional pressure on the child at this time. In such circumstances, the work at hand is to find common ground about what treatment can mean in alleviating some of the concerns about the child and how to shape a way forward that takes into account the different perspectives that often are rooted in a shared concern about the child's further development.

The structure of the assessment process

The assessment process in the present treatment approach moves through three stages, encompassing about eight sessions (see Table 5.1). In the first stage, we try to get started with all involved (parents, child, other important caregiving adults)

Table 5.1 Structure and objectives of the assessment phase

Stage	Indicative number of sessions	Objectives
1	3	Getting started with and clarifying needs of all involved (parents, child, other important caregiving adults) to develop an initial understanding of each person's main concerns, needs and reasons of referral, as well as their mentalizing abilities
2	3	Developmental assessment with the child to explore the child's functioning and dynamics, vulnerabilities and strengths
3	2	Formulating and sharing the case and focus formulation with the parents and the child

to develop an initial understanding of each person's main concerns, needs, and reasons of referral, as well as their mentalizing abilities. Stage 2 involves conducting the actual developmental assessment with the child. In Stage 3, we organise and synthesise the assessment information gathered into a coherent and accessible case formulation in which aspects of the child's development, both strengths and vulnerabilities, are adequately captured and placed in the context of prior and current environmental factors and dynamics. This dynamic and mentalization-based case formulation (Henderson & Martin, 2014; Muller & Midgley, 2015) affords us a tool to share our understanding with the parents and the child. In doing so, we aim to facilitate a shared understanding of the child's current problems and the underlying dynamics that lie at the heart of these problems. Based on this dialogue and exchange, we can decide together with child and family what next steps are best to take ('focus formulation').

Stage 1: getting started and clarifying needs

The first consultations (see Table 5.2) are meant to start building a working alliance with the parents and the child, to clarify what exactly has prompted parents to consult and what the child's perspective is on problems and needs. They also aim to develop an initial understanding about the quality of attachment relationships in the family and about strengths and difficulties in the family's capacity to mentalize (Muller & Midgley, 2015). It mostly requires about three sessions, usually two with

Table 5.2 Core tasks and strategies for assessment Stage 1

Establishing a working alliance with the parents	• Gain first impressions of the affective family atmosphere • Develop an initial understanding for the reasons for consultation and assess the severity of the burden on the family • Validate and explore the decision to consult • Help prepare themselves and the child for the next joint meeting
Meeting the child in interaction with their parents	• Start building a working alliance with the child • Observe the quality of the parent-child relationship • Address the child's understanding of the reason for consultation
Towards a further understanding of the problems of child and family	• Gain an understanding of the child's developmental history • Gain insight into vulnerabilities and resources in the family history as relevant • Chart the family's current social support network • Probe the parents' response to a 'trauma-informed' perspective on their child's developmental difficulties

parents and one with parents and child jointly, to thoroughly clarify what the needs and concerns are of the parents and the child in consulting. Sometimes, a phone call or a meeting with a referrer can be fruitful. This may be the case, for example, when the key foster care worker who knows the family well hears worrisome stories about difficulties at school and at home, raising questions about difficulties in the child's development and whether assessment and/or treatment may be helpful. Their observations and ideas can, then, be informative to the assessment in complementary ways to the child's and the parents' perspectives. Sometimes, this meeting can be held jointly with parents, also as a way of modelling the thinking-together process.

Establishing a working alliance with the parents and understanding how they view problems and needs

In this first meeting with the parents, we actively look for opportunities to validate and explore their decision to consult, underscoring the courage this requires. Helping parents to reconnect to courage and strengths is an important foundation for building a collaborative working alliance. From an assessment perspective, we aim to get first impressions of the affective family atmosphere, including the quality of the attachment relationships and the mentalizing capacities and difficulties in the family (see also Muller & Bakker, 2009; Muller & ten Kate, 2008). We also aim to develop an initial understanding of what is currently most destabilising and dysregulating for the family and to assess the severity of the burden on the family. Finally, we help parents to prepare themselves and their child for the next joint meeting.

At the first meeting, Jemal's adoptive parents talk about how they received some complaints from school about him acting 'negative and tough' and taking every opportunity to start an argument. The therapist learns that they only decided to contact the psychologist at the special educational needs school after Jemal's football coach phoned them, expressing his concern about Jemal being 'unmotivated'. They paint a picture of him showing behavioural difficulties at school and expressing anxieties and a depressed mood at home. Mother looks sad and tired when talking about Jemal's 'dark thoughts'. He sometimes asks her if life has any meaning. She understands that he needs her patience and presence when he feels depressed but she also says she feels hurt by 'the way he needs her'. She goes on to explain that Jemal has little appetite and is extremely selective about what he eats when he's 'in that hard place'. At times like that, he scolds his mum for being a bad cook or for never buying nice food. By contrast, when Jemal is relaxed, like during a holiday, he eats with visible appetite and seems to like anything his mum cooks. 'That's how I have learnt that his complaint that there is "nothing tasty in the house" actually means that he isn't feeling alright emotionally', Mother sighs.

In this first meeting, the therapist primarily listens to the content of the parents' narratives about the difficulties they face, and meanwhile – with a second ear – to the emotional impact these problems have on them and on the current emotional atmosphere in the family. In the case of Jemal's adoptive parents, we learn that they are profoundly worried. Both parents talk in a loving, empathic and concerned way about their adoptive son and his difficulties. They really seem to know who he is and what he needs to grow, and their efforts to give him all developmental chances are huge. They talk about Jemal as an individual with his own problems, vulnerabilities and needs, as well as strengths. In her notes after this first session, the therapist writes: 'These parents seem able to think about Jemal and his developmental needs, but I wonder if the patient and empathic way they try to remain loving parents to Jemal is at the expense of being in touch with their own needs'. The latter is something that was not voiced explicitly by Jemal's adoptive parents themselves and of which they are probably not aware (yet) but that the therapist sensed in listening to their story.

Parents may respond very differently to the challenges they face with their child. Sometimes, good parental mentalizing capacities with regard to a deeply traumatised child compromise a mentalizing stance towards one's personal needs as parents, as may be the case in Jemal's adoptive parents. Jemal's mum appears able to mentalize her son quite well, seeing how his comments to the food in the house may reflect something about his internal sense of well-being, but although she can name her own thoughts and feelings, she seems to struggle a bit more to make sense of them. In other families, negative or hostile utterances about the child can give a glimpse of parents being at the end of their energy and mentalizing capacities. Parents may feel over-solicited or personal vulnerabilities can get triggered. Some parents feel provoked by outbursts of aggression; others feel exhausted due to the never-ending claims. Sometimes, there are first signs that parents are losing control, for instance, when they speak in harsh, vengeful or bitter words about the child. The observation of impaired mentalizing capacities in parents during these first encounters thus offers ample opportunity to assess whether these poor skills are due to a mentalizing breakdown after a chronic period of difficulties with a severely traumatised child or, rather, reflect vulnerabilities in mentalizing capacity that have remained invisible as long as mentalizing capacities were not taxed too much. As a therapist, with time as our ally, we can only closely observe whether mentalizing capacities recover with the aid of mentalization-based parent work (see Chapter 7) and/or when the child's problems become less burdensome. In the same vein, we listen to the parents' concerns and anxieties about their child's and family's future and about their expectations about how to regain a sense of regulation and a feeling of mastery. Topics and questions that therapists can hold in mind can be found in the following box (pp. 101–102).

Later in the first consultation meeting, the therapist learns a bit more about what has brought Jemal's family to seek help and tries to assess the severity of the burden on the family:

Jemal's adoptive parents describe how they've got used to getting complaints from school about his behaviour. They learnt – from previous support – that their son is developing in an atypical way and this has helped them to remain patient and supportive, taking difficulties at school seriously though without expecting that these will really disappear in the long run. By contrast, what makes them anxious and even panicky is that Jemal seems to have lost his motivation in sports. The football coach's call was the wake-up call to take action, because sports has always been like a lifeline for Jemal and him being 'unmotivated' in sports is as if he has cut himself off from this lifeline. It makes them wonder if he is 'really depressed' now.

When asked what is hardest to bear for them, Mother talks about the way Jemal – particularly at difficult times – can't seem to accept any help from them. She wonders why he doesn't rely on them more. He can't stand them even asking how he is doing and responds in an irritated way to every comforting gesture. Although he suffers from sleeping problems, he never asks for or accepts a goodnight kiss. His decision to remove the drawings on the wall in his room and the stuffed animals from his bed, claiming to be 'too old for such childish stuff', makes Mother feel desperate. The only bright spot for them is when they see how Jemal can nestle against the dog and find some peace. Jemal's adoptive mother suffers from feeling powerless when seeing her child suffer and being kept at a distance.

In situations such as the one described here, even if problems have already existed for a while and development has not run smoothly so far, parents consult in response to a recent precipitating event – the proverbial drop that makes the cup run over. In other situations, parents' decision to consult follows a period of distressing experiences (e.g., a period of separation anxiety, nightmares and sleeping problems), a major dysregulating experience (e.g., a child running away from school or stealing a smartphone in a store) or a series of smaller negative events that keep repeating as a 'never-ending story' (e.g., seeking conflict at school, being disproportionally angry for every small frustration). Foster carers or adoptive parents, like Rebecca and Julian, are often prepared for difficulties or for developmental trajectories that do not fit in a narrow conception of what constitutes 'normal' development. They can often draw on myriad resources to support their child. The decisive moment to consult a child psychotherapist mostly indicates that an experience is overwhelming their resources. Understanding this 'drop' can teach us a lot about this family and may be put to good use as the 'port of entry' (Sameroff, 2004; Stern, 1995). Topics and questions that therapists can invite parents to talk about can be found in the following box (pp. 101–102). These questions aim to explore the way the parents look at the child's problems and development, attempting to see the child through their eyes, as a starting point. Additionally, in this early phase of getting to know the family, it is important to gain a first understanding of how severely the family's resources and skills are challenged by the child's problems and what the burden of suffering on different family members is.

Whilst listening and trying to understand, the therapist pays particular attention to validating and exploring the parental decision to consult:

> When asked how difficult it was to decide to consult a mental health professional about Jemal, his adoptive parents speak about their experience with Jemal's school psychologist. Mother talks in a warm and lively way about how they felt understood and supported and how they didn't hesitate long before contacting her again when new concerns arose. 'She told us that she has had good experiences in collaborating with your service here around children like Jemal, and we really trust her judgement'. For Jemal's adoptive parents, a previous experience of having felt helped and supported has clearly lowered the threshold to consult and talk about their family's experiences.

When parents decide to consult, needs are often high and help is much needed, yet, at the same time, parents usually don't want to have to turn to professional help. Therefore, in this very first encounter, making space for their perspective and validating their courageous step in undertaking this journey are important elements in building a working alliance. The key to feeling validated lies in the experience of being heard and taken seriously in relation to their concerns about the child as well as the suffering they experience in parenting by an open-minded and non-judgemental therapist. As such, empathic listening is the most important structuring agent in the early phase of treatment (Hoffman et al., 2015; Jaffrani et al., 2020). Additionally, being listened to in an empathic way helps parents to regain access to resources and potential strengths and for a perspective of hope to re-emerge. When parents return home after this first meeting with a feeling of being heard and understood, a first hurdle has been taken and the chances for a further engagement in the challenging journey of treatment have increased (see also 'epistemic trust'; Fonagy et al., 2019). Sometimes, it can help to explore by asking explicitly what seeking professional help means to parents and how consulting with regard to their child's vulnerable development influences their feelings and experiences.

Particular feelings or experiences parents have had may heighten the threshold and make them more careful and reluctant to ask for help. Sometimes, parents struggle with feelings of incompetence, which further undermine their parental capacities as well as their relationship with the child. Or parents may have received critical comments in the past about their parenting and feel held responsible for their child's difficulties. Therefore, for many parents, it is helpful to have the therapist address these feelings and experiences early in the consultation process. Topics therapists can hold in mind to invite parents to talk about regarding their decision to consult can be found in the following box.

During and certainly at the end of this first meeting, the therapist should pay particular attention to helping parents prepare themselves and their child for the next meeting meant for them jointly as a family (see box). Some parents will need little preparation, in that they have already thought and spoken about it among themselves, they have already mentioned it to their child or they feel confident in talking to their child about coming to the therapist. Other parents may need some help in finding the 'right' words to talk to their child in an age-appropriate way about something that is important to their family without eliciting too much pressure on or anxiety in the child.

Topics to hold in mind during intake session with parents only (Session 1)

1. To get first impressions of the affective family atmosphere, including the quality of the attachment relationships and the mentalizing capacities and difficulties in the family

- In what kind of affective wording do parents speak about their child? Can you hear love, empathy and concern despite the intense difficulties? Or, are these first stories primarily accompanied by feelings of misunderstanding and anger or of tiredness and despair? Are there signs that parents/carers are losing control, for instance, speaking in harsh, vengeful or bitter words?
    - Is there still curiosity and interest in the child's particular perspective?
    - Is the child seen as a person with their own needs, problems, vulnerabilities, driven by wishes and sorrows?
    - Are parents/carers still able to think and talk about what they themselves are in need of emotionally?
    - What are parents concerned about, what are they afraid of, when looking to the future of their child within their family?
- How do they think about regaining a sense of regulation and a feeling of mastery and control in the family?

2. To explore the way the parents look at the child's problems and development and to assess the severity of the burden on the family

- What kind of experience is perceived by parents as beyond their abilities, as the 'too much to bear' and a reason for consulting? Why and why now do they seek help? What are the child's symptoms they are seeking help for?
- When did they notice these symptoms/behaviours for the first time, and do they have any thoughts about precipitating factors?
- How long have these symptoms/problems existed, and how have they evolved over time (fluctuations, worsening)?

- Who is suffering from what?
- How do the parents experience their child's suffering, their own, that of siblings, other family members?

3. To validate and explore parents' decision to consult

- What were thresholds to contact mental health services?
- What are (positive and negative) feelings and attitudes towards seeking help for the parents and for the child?
- Who referred this family for consultation and what kind of explanation for referral did the parents receive?
- Who has been informed about the problems that the family is dealing with? Are parents surrounded by people who support them in helping a vulnerable child grow up as constructively as possible? Or do people surrounding them make parents feel responsible for the child's problems?
- How does the family's environment perceive the step to consult? Who has been informed about the consultation? What kind of reactions did the parents get and how do they feel about these reactions?

4. To help parents prepare themselves and their child for the next joint meeting

- Have parents already explained the consultation to the child?
- How do parents imagine their child's reaction?
- Do they feel somewhat confident to talk to their child about coming to the therapist together?

Meeting the child in interaction with their parents

In meeting the child for the first time, in the presence of their parents, we aim to start building a working alliance with the child and to observe the quality of the relationship between child and parents as well as the way they talk to and think about each other in a new, somewhat anxiety-provoking situation. We also pay specific attention to addressing the child's understanding of the reason for consultation.

In the first meeting with Jemal in the presence of his adoptive parents, the therapist invites them to each choose a picture card that they feel matches with their family in some way. Jemal takes the card of a sheep and says: 'This is what my mum does: "Mè, mè! Jemal, you have to go to bed! Jemal, it is 10 o'clock!"' Later on, his mum picks out a sun, saying: 'Jemal is the little ray of sunshine in our home'. Jemal immediately replies: 'I'm no ray of sunshine at all, and it's always boring at home!'

Later on, elaborating on his mum's squiggle, Jemal completes the drawing as a surfer on the sea. He talks about a surf camp he attended. He wanted so eagerly to learn to surf that he was courageous enough to go by himself – 'without any friends' – his parents emphasise. Jemal leans towards the therapist and whispers: 'But the last two days, I really missed my mum'.

Therapist (whispering in the same way):	'And that seems to be something we can only talk about very, very quietly?'
Jemal:	'Yes, because it's really embarrassing'.
Therapist (still whispering):	'Really? For me, it's hard to imagine what the embarrassment could be about; I think it's brave for children to dare to talk about missing someone'.
Jemal (still whispering too):	'I even missed her voice, (in his sheep-like voice) "Jemal, do this, Jemal, do that . . ."'

Although the therapist feels struck by the harshness with which Jemal talks about his mum, she decides to leave this more difficult theme for a later moment – when a working alliance is a little bit more established – and first explores how Jemal experiences bedtime. Jemal says it is very difficult for him to go to bed, he is a 'bad sleeper' and he hates the moment he has to go upstairs to prepare for bedtime. With some humour, the therapist suggests that he is lucky that his mum keeps insisting that he does go to bed, because maybe otherwise he would never reach his bed. His parents join the conversation and talk about how they try to help Jemal with his sleeping issues.

Coming to meet the therapist is far from a neutral event to children. They often more or less grasp the fact that it is their behaviour that is the reason for referral by their parents or other caregiving adults. Sometimes they fear to be accused, punished, judged as weird or naughty. This is certainly the case for children whose behaviour is driven by complex traumatic dynamics, which is yet to be understood by the child themselves and their caregiving environment.

The least children may expect is to be addressed in their own 'language'. Addressing the child as an equal partner in the interaction by trying to tap into the child's preferred ways of communicating can be done by offering the child some tools, such as a box of pictures, drawing materials or age-appropriate toys (e.g., dolls to express thoughts and feelings about their family). Also, we often make use of a squiggle (Ensink et al., 2017; Winnicott, 1971) or another game or task, as a way to facilitate interaction between child and parent(s) and to get to know them in how they interact with one another. Meanwhile, we try to remain mindful for signs that the child is becoming anxious about too much attention. In the previous vignette, Jemal is able to make use of these means to communicate about his experiences, which allows the therapist to take an inquisitive and interested stance to following his communications. The therapist participating in his whispering enables him to talk about feeling embarrassed when he misses his mum. This first meeting with the child often provides an opportunity to observe how they cope with first and cautious explorations of their inner world, in the safety of the parents' presence (see box p. 106). In Jemal's case, we learn a lot about his perspective on important and vulnerable aspects of his life. In this way, we aim to get a first impression of how the child experiences the consultation and the new relationship.

Throughout this first joint meeting, there is an opportunity for observing the relationship between child and parents:

> Upon entering the room, Jemal takes a seat near the (new and unknown) therapist and doesn't seek any comfort from his adoptive parents to deal with this new situation, either by seeking physical proximity or by checking-back through eye contact.
>
> It strikes the therapist that while Jemal seems to feel free to talk about how he experiences his adoptive parents, he does so in a rather harsh and stand-offish way, even in their presence, as if he doesn't really take into account how his words may impact them emotionally. His adoptive parents remain positive and warm; they are able to speak in a growth-promoting way with him, about how brave he was to attend a surf camp by himself as well as about how they try to help him with his sleeping difficulties.

The consultation setting constitutes a new, unusual and potentially anxiety-provoking situation for the child, and the therapist is perceived as a new and strange person to relate and entrust oneself to. This offers opportunities for observing the child's reactions to this specific context. We can catch glimpses of the quality of the relationship between the child and their parents from an attachment and mentalization-based perspective (see box p. 107). In the previous vignette, Jemal shows his difficulties with being near to his adoptive parents and seems to avoid any experience of being dependent on them. Rather, he expresses his distant and even negative attitude and seems not to concern himself with how that may make them feel. In attachment terms, Jemal seems to be resorting to a rather avoidant style, deactivating the significance of others or relationships to himself, as a means of coping with attachment-related stress.

As the session progresses, there are usually opportunities to address the child's understanding of the reason for consultation:

> Towards the end of this session, the therapist has got to know Jemal as a child with some insight into why his adoptive parents are asking for help. She ends the session by summarising what she has learnt (directed towards Jemal): 'I've learnt about you that sleeping is a big problem, and that you maybe feel embarrassed when you miss your

mum'. Before she can go on, Jemal adds 'And I hate to admit when something is difficult'.

Therapist: 'Ah, that seems to be something interesting that you know well about yourself. So, tell me what that looks like, when you hate to admit when something is difficult'.

Jemal (thinks for a moment, and then says in a softer voice): 'Like this morning, when I was shooting hoops on the driveway, and Mum came to ask whether I wanted some lemonade. . . . I snapped at her . . . but actually I did want lemonade . . . but not until I could get the stupid basketball through the hoop. . . .'

Therapist: 'Wow, it seems to me you have a fairly good idea about what happened inside-and-out this morning. But I also get the sense that you're still bothered about what happened, maybe feel embarrassed that you snapped at your mum?'

Jemal (in a stronger voice): 'I don't mean to! (and then softer again) But it comes out . . . and then everything is ruined again. . . .'

In the first meeting with the child, we aim to create a joint space in which parents and child can communicate about their perspectives on the reasons for consulting and find common ground. Again, we try to bring the child's perspective to the fore by adopting a genuinely curious stance when inviting the child to talk about things (see box p. 107). Such questions offer a starting point to communicate about the child's level of awareness of problems, as well as about how some of these problems could be alleviated. Moreover, they offer the therapist a first glimpse into the child's mentalizing capacity. The therapist can get a sense of whether the child has any notion of a problem yet, of something they experience as difficult, even if this doesn't necessarily coincide with other people's main concerns. Often, traumatised children experience being 'different' from other children: they notice having more conflicts or realise their siblings never experience the kind of overwhelming nightmares they have. Some of them have ideas about themselves as weird or naughty, because of having more fights with others or unpredictable temper tantrums. The therapist can also listen for cues whether the child feels 'driven' by behavioural impulses and outbursts, as if they have no control over them or, rather, whether there are preliminary thoughts about reasons for behaviour, about an affective inner world that directs behaviour. For example, some children can – with a little help – start to link their behaviour (e.g., running away) with an inner experience (e.g., 'I was so angry because he accused me of taking his pencil case'), while for other traumatised children, this will be part of the work in treatment. In the vignette earlier, Jemal needs little invitation or support to recognise how an inner experience (hating to admit when something is difficult, like shooting hoops) may be linked to his behaviour (snapping at his mum) and even how his behaviour then complicates relationships and strains his sense of self. Yet, learning to gain control over behaviour that 'just comes out' will be part of the work in Jemal's treatment.

We pay specific attention to attempting to convey to the child (and parents) something of this common ground of why the child will be coming to the therapist for a few times. The therapist might suggest something about how the child's temper tantrums, terrifying nightmares or their urge to run away teaches us that they're going through a rough patch and that they possibly can use some help to make things go more smoothly. Jemal's therapist, for example, related something back about how he could get help with 'his difficulty to admit that something is hard, which sometimes makes him push away people harder than he means to, and makes him feel that he has ruined everything' and how his parents and teachers could be helped to better understand and manage that part of him. We also discuss and agree on what 'coming to the therapist for a few times' will look like (how many times, what dates and times, in which room, what they will do with the therapist, etc). This is important to foster feelings of mastery and control, which is so often lacking in children who have experienced complex trauma.

Topics to hold in mind when meeting with the child in the presence of the parents (Session 2)

1. *To start building a working alliance with the child*

   • What are the child's preferred ways of communicating?
   • How does the child react to the new situation and the new relationship?

2. *To observe the quality of the relationship between the child and their parents from an attachment and mentalization-based perspective*

   • How does the child negotiate the balance between seeking proximity and comfort in this new situation and being able to explore the new situation (room, toys, therapist)? Does the child remain in contact with (one of) their parent(s) while exploring?
   • How does the child regulate affects (e.g., anxiety, excitement)?
   • How do the parents respond to the child's way of behaving and relating during this session? Are they able to take the child's perspective, understand the child's reactions and act upon that understanding (e.g., support the child in negotiating proximity and distance)?

3. *To address the child's understanding of the reason for consultation*

   • Are there things the child would like to change in their life?
   • What does the child already know about the parents' reasons for consultation? What have they told them?
   • Can the child understand or at least relate to the parents' concerns?
   • What does the child think (and phantasise) about the reason for consultation and the parents' concerns?

Towards a further understanding of the problems of child and family

In this first stage of getting to know the child within their family as well as within their broader social context, we also want to explore the background of the current problems at a deeper level in a further explorative session with the parents. In cases of complex trauma, we thoroughly chart the historical and contextual aspects of the child's specific developmental difficulties, in order to be able to gain an understanding of the current developmental issues and mental health needs. To this end, we invite parents to share their views and experiences with regard to the child's history as well as their own, their family's current social embeddedness and how they have experienced these first few meetings with the therapist(s) (for topics the therapist can hold in mind, see box p. 110).

As a new-born, Jemal was abandoned near a police station in a small town in Ethiopia. After he was found, he was put in a cardboard box and brought to an orphanage in the neighbourhood. At one year of age, he was moved to another orphanage. When he was three years old, Julian and Rebecca travelled to Ethiopia to adopt him. When they saw him for the first time in the orphanage, he was a small but fat child, 'at least, he had been fed well', the parents remembered thinking. He was really attached to his nursery nurse. He immediately made good contact with his adoptive parents, was easy to hold and to comfort. Once in their family, he asked for food frequently but slept well and was a happy, open and joyful child. He liked to go to preschool and to be with friends.

For his adoptive parents, everything changed when Jemal started elementary school, 'as soon as the scholastic demands appeared in his life'. It seems as if learning is very stressful for him – is it about a fear of failure? his parents wondered. From that point on, Jemal suddenly stopped sharing what was going on in his mind. 'Sometimes, we found him in bed in the middle of the day, and when we asked what the problem was, he didn't speak for hours. That's why we contacted the school for special education. He went there for two years, and there he started to flourish again. We felt he related to us again, he could talk about his experiences again'.

In inviting parents to share what they know about the child's developmental history, we aim to gain insight into how the child came to be the way they are. Therefore, we pay particular attention to what parents tell us about the child's symptoms and their impact in different contexts of the child's daily life; the child's developmental history, since they became a member of the family and what is known about the child's history prior to placement. In doing so, we try to listen with a specific focus to how constitutional and prior as well as current environmental factors potentially interact with one another (Greenspan & Thorndike Greenspan, 2003).

Rebecca and Julian talk about the loss of a child before Jemal came into their life. Prior to the decision to engage in an adoption process, Rebecca easily got pregnant and gave birth to a girl who was severely disabled. She only lived a few weeks. Later examination revealed a hereditary disease and a large risk for a new child to also have this life-threatening disability. 'This was the first time we were confronted with a psychologist', Rebecca says. 'The ward psychologist was an unexpected golden gift in difficult times. She really helped us think and talk about our experiences, it was a mourning process that required a lot of energy, but it really brought us nearer to each other. It was during those conversations that the word adoption was mentioned for the first time'.

As far as is relevant to understand the current problems, we aim to gain insight into vulnerabilities and resources in the family history. To this end, the therapist might invite parents to talk about important moments in their lives with regard to 'becoming parents'. Jemal's adoptive parents talk about giving birth to and losing a child with a severe disability and how this impacted their life. Moreover, parenthood may be influenced by earlier life experiences in one's family of origin. Making use of a genogram may be helpful in this context, because it can convey to parents the therapist's genuine interest in how they feel about the different members of their family. This may help to gain insight into important aspects, such as how the parents negotiated prior challenges (e.g., experiences of loss). In this regard, we want to highlight that it is as helpful to make an inventory of parental strengths and resources as it is to gain insight into parents' anxieties and vulnerabilities.

Jemal's adoptive parents are surrounded by a warm and caring family. Both sets of grandparents live near them, and Jemal can easily and safely cycle between their houses by himself. Rebecca and Julian feel supported by their parents' caring presence. Sometimes, the grandparents will take Jemal along on a holiday, which helps Rebecca and Julian recover after an especially tiring period. Both parents feel a great deal of acceptance for Jemal's atypical development in their respective families. Furthermore, Aunt Evelyn, Julian's older sister who recently retired, comes in twice a week to help Jemal with his homework. This idea arose following a period of intense conflicts between Jemal and his parents about homework.

Of major importance to a family's ability to manage a vulnerable child's developmental and behavioural difficulties is the social support which the family can rely on. Therefore, we also invite parents to talk about who they feel are important 'partners' in raising this child in the family, school or leisure environment and what kind of support or assistance these partners offer. Sometimes, this is the first time parents have been invited to reflect upon 'social support', as they haven't thought about 'asking for help' or see it as a sign of weakness and shortcoming. In other families, asking about their supportive network evokes anxiety about the lack of support or even the abundance of highly critical family members. In these cases, inviting the broader family or organising a psycho-educational meeting to talk about raising a traumatised child can be of major help (see Chapter 8).

 In the special educational needs school Jemal attended, phrases such as 'vulnerable development' and 'deeply hurt early in life' had already been introduced to his adoptive parents. However, Rebecca and Julian seem to not fully grasp the breath nor the depth of what this implies for their son's development. They seem intensely absorbed in helping and supporting their child to develop and to achieve things 'as normally as possible', as if they cognitively understand about atypical development though it seems difficult for them to also emotionally come to terms with the profundity of the impact of trauma. The therapist makes a mental note that she will need to explicitly help Rebecca and Julian with that.

These early treatment processes and the information gathered in these first sessions are meant to enable the therapist to formulate a preliminary and shared psychodynamic understanding of the child's problems, which will guide the further assessment phase. At this stage, it is important that the therapist probes the parents' reaction to a 'trauma-informed perspective' on their child's developmental vulnerabilities. In reality, this might differ quite a bit among parents. For some parents, for instance, when they've had prior experience with mental health professionals or have followed a parenting programme, phrases such as 'atypical' or 'vulnerable development' or even 'trauma' will not be completely new, such as in the case of Jemal's adoptive parents. For other parents, however, the therapist will sense that it is likely too soon to use such words for these to be experienced as helpful by parents at this point and that it might be wiser to use 'more acceptable' phrases such as 'social-emotional difficulties' until these parents' process is further along. Often, as in the case of Jemal's adoptive parents, it is not even this 'black-or-white', with parents having some prior knowledge but not yet emotionally grasping the full extent of the impact of trauma. Then, the latter will often be at the core of the work conducted with the parents during treatment (see Chapter 7).

Topics to hold in mind when gaining a further understanding of the problems of child and family (Session 3)

1. To gain insight in how the child came to be the way they are

- What can parents tell us about the child's symptoms and their impact in different contexts of the child's daily life (family, school, leisure)?
- What can parents tell us about the child's developmental history, since they became a member of the family?
- What is known about the child's history prior to placement (including possible difficult or negative experiences)?

2. To gain insight into vulnerabilities and resources in the family history

- What can parents tell us about important moments with regard to 'becoming parents'?
- What can parents tell us about relevant life experiences in their families of origin (e.g., experiences of loss)?

3. To map the family's current social embeddedness

- Are there important 'partners' in raising this child in the family, school or leisure environment? What kind of support or assistance do these partners offer?
- What seems helpful in the parents' eyes?

4. To get a sense of parents' understanding and preliminary acceptance of a 'trauma-informed' perspective on their child's developmental vulnerabilities

- How do parents react to first ideas or phrasing in terms of 'vulnerable development' or 'traumatic experiences'?

Stage 2: conducting the developmental assessment with the child

In three (or four) assessment sessions, we aim to get to know the child in different aspects of their social and emotional functioning. Particular attention is paid to the child's preferred ways of communicating and relating, the child's strengths and vulnerabilities from a developmental perspective, the child's readiness and suitability for individual therapeutic work and the possible ports of entry for a therapeutic process.

A preceding session to assess the child's intellectual capacities and observe their skills with regard to structured cognitive tasks, such as in an intelligence test, is often warranted, as it may not only inform what may be expected in terms of educational attainment but also provide insight into the interplay among intellectual/cognitive and social-emotional capacities. For example, some traumatised children, despite average cognitive capabilities, seem to continually underperform at school. This might have to do with a lack of self-confidence or with a hyperalert stance due to an over-sensitive stress response system. Other children may have been overestimated with regard to their cognitive capabilities because they have been tiptoeing and exhausting themselves up till a thorough intellectual assessment opens up new avenues to be considered in terms of scholastic decisions. In still other situations, a child's disharmonious intelligence profile may make understandable to themselves, parents and teachers how their insecurity about their own abilities may have come about.

These assessment sessions with the child take about an hour each, but can range from 45 to 90 minutes, as the duration may be adapted flexibly to accommodate the child's pace. Some children are slow to warm up and need some time, whereas others adapt rapidly, only to become more anxious as they begin to communicate about inner experiences.

A developmental assessment with any child but with a traumatised child in particular draws on as wide a range of data as possible (Midgley, 2011) and thus requires a setting that maximises the amount of information that can be observed (Greenspan & Thorndike Greenspan, 2003). A mixture of methods – both structured and un-/less structured – invite the child to symbolise through drawing, playing or talking and to express themselves on a wide range of themes. There is no prescribed protocol for these assessment sessions, but it can be helpful to make use of a relatively 'fixed' set of instruments and methods within a team. Not as a rigid protocol to be followed to a tee but rather to enable a team to gain experience with how these children cope with this set, while also remaining mindful of any child's idiosyncratic response to any instrument offered that may warrant the therapist to decide to 'deviate from the standard set'. Inviting the child to engage with these instruments in a predefined order should in no way interfere with the therapist's sound judgement about what is appropriate and suitable for a particular child. For instance, if a child gets upset in response to the content of drawings or narratives, the therapist should rely on their clinical skills to decide how to proceed, when to stop and how to help the child to round things up in a containing way.

One way of structuring this assessment phase can be the following. In a first assessment session, the Four affect drawings and the Family as animals drawing can be useful in gaining first impressions about the child's affective world and representations about their family as well as about the child's skills to express aspects of these emotionally charged themes. In the second assessment session, the child's responses to a set of narrative story stems can reveal more in-depth attachment representations as well as affect regulation strategies and relational skills. In the third assessment session, a semi-structured interview, including a life history and inviting the child to play freely, may help to further deepen the insight into their inner world while the child is engaging in the relationship with the therapist on a more personal level. More information about and some guidelines for administering each of these instruments of this set can be found in the following box.

Four affect drawings

We first invite the child to draw what makes them the most anxious, the most angry, the most sad and the most joyful. After each drawing, we invite the child to tell us something more about it.

Follow-up questions/probes after each drawing:

'What is going through your mind (when you are most scared/angry/sad/happy)?'

In case the child draws and/or talks about a situation involving others:

'What are others feeling?'

'What are they thinking?'

Rule of thumb if the child is struggling to elaborate: repeat a child's spontaneous statement and then repeat the question/probe once.

Family as animals drawing

We invite the child to pretend that each of their family members could be turned into an animal and to draw them as animals. Afterwards, we invite the child to elaborate verbally on their drawing, for example, by asking what they like and dislike about each animal.

It is important to guard the aspect of displacement, i.e., to talk about the animal figures and not directly about the family members as individuals.

Narrative story stems

We invite the child to tell and show, using dolls and props, what happens next in the story of the stems that we as therapists have introduced.

Semi-structured interview

We introduce the interview to the child as not being a test but 'a wish to know what things are like for you, from your point of view'. In order to scaffold representational capacities and to ensure a correct understanding of the child's perspective about their family and their life history, three sheets of paper and a pencil are offered to draw (a) a family tree, (b) a timeline and (c) the child's wish for the future.

(a) 'I wonder if you could start by telling and drawing me a little bit about your family and yourself'.

   Follow-up questions/probes:
   'Who is part of your family?'
   'What are they like?'
   'Where do you live?'
   'What do you do together?'

(b) 'If this line represents your life course, can you indicate and tell me about your life and important things that happened to you from birth to now?'

   Follow-up questions/probes:
   'How old were you?'
   'Where were you living, and with whom?'
   'What exactly happened at that time?'
   'How did you feel?'

(c) 'If you could make a wish when you are older, what would that be?'

Free-play observation

We invite the child to play without constraints with a variability of materials, affording the child some time to get somewhat acquainted to the new setting and the new relationship.

Moreover, it is helpful to make use of the transition moments (waiting room) as opportunities to observe separation and reunion between parent and child (Hoffman et al., 2015), as well as with the therapist. Finally, it is important to contact the school and/or other relevant network partners to hear their thoughts and observations about the child's strengths and problems (Muller & Midgley, 2015). In some cases, an observation at school may be a helpful add-on.

Drawing on all the information gathered from multiple perspectives and multiple informants allows us to form as comprehensive an image as possible of the child's social and emotional functioning across the four developmental domains (for core topics to gather information on, see Table 5.3). Of course, these 'categories' do not emerge spontaneously from the material; it will require the clinician's analytical and, subsequently, synthesising skills to 'bring together' the material to paint a nuanced though coherent picture. How the clinician may go about this is illustrated in the following subsections using material from the assessment sessions with Jemal.

Table 5.3 Core topics in the developmental profile of the child

Developmental domain	Core topics to gather information on
Cognitive capacities and executive functioning	• Intellectual capabilities as assessed in intelligence test or other structured cognitive task • Academic progress and difficulties
Representational capacities	• Capacity to be playful, to express themes and to symbolise • Content of play and symbolisation • Capacity to mentalize
Affective development and regulation strategies	• Overall mood and emotional tone • Acknowledgement and expression of drives and affects • Central affects • Affect regulation strategies
Attachment development and relational capacities	• Basic sense of safety • Representations of caregiving relationships • Representations of self-in-relation-to-others • Relationship qualities in relation to significant others • Relational capabilities in relation to the therapist
Sense of self and identity	• The vital spark • Ability to experience and express loss and mourning and opportunities for growth • Ability to acknowledge and come to terms with being an adopted/a fostered child • Ability to construct a coherent life narrative

Affective development and regulation strategies

When asked to draw what makes him feel most scared (Session 1, Four affect drawings), Jemal remains silent for a full minute. He looks around, his face tense, but nothing seems to come to his mind.

Therapist (in a reassuring tone, attempting to normalise 'feeling scared'): 'Everyone – children as well as adults – is scared of something, just take your time to think about what that might be for you'.

Jemal (whispering): 'I used to be scared of vampires, I was convinced they really existed. Then, Mum put an onion beside my bed, she said that it would help against vampires as well as against a cold'. Then, Jemal draws a lion and says: 'he can roar loudly; he's a meat eater and a wild animal. Imagine that the gate is open, then the lion could eat me. I'm also scared of crocodiles, but they're harder to draw. And I'm scared of killer clowns; they scare people every day, and at night on the streets, not only on Halloween! They can kidnap you or knock you out'.

Therapist: 'Do you often feel scared?'

Jemal: (nods affirmatively) 'Sometimes, I'm scared in the dark in my room, and when I hear scary noises. Then, I take my Nintendo and turn my headphones on loud. When I pretend that everything is fine, it sometimes passes'.

Getting a sense of what the child's emotional world looks like and how feelings are experienced, regulated and processed is especially important in therapeutic work with children who have experienced complex trauma. Having been subjected to a large amount of negative, neglectful or traumatising experiences, these children more often than other children lack a basic positive mood. For some of them, like Jemal, their *overall mood and emotional tone* ranges from rather vulnerable, flat and sad (e.g., whispering and speaking with a soft voice, expressing embarrassment about missing his mum) to a rather distant and even slightly 'arrogant' attitude (e.g., speaking in a monotonous way and commenting on a lack of interesting stuff in the playroom). With such children, it is particularly important to remain alert to observe when their eyes and face clear up, for example, when they talk about hobbies or sports or about friends. Getting to know their 'vital spark' (see also later – 'Sense of self and identity') and scaffolding interactions and activities that can bring brightness and lightness in their sometimes 'dark' and 'heavy' inner worlds is as important as it is to address the difficult and sad feelings. In other children, there is an explicit negative or hostile basic mood, or their inner life is dominated by mood swings. Then, emotional expressions can be intense and highly observable or they can be small requiring a good observer. Still other children seem to express a positive mood, however, it lacks a genuine feel to it: the therapist somehow senses that positivity is a façade, masking much more difficult affect.

Moreover, it is important to get to know the child's way of *experiencing, expressing* as well as *regulating basic affects* such as anxiety, anger, sadness and happiness. Is the child able to live through and name these affects? Can they talk or play about them when explicitly evoked (e.g., in affect drawings) or spontaneously? Some children, like Jemal, can acknowledge being *scared* (of vampires, of lions or crocodiles that could escape in the zoo and eat you, of killer clowns and being kidnapped, of darkness). Sometimes, children express being aware that these fears are rather primitive or age-inappropriate, calling them childish or weird and/or trying to hide them from others, like Jemal in the beginning. Others are unable to name what they are afraid of, or become overwhelmed by anxiety as soon as they start talking or drawing about it. *Anger* is often a difficult emotion to acknowledge and to talk about, as is *sadness*. In children who have experienced complex trauma, anger and sadness may have acquired a particular meaning or affective load, linked to their early experiences. When asked what makes Jemal feel most sad, he talks about a movie 'about a child who lost his parents, that made him cry and cry' (see later). Having been abandoned at a young age, watching a movie about a child 'losing parents' elicits a deep and pervasive sense of being hurt and having suffered losses. Even the feelings of *happiness* or contentment that may seem 'easier' at first sight can be more complex or difficult for children who have experienced complex trauma. Jemal, for example, never once expressed a moment of real joy or happiness during the assessment sessions. When asked what makes him most happy, he draws what he finds funny instead. He says he really laughs when funny things happen: one of his friends with messy hair or toddlers arguing in the playground at school. 'When I don't have to go to school, I'm happy. But I don't feel happy often'. Some children show a rather narrow range of basic emotions; others express a broader range and are able to also express more sophisticated emotions such as shame or disappointment.

With regard to *affect regulation strategies*, particular attention during the assessment sessions is directed towards whether the child has strategies to remain in a relative state of regulation and emotional balance while thinking or talking about feelings or affective themes. Some traumatised children lack the capacity to express feelings in play, drawings or words and show them through their body, in immediate action. Some children's primary way of coping is denying any disturbing affect or feeling, 'pretending that everything is fine' and hoping it will pass, like Jemal. For others, emotions are mainly experienced as 'forces that steer their (motor) behaviour', which they feel they have little or no control over. The fact that their behaviour is continually commented on by the adults or peers around them, of course, does not remain without consequence to these children's sense of self (see later).

In considering the pre-therapeutic value of the assessment phase, it is not only important to get to know the child's affective world and regulation strategies but also to acquire first-hand experience about what is helpful versus dysregulating in interactions between child and therapist. In the vignette earlier, seeing the tension on Jemal's face when she invited him to draw what makes him feel scared, the therapist reflects on whether it would help him if she normalises feelings of anxiety. In an attempt to find out what may be helpful, she therefore adds that 'everyone is scared of something'. Jemal's response – although in a whispering voice – reveals that the therapist's intervention was helpful to reduce the tension to a level that allowed him to express aspects of being scared. It also shows that the theme of 'being scared' evokes in Jemal rather unrealistic images of vampires, crocodiles and killer clowns, giving a glimpse of the deep and almost tormenting levels of anxiety in his inner world.

Representational capacities as expressed in play and narrative

When asked what makes him most sad (Session 1, Four affect drawings), Jemal thinks for a while. 'Ah yes, there was a movie that was so sad that it made me cry for half an hour . . . Peter and the Dragon the movie was called'. A detailed but difficult-to-follow account of the movie's storyline follows: 'and Peter's parents were dead, and the dragon chases the wolves, and there was a hole in the bridge and a car drove over with a lady and a child sitting in it. . . .' Jemal recalls fragments of the movie, seemingly without any awareness of what information would be relevant to the therapist, indicative of a sense of overwhelm while recounting the experience.

Therapist (in an attempt to co-regulate by scaffolding symbolising and slowing down): 'Could you draw something about how you felt watching *Peter and the Dragon*?'

Jemal: (nods) 'Do I have to draw all the seats (referring to the seats from the movie theatre)?' He also adds tears. He says this was the first movie he went to. 'I also have tears sometimes when I'm in pain'. A detailed account of all his injuries follows: 'Once I fell on rust and iron and I have a big scar. I've also walked into a wall and then the teacher put a band aid on the wound. I've already fallen on my back, my stomach, my chest, basically everywhere. I also fell with my bike, then I had a scar on my head but that's gone now. But I'm not really sad often'.

The ability to express aspects of one's inner world in play, drawings and words underpins the development of mature mentalizing capabilities. Therefore, assessing a child's strengths and vulnerabilities in the domain of representational skills is a major focus of attention during assessment sessions. Jemal is able to share some thoughts about 'having been deeply sad and moved to tears'. Surprisingly, when invited to draw about this feeling, he doesn't draw anything about the content of the movie that made him feel sad, but he draws himself as a child crying in the movie theatre. The drawing is more about the outside of a sad child (the tears, the movie theatre and the seats) than about the inside (the child mourning the loss of their parents), possibly because the inside is still too threatening to 'let it all out'. At other moments, Jemal is able to express something more about a feeling state 'from the inside-out'. For example, when he plays about knights in a castle 'being prepared for the attacks, not knowing where these will come from', referring to his hypervigilant state of mind or when he draws about a surf camp, it allows him to talk about being brave enough to choose something one eagerly wants to learn, even if that means one has to attend without knowing any of the other kids.

Assessing the child's representational abilities thus always also includes gaining insight into fluctuations or complex particularities in this domain. Some children show good capacities to express and represent specific affective topics but not other themes. Others require support through actively being invited to draw or respond to a story stem about a particular theme (semi-structured methods). Often, children who have experienced complex trauma are able to tell narratives that vary from rather well-structured ones about some of the mildly stressful events (e.g., about feeling scared) to less structured and less comprehensible ones about other possibly more anxiety-provoking situations (e.g., about a profound sense of loss), like in Jemal's case. In this context, it is important to remember that a situation of free play appeals to relatively strong capabilities of remaining regulated and finding words or images to express oneself. When invited to play freely, some traumatised children then get stuck in opening and closing cabinets, commenting that 'there's not much to play with'. Or they start to play with something without really engaging in that play, as Jemal did when he started to play with the castle in a flattened and distant manner but disengaged again rather quickly. The therapist's support to unfold his play, by asking what might be happening in the castle, subsequently leads to the castle getting completely destroyed and everyone who lives there dying, attesting to Jemal's inability to regulate himself when finding himself confronted with coping with themes of aggression and failing protection.

Aside from the more indirect semi-structured or unstructured methods to assess the child's representational skills, the therapist can ask the child direct and straightforward questions about real life, inviting the child to use a genogram or a life history method, for example, to talk about their life. Some children, like Jemal, are unable to complete a genogram or a timeline representing their life history. Jemal seemed not to know or to understand who belongs to his family and froze when invited to complete the timeline of important events in his life. Other children get lost in a 'wood of people' without understanding who belongs to which family, where they themselves belong and how families are related to each other.

In sum, most traumatised children seem to have acquired some basic representational capacities, but the ability to use these to express something about their inner world is mostly variable, dependent on the situation and the affective charge of the theme. Especially when external impulse or structure is lacking, these children's difficulties to engage in play and playfulness become visible, with play that is poor, joyless and non-reciprocal. A profound understanding of the child's abilities to play and otherwise represent experiences – and of how these are (under-)developed and/ or may be taxed by internal or external experiences – is informative to the therapist. It helps to tailor the treatment approach from the outset in terms of challenging the child's abilities enough while being mindful not to overburden the child with highly strung and unrealistic expectations. Only within a well-attuned therapeutic relationship that takes into account the child's particular developmental profile will the child be enabled to start to create their personal therapeutic journey.

Attachment development and relational capacities

 The therapist starts telling a story (Session 2, Narrative story stems) with a mother and a child protagonist, called Bob, in the kitchen. Mother warns Bob not to touch the hot stove. When Bob nevertheless burns his hand, Jemal, invited to complete the story, continues:

Mother: 'That's what happens when you want to eat right away. Now, make new food'.
Bob: 'Okay. May I open this (oven)? That's a bit safer' (puts a pan in oven).
Mother: 'Bob, get out of the kitchen, you'll get burnt and then. . . .'
Bob: (leaves) 'Okay, Mum'. (Then Jemal gestures that the oven explodes, flying through the air). 'It's on fire. Mummy, Daddy, come here. The kitchen is on fire'.
Mother: 'We have to buy a new kitchen and Bob may never cook again. When is dinner ready? Five more minutes'. (shouts) 'Dinner is ready! Here are the pancakes'.
Bob: 'I'm going to eat' (cheers).
Mother: 'Bob, you ate everything'.
Bob: 'Sorry!'
Mother: 'Hah, did you fall off your chair again?'
Bob: 'The chair was here. . . . Ouch, I'm sitting so low, where is my chair, I'm sitting on the floor. The end'.

Traumatised children's *representations of caregiving relationships* – as expressed in their play and narratives – are more often negative, contradictory or highly volatile, requiring them to be assessed in a particularly sensitive way during the assessment sessions. Responses to story stems that evoke attachment representations are often stories about children avoiding or even warding off parental care, as well as stories about neglectful or maltreating caregivers who do not help when the child is afraid or in need of care or comfort, who frighten the child or who cannot help or protect the child or uphold adequate limits and boundaries. As illustrated in Jemal's response to the 'Hot Gravy' story stem, the parent blames the child figure for causing the accident, expects him to solve the problem by himself ('make new food') and/or reacts in an overly punitive way ('Bob may never cook again'). Sometimes, the child protagonist is represented as clumsy and foolish, as acting dangerously and greedily in the eyes of the parental figures; in other stories, the parent figure is the one who is helpless and needy and needs the child figure to take the lead and solve the problem. Such negative or role-reversed caregiving representations are often difficult to contain in traumatised children, leading to ever-more escalating scenarios in their stories and/or bizarre 'resolutions', such as in Jemal's case (the oven exploding, causing a fire; the child falling off their chair, and Jemal abruptly ending the story at that).

In the same vein, traumatised children often show negative representations of parental figures across assessment methods. For instance, depicting a parent as a snail spreading slime in the Family as animals drawing or a mother as a duck who always nags. However, stories and play often also show positive elements and representations of others, rendering their inner world more complex and unpredictable for themselves as well as for others. A similar fluctuating dynamic often characterises the child's parallel *representations of self* (self-in-relation-to-other), with indications of a negative sense of self alternating with representations of a good, talented or more confident child. Sometimes, the child might even present initially as rather confident, with a positive or even a somewhat inflated sense of self, expressed in, for example, an 'anti-dependent' or 'arrogant stance' as was the case with Jemal. Yet, in many cases, this is merely a façade to mask more negative or insecure feelings about oneself, which often break through easily. In the meetings with Jemal, we can sense his longing to be seen as a 'normal' child with talents: when invited to talk about things he's good at, he asks his adoptive father in a soft tone of voice, 'Do you really think I'm good at anything?' School demands seem to be stressful, and the 'arrogant stance' some teachers point to may be a way for Jemal to hide more profound feelings of insecurity. The therapist calls him 'vulnerable' in her notes, referring to his fragile sense of self and self-worth.

With regard to *friendships*, some children have huge difficulties engaging constructively in relationships with peers, resulting in them not having many friends or only being able to hold on to friendships in a very volatile manner. Other children, like Jemal, are able to maintain close friendships. Jemal seems to feel much more confident in the presence of his friends; he meets them daily after school, they do sports together, sleep over frequently. While his adoptive parents do feel disappointed by the inability to build up a warm and mutual relationship with Jemal themselves, they offer him ample opportunity to be with friends, invite them over . . . allowing him to enjoy and to grow in these relationships because they see that relationships with friends seem more relaxed. Although there is a large family network supporting the parents as well as Jemal, Jemal doesn't refer to any one of these adult family members during the assessment sessions. It seems that relating to same-aged peers is somehow much less anxiety-provoking or affectively laden to Jemal than engaging in relationships with adult carers.

In assessing relational capacities in children who have experienced complex trauma, we pay particular attention to the child's *basic sense of safety* and the precariousness thereof. Does the child show any confidence in being connected to others, as a basis from which to engage in exploration of the world and in relationships outside the family? Jemal, for example, only reluctantly accepts others coming close when he is really relaxed, for instance, during holidays. Therefore, his adoptive parents go on holiday with him rather frequently and often look for places where Jemal can engage in sports activities. Jemal only hesitantly acknowledges separation and separation anxiety (e.g., talking about missing his mum); he mostly avoids and denies any conflict, distress or closeness. In this regard, the therapist also closely observes the relational dynamics in *the therapeutic relationship*. While the child is playing, drawing and talking, the therapist can observe their abilities to make use of the therapeutic relationship: does the child engage the therapist as an audience, someone who witnesses what the child wants to show? Or does the child engage the therapist as an actor who facilitates the understanding of what the child thinks and feels? Or does the child invite the therapist to be a co-constructor who actively participates in the child's play? Jemal now and then was able to make use of the therapist as an audience, watching how a castle is destroyed and the people get killed. At other moments, he needed her as a co-constructor of a story. Similarly, the therapist can get a sense of what's happening in terms of feeling connected, engaged, trusted. In observing closely and allowing oneself to feel what is to be felt in the countertransference, the therapist can assess the extent to which the child is allowing themselves to open up to and use the therapeutic relationship in service of developmental recovery and personal growth – the therapist becoming a 'developmental object' (Hurry, 2018) and a transference figure to the child. The therapist, feeling Jemal's reluctance to fully engage in the relationship, writes in her notes that after three assessment sessions she experiences some small islands of openness, but she still doesn't feel genuinely connected to Jemal – a feeling resonating with his adoptive parents' experience. This experience is both a reason to be hopeful – as Jemal will probably be able to open up to and thus benefit from a therapeutic relationship – and a reason for concern, as this will take time and patience.

Sense of self and identity

When invited to complete the timeline of important events in his life (Session 3), Jemal remains quiet for a while. Then, he says he doesn't know anything about it. No matter how much the therapist supports and encourages Jemal, nothing appears on the sheet of paper. Jemal says that he has forgotten it all and that there is nothing important enough in his life to put on paper. He gives a somewhat sad impression when he says this. The timeline remains empty.

The therapist then invites Jemal to draw and tell about the three things he would wish for. Now, Jemal comes up with an idea much faster. He draws a Lamborghini, saying he wants a sports car when he grows up.

Jemal doesn't think his first sketch is good enough and starts over. His drawing is small, simple and without much detail. When the therapist asks him where the sports car would like to drive to, Jemal replies: 'he doesn't really want to go anywhere, he wants to be in Germany because there he can drive as fast as he wants; preferably all alone on the road'.

Then, for his second wish, Jemal wants a villa, with a helicopter on the roof. At night, police helicopters guard his house. The villa has a gym, an outdoor pool with lounge chairs, and an art gallery of gnomes. Jemal also told this during show-and-tell in class. When the therapist asks him who lives in the villa, Jemal first says that only he does, alone. When the therapist enquires about possibly feeling alone or lonely, Jemal replies that there is also a butler and a servant. He continues to say that he would buy a friend to live with him; the butler has to search for a friend because he doesn't want to do that, and if the friend isn't nice, then he will be discarded and a new one will be sought. In the meantime, Jemal just wants to hang around in the sauna and at the pool because 'it's boring to find friends'. Jemal gives a lonely and gloomy impression while telling this story.

When the therapist enquires about the third wish, Jemal says his third wish is to have three more wishes, so that he can go on forever. He goes on to say that whatever he wishes is never-ending: the dog, the cat, a horse, the rabbit, the earth and the sun that never explodes, 'and myself', he adds at the end.

A fragile or essentially negative sense of self and a fragmented, incoherent life narrative often characterise children who have experienced complex trauma. Therefore, this important domain of developmental recovery warrants thorough assessment so as to inform the subsequent treatment approach. From the meetings with Jemal's adoptive parents and Jemal himself, we learn that core themes and domains of interest and of joy in Jemal's life have to do with sports. Talking about sports brings a *vital spark* into his facial expression, making understandable why his coach's message that he seemed to be losing his motivation worried his adoptive parents. With his adoptive father, Jemal shares an interest in cars, and together they attend car shows. He dreams of becoming a car salesman and driving fast sports cars.

Both indirect and more direct methods of assessments allow insight into the child's sense of self and identity. With Jemal, for example, *experiences of loss and mourning* remain unimaginable at a more conscious level (life history); yet, talking about sadness brings Jemal to list all the physical injuries he has sustained in life (Four affect drawings). 'Home' seems to be associated with destruction (the castle is destroyed; the kitchen burns out due to an exploded oven) and has to be protected (when he grows up, Jemal wants a villa, guarded by a police helicopter). No explicit references are made to phantasies about conception, birth and the circumstances of his adoptive placement or to any other aspects of 'being an adopted child'. However, the impossibility to talk about life events, evoking a sad silence, brings to the fore how difficult it is to try to make sense of his life history, compromising the 'telling' process of his life story. The one exception concerns a preoccupation with owning things which money can buy. Only when Jemal is invited by the therapist to explicitly consider what human relationships may offer, he adds people to his wishes in life – but only in a functional way: a butler and a servant, a friend who the butler has to search for and buy and who can be easily replaced if not serving his function. It seems that Jemal has little awareness or confidence that human relationships can offer anything of added value to enrich his life, and, although he surrounds himself with materialistic and functional riches, Jemal paints a gloomy picture of being doomed to end up alone and lonely.

In the context of assessing the traumatised child's sense of self and identity, it is important to remember that for internationally adopted and foster children, experiences of loss and mourning include all experiences of discontinuity in (sub-)culture and the accompanying feelings of 'being different' from the people in their new (sub-)culture. Therefore, the child's adoptive or foster status, their being 'of colour', their struggle to reconcile the (perceived) expectations from two sets of parents (adoptive/foster vs. biological) and other relevant issues of diversity require explicit addressing by the therapist. The child's and the parents'/carers' readiness at an early stage to have such issues addressed will, of course, differ and need to be respected. In Jemal's case, the therapist assessed this to be too soon, as Jemal was unable even to talk about events that have been important in his life; however, she did keep this actively in her mind to possibly address at a later stage in Jemal's treatment, and she knew that her colleague working with Jemal's adoptive parents would do the same (see Chapter 3).

Stage 3: in search of a shared understanding and a shared treatment focus

Based on all the information gathered in the previous sessions, we aim to construct – as a further step in synthesising and integration – a psychodynamic case formulation and an accompanying focus formulation to be shared with parents (Session 7) and child (Session 8), in order to facilitate thinking together about the 'best' next step(s) to take. A case formulation is meant to explain, in an accessible and recognisable way, how the therapists understand the presenting problems in their contextual, historical and developmental perspective. Building on this, a focus formulation phrases the focus of treatment in a way that parents and child can understand and that makes sense to them and, in that sense, fosters their engagement in the subsequent treatment phase (Midgley et al., 2017). Sharing insights and ideas stemming from the assessment sessions aims to facilitate the meaning-making process about the assessment phase, by discussing and drawing shared conclusions about the content as well as the relational dynamics which were observed during the assessment sessions and to introduce the new treatment phase.

Constructing the case and focus formulation

A case formulation summarises the information gathered so far into a coherent and meaningful story (Henderson & Martin, 2014) and helps to understand the intrapsychic and interpersonal dynamics and the transactions between these which underpin the current problems and the child's current clinical presentation. A helpful way to organise assessment information about the child within their family is in a developmentally based diagnostic profile. In developing such an assessment profile for the present treatment approach, we have been inspired by the diagnostic profiles of Greenspan and Thorndike Greenspan (2003) and A. Freud (1965, as described in Davids et al. (2017)), which we have adapted and tailored to the developmental domains which have been found to be particularly implicated in vulnerability to psychopathology in children who have experienced complex trauma (see Chapter 2).

One way of structuring the assessment profile can be the following (see next box). In a first part, several strands of background information are presented. A first subsection concerns a dynamic definition of the problem, specifically, the history of the problems and complaints with which the child has been referred and how these problems may be understood from a dynamic perspective. A second background information subsection contains a factual account of the child's history prior to placement, aimed to help to contextualise the child's current problems and dynamics in light of any experiences of early adversity and discontinuity in their life prior to placement and the circumstances of these discontinuities. Following that, an account of the current family constellation and family life provides information about the composition of the current family, the nature of the family system and the place of the family system in its community. Finally, the child's school and leisure environment are described.

In a second part, in order to chart the child's strengths and difficulties in different domains of life, we synthesise the child's material that has been gathered throughout the assessment phase. This material is structured according to the four developmental domains which may be considered the components or building blocks of the present treatment approach: representational capacities, affective development and regulation strategies, attachment development and relational capacities and sense of self and identity. In taking on an explicit trauma-informed developmental psychopathology perspective, we try to gain insight into the past as well as the current environment and its potential transactional relations with the child's development.

In the final part of the assessment profile, we summarise what has been found to be the core intra- and interpersonal dynamics which underpin the child's current clinical presentation and based on this what focus for future work could be considered. The focus formulation thus coherently and logically follows from the case formulation and points to the work that lies ahead in the subsequent treatment phase. A focus formulation is preferably phrased in the child's language and can make use of an expression, a metaphor or an image the child used or evoked during the assessment phase. As such, we aim for the treatment focus to be concrete and recognisable, easy to understand, and invite both parents and child to think along with the therapist. When a focus formulation is well designed, it evokes recognition and curiosity, communicates hope and fuels resources and a wish for change (Haugvik & Johns, 2008; Midgley et al., 2017).

I. Background information

1. Dynamic definition of the problem

Section on the history of the problems and complaints with which the child has been referred and on how these problems can be understood from a dynamic perspective. Information included relates to:

- the referral (e.g., why is the child referred, why now)
- the phenomenology of the symptoms and problems (e.g., onset, precipitating factors, duration)

2. The child's developmental history

Section on the child's history prior to placement

- Early separations or death of a family member, exposure to parental mental or physical illness, long-standing parental disharmony and/or divorce, accidents or severe illness in the child, institutional care and description of that care, genetic vulnerability and/or exposure to severe social problems (e.g., extreme poverty, community violence) in the family of origin

3. Current family constellation and family life

- Composition of the current adoptive/foster family
- The nature of the family system
- The place of the family system in its community (presence of social support)

including (when relevant) a description of environmental factors relating to physical and emotional safety, presence of the parents as safe attachment figures, pedagogical and structured family environment and parental mentalizing capacities

4. The child's school and leisure environment

including an account of how the child and their functioning is perceived in these environments

---

II. Developmental profile (see Table 5.3)

1. Cognitive capacities and executive functioning
2. Representational capacities
   3. Affective development and regulation strategies
   4. Attachment development and relational capacities
   5. Sense of self and identity

III. Diagnostic statement and recommendations

- A dynamic understanding of the child's presenting problems
  - Specifying the nature of defects, conflicts and deficits that underlie the child's symptoms, which addresses the (intrapsychic, biological, and family/systemic) etiological factors
  - Framing the child's developmental difficulties in terms of the continuum between normal and pathological development, giving an understanding of to what extent the child's development is being interfered with
- A clear statement of the recommendations
  - Specifying the aims of the recommended treatment
  - And some kind of prediction about what may be achieved by it

Often, it proves useful and helpful to write up this assessment profile as a report. An actual write-up helps to structure the assessment material and facilitate the meaning-making process thereof and thus aids in formulating a coherent case and focus formulation to share with parents. Moreover, the resulting report can be handed to the parents at the end of Session 7, as thoughtful words that one can look back on and which can function as a starting point for further reflection and discussion (see later). As we keep this in mind, we pay particular attention to using language which is respectful as well as accessible.

Another important issue of consideration is that a case formulation is meant to generate hypotheses and is therefore iterative. As new information, a proceeding relationship and so on reveal further layers of functioning and thus a better understanding of the child's inner world, the case and focus formulation should similarly evolve and be adapted accordingly over time (Henderson & Martin, 2014). Hence, a case and focus formulation should be considered a momentary insight and a 'work-in-progress', rather than a static or rigid statement to pin the child or the family down on.

Session 7: sharing the case and focus formulation with parents

In Session 7, ideally with both parent worker and child therapist present, we aim to relate back to parents how the problems leading up to their seeking help for their child may be understood from a mentalizing perspective, in which symptoms are

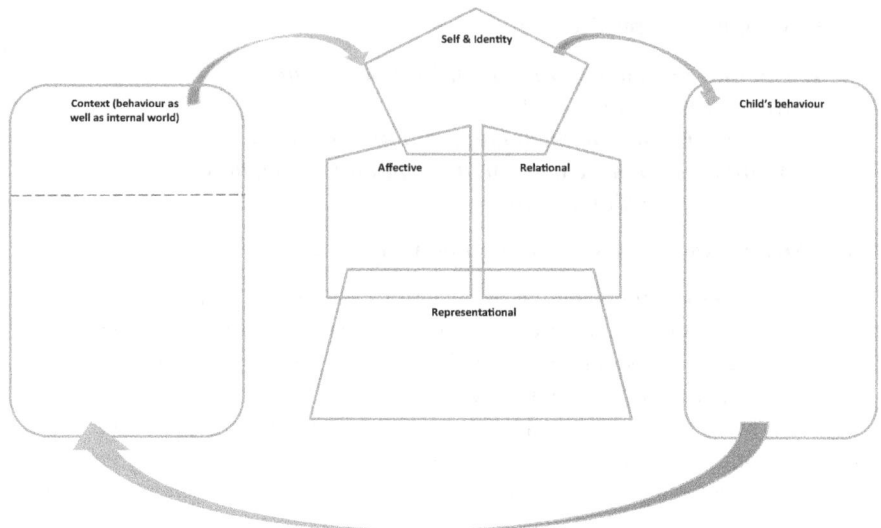

Figure 5.1 Template for visualising and sharing the case formulation.

considered as reflecting the child's inner world of motives, anxieties, desires and so forth, interacting with particular life events. Specifically, using a 'draw-and-tell' technique inspired by the work of Maurer and Westermann (2006, 2018), we construct with and present to the parents an image of how we have learnt to know the child in the context of their family, as represented in the case formulation (for a template, see Figure 5.1). Subsequently, we also share the focus formulation as a port of entry to start discussing the therapeutic work that lies ahead.

The following vignette is an example of what a line of thinking and speaking may look like. For readability, it is more a summarising line of thoughts, leaving out all the twists and turns a real conversation may take. Therefore, this vignette reads as much more straightforward and one-directional than this kind of conversation would play out in reality. However, we hope that it gives the reader a sense of the manner and the language that may be used to convey a case and focus formulation to parents.

 While starting to draw (see template), the therapists remind Jemal's adoptive parents of their main concerns when they first met: how Jemal's decision to let go of sports, the school's stories about negative behaviour, the dark thoughts and bad sleeping and eating at home (Jemal's behaviour) led to the parents (as well as the teachers) being worried about his emotional well-being and deciding to consult (context). Rebecca and Julian nod in recognition. The therapist continues: 'Jemal is fortunate to have you as his parents, being so attentive to his well-being and his emotional development. Just like you could see Jemal's loss of motivation at football practice as a sign of something more inside of him going on, we found it a telling moment when Jemal asked you (father) whether he had talents, as if he has lost any connection to the good and strong parts within himself (identity development)'. Father recalls that that was indeed a very moving moment and a difficult one, being confronted with his adoptive son feeling 'worthless'. The therapist agrees but adds that it was also very moving to witness how Jemal allowed father to offer comforting words ('I wish you could believe that') and gestures (putting his hand on Jemal's shoulder). The therapist notices how Jemal's adoptive parents exchange a faint smile. She continues that she also knows from their stories how rare such moments at home are, how Jemal mostly wards off any comfort and nurture they so dearly want to provide and how difficult this must be for them. 'Not knowing who you really are and whether there is "any good" in you is a really scary place to be. Like the flat affect and dark thoughts you (mother) talked about noticing at home, during the sessions here, Jemal showed many signs of struggling with feelings of emptiness, loss and also fear and sadness. And, for some children, like Jemal, it then makes sense to push others away and act tough and negative: in a sense, it's "easier" to act all grown-up and not to need anyone than to be confronted with your own vulnerability' (affective development). . . . 'We were happy to learn that relating to age-mates seems to be much easier for Jemal. This is a really good thing, for his sense of self now as well as for his future development. Strong friendships will really provide him a lively network in which he can grow socially and emotionally and nourish his feelings of being someone' (relational development). The therapists take time to, again, explicitly validate how Jemal's adoptive parents already support him in maintaining his friendships, for example, by allowing him to have friends over frequently. 'What we, like you, are really concerned about is the way Jemal seems to close down in relationships with adults, with you at home but also with teachers at school. We can see you are extraordinarily patient parents, who try time and again to remain understanding and reconnect with Jemal, but at school, he seems to be losing credit because of an attitude that is perceived as negative and arrogant'. The conversation turns to parents recalling something they've also talked about during the previous sessions: how Jemal always seems to open up again when scholastic demands are less tense, like when they go on holiday, especially when they do sports activities (like walking, biking or skiing). At such times, Jemal becomes more talkative again, talking about school and friends, and he sleeps and eats much better. Parents also recognise how once at home again, Jemal closes down again. 'Sometimes, it seems as if he can only find calm and recover in being close to the dog', Mother adds. The child therapist talks about how she has experienced similar things in her relationship with Jemal during the assessment sessions: how he is able to talk or play or draw about some topics about himself – often with some support from her – but how she has struggled to really feel connected to him and his inner world as well as how he seems to shut down when the topic becomes too tense or difficult for him, for example, talking about his past (representational development). . . . As the therapists feel that they have addressed the most important aspects of the case formulation with Jemal's adoptive parents, they turn the conversation to the focus formulation: 'So, if we take this together, I think we could agree that Jemal needs some support to reconnect to who he really is or wants to be inside, as well as to learning that it's okay to rely on adults when he's feeling distressed or in need of help'. . . . 'And we've seen some good signs here that Jemal can make use of a reliable relationship with a trustworthy adult to start that process'.

In this context, it is important to remember that having a case and focus formulation about their child and family being related back to them is an affectively charged event for many parents. Often, the ambivalent feelings around consulting and seeking professional help get re-activated as this final stage of the assessment phase approaches. Therefore, it is not because we strive and aim towards recognition and collaboration in sharing and discussing the case and focus formulations that the messages implied in it will be easily taken in and processed by parents. It is not uncommon for parents to need time to fully grasp all aspects and implications of the image we have shared. Often, this processing will be at the core of the parent work conducted in the treatment phase (see Chapter 7). Nonetheless, it seems important to allow parents enough time to let things 'sink in', talk about it among themselves, get back to the therapist(s) with questions or concerns and have these addressed appropriately. Ideally, if this process goes well, there is some basic sense of a shared understanding and of a shared plan of how best to proceed, as well as an idea of how all this will be shared with and conveyed to the child. Moreover, relevant people in the child's and family's network will equally need to be informed and involved.

Another important point to consider is that although we try to convey a hopeful perspective in terms of what treatment can mean to the family in terms of recovery in child development and in relationships, we tread carefully in the language we use to talk about treatment goals. A well-designed focus formulation encompasses the treatment goal(s) we hope to achieve with this child and this family. Yet, particularly in the case of a traumatised child, the pathway towards these goals is often not one of linear progression, and obstacles along the way are often difficult to predict. The therapist might, for example, say:

Traumatised children have often developed ways of reacting to particular situations that have become habits and patterns. It takes some time to get to know these habits and patterns, to understand their meaning in the child's functioning and to bring about new, more adaptive ways of being and responding. You can compare it to learning something new at school: one needs some time to practise before one feels that one has really mastered the new knowledge or skills. In our experience, it takes the time of about a school year or two before changes can really take hold.

Moreover, it can be helpful to reassure parents that change becomes visible not only in big leaps but often in small steps long before anyone is thinking about the end of treatment and that we will work together to observe the smaller and larger signs of change and to think about what this change means with regard to daily life as well as to future developments. For example, the therapist might say something like:

This doesn't mean that you'll have to wait a year before change happens. As parents, you will often notice it when changes start to happen. It is important to share what you see and feel with regard to your child, because early change can take very different forms. Sometimes, a child opens up their mind in relation to people in their environment, or they show they are feeling more connected. Change can also start with expressing more what they want or how they feel. This might involve showing anger or anxiety or the "weirdness" the child is experiencing inside. So, it happens that first change is not synonymous to "feeling or behaving better". Then, it's important to remember that this change is more a kind of a starting point, not the endpoint. So, it would be good if you also share it here when you notice that happening.

Or:

You won't be alone in trying to figure out whether change is happening. We will do our utmost to do this together, and to think together about how this relates to some of the things we've discussed to focus on in treatment. So, this will definitely be something we will refer back to and talk about regularly.

As such, we aim to pay particular attention to conveying hope in a realistic sense, this is, with no guarantees of objectives achieved but all the more with the guarantee of standing by and guiding the parents as they grant their child and their family this journey towards more constructive development and healthier relationships. This includes regular and timely assessments of whether treatment is 'on track' or whether 'a change of plans' is warranted. A realistically hopeful treatment plan also means that parents of traumatised children will often be confronted with feelings of loss and mourning as they start to realise that some vulnerabilities will persist throughout their child's life. This mourning process takes time and will need to be revisited in the further work with parents (see Chapter 7).

Session 8: sharing the focus formulation with the child and transitioning to the early phase of treatment

In Session 8, the therapist shares with the child their understanding of the child's strengths and vulnerabilities in a way that is adapted to the child's level of functioning, particularly, their mentalizing abilities to grasp something about themselves as a person. We purposefully keep this sharing of part of the case formulation brief, recognisable and easy-to-understand and take more time to share and discuss with the child what the next step(s) will be in aiming to relieve some of the child's most pressing suffering (focus formulation).

'So, Jemal, as you know, I've met with you and with your parents, to get to know you and to see whether we could help your family with some of the things you're struggling with. So, we'll be talking a bit about that today, but I just wanted to check in with you first whether you would like to share something about what it has been like for you to come here?' Jemal looks away and shrugs his shoulders. 'That's quite alright, maybe later. Would it be okay if I share some thoughts on how I've got to know you in our meetings?' Jemal starts doodling on a piece of paper and nods. The therapist feels space to tell something about her perspective on what is going on in his mind: 'what has struck me most is how you really want to be big and strong. That's really an excellent quality; it helps you to dare to go to a surf camp without any friends'. Jemal nods again. 'You know, sometimes the things that make us strong can also get in the way of other things that are equally important in growing up. Like when you said that you hate to admit when something is difficult, and you don't want anybody to see it, you want to solve it by yourself, and sometimes you then push other people away who try to offer help'. Jemal stops doodling for a moment, as if thinking about what the therapist has said. Then he continues doodling, as if in agreement with the therapist. The therapist continues: 'Sometimes, when you do show other people that it's tough, they can help in some way. Remember when you doubted whether there was anything you're good at, Dad was able to reassure you?' Jemal hums barely audibly. 'In growing up, it can be helpful and even brave to feel little now and then and to be able to admit some things are difficult and ask for help . . . because some things are really difficult without help'. Jemal shrugs. 'Not an easy task to think about', the therapist translates this gesture. Jemal focuses further on doodling and a male figure emerges on his sheet of paper. The therapist gives some space for his drawing. After a while, she tells him about this playroom as a space for children to figure out how they think and feel about things in their life by playing, drawing and talking about it. 'How would you feel about coming to do that here once a week?' 'As long as I don't have to talk too much', Jemal replies. With an understanding smile, the therapist says: 'maybe, we've already been talking too much today! How about taking a look at the drawer I have for you? You know, all the stuff in the playroom is for all the children who come here, but this drawer is only for you for the time you will come here. I've already put some stuff in to draw and craft with. We can think about how you want to let the other kids know that this drawer is yours or what you want it to look like'.

In the case that direct work with the child is indicated, the therapist will want to listen carefully to any thoughts that the child might have and talk with them about what it has been like so far to come to the service. Whereas the therapist aims for a gradual and relatively smooth transition from the assessment phase to the early phase of treatment, this transition should nevertheless be marked, highlighting some changes with regard to the setting as well as to the therapeutic relationship. First, the therapist explains to the child when and where they will meet for this new phase of treatment, as well as how long the grown-ups think therapy might take. A set time in the therapist's agenda that begins and ends at a prearranged hour helps to define the therapeutic work and is meant to 'hold both the child and the therapist when they are experiencing and exploring the turbulence of their relationship' (Blake, 2008, p. 193). If the child seems to have questions about the time frame – which is not unusual as this is quite a bit longer than the assessment phase and might be more than the child had bargained for – the therapist can say something like:

Children who went through a lot early in life have often developed ways of reacting that were helpful at the time. Remember you talked about feeling too big to be close to your parents and to need them to help you with some things? Maybe when you were a small child, that was a good idea because there weren't a lot of adults around whom you could turn to. But sometimes, what was a good idea once is not so helpful anymore, but it's difficult not to react in the same way because you're so used to it. In therapy, we can take time to get to know how these things work inside of you and also to find out together about new ways of reacting that might feel more helpful to you now. It's a bit like learning to ride a bike: if you've always only learnt to take right turns, it needs some time to practise left turns too, and to be able to decide almost automatically which turn to take to go where you need to be quickly and safely. From working with kids like you, we've learnt that therapy can take the time of a school year or so.

Furthermore, the therapist explains to the child that the colleague (as known by the child) will also attempt to help the child's parents to better understand and support them by meeting with them at regular times and that, in fact, all important grown-ups in their life will meet regularly in service of thinking and talking together about the child's needs and how best to meet these.

As illustrated at the end of the vignette, each child is also offered a personal drawer or box that can be closed, as a safe place for their personal creations in therapy. A containing space for the child's drawings, writings and other creations symbolises the therapist's containing mind in which thoughts, feelings and experiences will be held together. Furthermore, being offered a drawer or box that can be filled as well as a blank sketchbook symbolises the start of a new experience in the child's life. In filling a container and preserving the content of it, the child can experience how aspects of history can grow and be held together. Finally, it is helpful for the child to have the opportunity to personalise the drawer or box and sketchbook, scaffolding preliminary notions of a sense of self.

In this regard, it is also important that the therapist introduces something about 'the new phase in the slightly changed relationship'. Due to the more structured quality of the assessment phase, the therapist took a more active and directive stance, whereas from the early phase of treatment onwards the therapist will follow the child's lead where possible, with an actively open and genuinely interested mind, 'being there to receive the child's communications and enabling the child not only to project his inner world to the toys in the therapy room, but also on the therapist' (Blake, 2008, p. 200). Hence, the therapist invites the child to explore, choose from and play with the materials provided in the room, as a port of entry to the child's inner world.

Beyond the three-track approach: when something more or other is needed

As mentioned in Chapter 4, we keep open the perspective that the outcome of the assessment phase may be that something other than the three-track treatment approach will be most helpful to a particular child and their family or that, in addition to what the present three-track approach may offer, the child and/or the family may be in need of additional support (e.g., medication, home-based family support work). In any case, we advocate this to be discussed openly and clearly with both the adults involved (parents as well as relevant network partners) and the child in preparing for this next step.

In the case that the outcome of the assessment is that, at this time, further treatment is not the most adequate answer to this child's/family's problems, it needs to be discussed with and explained to the parents and the child what will happen next and why. This may be the case if other questions or problems with regard to the child's functioning need to be cleared up first, for example, if during the assessment questions arise with regard to a learning disability (e.g., dyslexia), a physical problem (e.g., a motor or perceptual problem) or a potential 'comorbidity' (e.g., ASS). Then psychotherapeutic treatment may be indicated at a later moment, when a more comprehensive understanding about what is at stake in the child's clinical presentation has been reached. In this/these conversation(s), the therapist tries to probe any questions or concerns the parents or the child might have. Additionally, they are invited to look back on the past process and share these experiences with the therapist. As such, we aim to help the family members go through the rounding-up process in a containing way, which can hopefully be experienced as a good-enough experience in light of the sometimes traumatising experiences of loss and separation that a child suffering from complex trauma has been subjected to previously.

Concluding thoughts

Gaining a thorough understanding of the child's functioning 'in context', as conceptualised in the present treatment approach, is often experienced as a complex – even arduous – task. Yet, in working with families with a traumatised child in particular, the assessment phase is equally considered as indispensable to the 'success' of the further treatment trajectory. First, modelling and scaffolding a genuine, non-judgemental curious stance towards how the child's and the parents' minds are 'at work' paves the way for becoming a collaborative mentalizing system that is concerned about each other's inner world. Moreover, in attempting to create a shared understanding of the complex interplay between the child's development and prior as well as current environmental factors, the 'outcome' of the assessment phase, as expressed in the case formulation, aims to inform the tailoring of the further treatment trajectory to the child's and family's needs (focus formulation). As so aptly phrased by Melandri (2017), the value of the assessment work conducted lies in providing

> a framework from which to begin the process of meeting the child patient and his parents where they are. Our capacity to scaffold the treatment is founded in our way of organizing the evidence in front of us with the purpose of guiding our interventions and main clinical goals.
>
> (p. 173)

In other words, if the assessment work receives the attention and the time it requires and is conducted in the intended way (that is, from a trauma- and developmentally informed as well as a pre-therapeutic perspective), this should go a long way in guiding us towards what the best next steps are in meeting a particular child's and family's mental health needs.

References

Allen, J. G. (2013). *Mentalizing in the development and treatment of attachment trauma.* Karnac.

Blake, P. (2008). The setting, physical and mental, and limits. In P. Blake (Ed.), *Child and adolescent psychotherapy* (pp. 193–209). Karnac Books.

Catty, J., Cregeen, S., Hughes, C., Midgley, N., Rhode, M., & Rustin, M. (2017). *Short-term psychoanalytic psychotherapy for adolescents with depression: A treatment manual.* Karnac Books.

Davids, J., Green, V., Joyce, A., & McLean, D. (2017). Revised provisional diagnostic profile: 2016. *Journal of Infant, Child, and Adolescent Psychotherapy, 16*(2), 149–157. https://doi.org/10.1080/15289168.2017.1309208

Ensink, K., Leroux, A., Normandin, L., Biberdzic, M., & Fonagy, P. (2017). Assessing reflective parenting in interaction with school-aged children. *Journal of Personality Assessment, 99*, 585–595.

Fonagy, P., Luyten, P., Allison, E., & Campbell, C. (2019). Mentalizing, epistemic trust and the phenomenology of psychotherapy. *Psychopathology, 52*, 94–103. https://doi.org/10.1159/000501526

Freud, A. (1965/1980). Diagnostic profile. In assessment of pathology. Part 1. Some general considerations. In *Normality and pathology in childhood: Assessments of development*. The Hogarth Press and the Institute of Psychoanalysis. (Original work published 1965).

Greenspan, S. I., & Thorndike Greenspan, N. (2003). *The clinical interview of the child* (3rd ed.). American Psychiatric Press.

Haugvik, M., & Johns, U. (2008). Facets of structure and adaptation: A qualitative study of time-limited psychotherapy with children experiencing difficult family situations. *Clinical Child Psychology and Psychiatry*, *13*(2), 235–252.

Henderson, S. W., & Martin, A. (2014). Case formulation and integration of information in child and adolescent mental health. In J. M. Ray (Ed.), *IACAPAP e-Textbook of Child and Adolescent Mental Health*. International Association for Child and Adolescent Psychiatry and Allied Professions.

Hoffman, L., Rice, T., & Prout, T. (2015). *Manual of Regulation-Focused Psychotherapy for Children (RFP-C) with externalising behaviors*. A psychodynamic approach. Routledge.

Hurry, A. (Ed.). (2018). *Psychoanalysis and developmental therapy (Psychoanalytic Monograph No. 3)*. Routledge.

Jaffrani, A. A., Sunley, T., & Midgley, N. (2020). The building of epistemic trust: An adoptive family's experience of mentalization-based therapy. *Journal of Infant, Child, and Adolescent Psychotherapy*, *19*(3), 271–282. https://doi.org/10.1080/15289168.2020.1768356

Maurer, J., & Westermann, J. (2006). *Beter communiceren in de hulpverlening: Het dialoogmodel als leidraad. [Enhancing communication in mental health care: The dialogue model as guideline.]* Bohn, Stafleu & Van Logum.

Maurer, J., & Westermann, J. (2018). *Praktijkboek gedeelde besluitvorming in de GGZ. Kracht van verhalen, beeld en dialoog. [A practical guide for shared decision making in mental health care. The power of narratives, images and dialogue.]* Bohn, Stafleu & Van Logum.

Melandri, F. (2017). Milk and tears: A very difficult beginning: The assessment and treatment of a young boy with atypical presentation. *Journal of Infant, Child, and Adolescent Psychotherapy*, *16*(2), 158–174. https://doi.org/10.1080/15289168.2017.1309133

Midgley, N. (2011). Test of time: Anna Freud's Normality and Pathology in Childhood (1965). *Clinical Child Psychology and Psychiatry*, *16*(3), 475–482.

Midgley, N., Ensink, K., Lindqvist, K., Malberg, N., & Muller, N. (2017). *Mentalization-based treatment for children. A time-limited approach*. American Psychological Association.

Muller, N., & Bakker, T. (2009). Oog voor de ouders. Diagnostiek van de hechtingsrelatie tussen ouders en kinderen en het mentaliserend vermogen van ouders. [Keeping an eye on parents. Assessment of the parent-child attachment relationship and parental mentalizing capacities.] *Tijdschrift van de vereniging voor Kinder- en Jeugdpsychotherapie*, *39*, 65–79.

Muller, N., & Midgley, N. (2015). Approaches to assessment in time-limited Mentalization-Based Therapy for Children (MBT-C). *Frontiers in Psychology*, *6*, 1063. https://doi.org/10.3389/fpsyg.2015.01063

Muller, N., & ten Kate, C. (2008). Mentaliseren Bevorderende Therapie in relaties en gezinnen. [Mentalization-Based Treatment in relationships and families.] *Tijdschrift Systeemtherapie*, *20*(3), 117–132.

Sameroff, A. J. (2004). Ports of entry and the dynamics of mother-infant interventions. In A. J. Sameroff, S. C. McDonough, & K. L. Rosenblum (Eds.), *Treating parent-infant relationship problems* (pp. 3–29). The Guilford Press.

Stern, D. (1995). *The motherhood constellation. A unified view of parent-infant psychotherapy*. Basic Books.

Winnicott, D. W. (1971). *Therapeutic consultations in child psychiatry*. The Hogarth Press and the Institute of Psychoanalysis.

Chapter 6

Direct work with the child

Direct work with the child plays an essential role in the recovery from the developmental sequelae of complex traumatic experiences. It offers ample opportunity to address the issues which have been identified in the assessment phase to underlie the problems which have brought the child's family to seek professional help. In this chapter, we describe how the basic principles and attitudes underlying the present treatment approach can be applied in the direct work with the child. Specifically, in a first section, we discuss therapeutic attitudes that aim (a) to establish and maintain a solid but flexible frame for therapy, as a prerequisite for further growth and development; (b) to support children in establishing and maintaining safer and more positive relationships with caregivers; and (c) to keep a mentalizing stance front and centre (see Table 6.1). In the second section of this chapter, we describe therapist interventions aimed to foster recovery in the four developmental domains set out in Chapter 2.

Mindful relationships inside and outside therapy as the backdrop for developmental recovery

A solid but flexible therapeutic frame: creating time and space to help connect to one's inner world

A 'good-enough' therapeutic frame to get in touch with 'bad' care representations

Session after session, Lisa wants to play 'hairdresser'. She fully engages in pretend play: she enters the barbershop with her purse in her hand and asks the therapist-hairdresser to wash, cut, colour . . . her hair over and over again. The therapist-hairdresser carefully tries to meet Lisa's seemingly endless requests: a little bit shorter, darker. . . . Yet, time after time, Lisa decides it's just not good enough and asks for a new treatment. During several sessions of this kind of play, the therapist feels overwhelmed by uncertainty and incompetence, of doing things wrong and never being able to meet Lisa's needs.

DOI: 10.4324/9781003044918-9

Table 6.1 Core attitudes and related tasks in direct work with the child

A solid but flexible therapeutic frame	• Provide predictability and continuity through a (relatively) stable frame: time, space and frequency of sessions • Offer a relationship characterised by benevolent and genuine curiosity in the child's inner world and do so attuned to the child's preferential ways of communicating • Pay specific attention to how moments and experiences of separation are negotiated • Pay specific attention to how the child makes use of their personal drawer or box • Take particular care in considering 'adjustments' to the therapeutic frame
A continuous focus on relatedness	• Be alert to how the child's representations of caregivers come to the fore and become visible in and are of influence on family relationships • Take particular care in managing and responding to stories about 'bad' care
Keeping a mentalizing stance front and centre	• Balance between fostering mentalizing capacities (process) and facilitating narratives (content) • Balance between support and exploration • Actively scaffold or provide words and images as appropriate

The weekly sessions, lasting approximately 50 minutes, of the child with the therapist at the same time in the same playroom with the same play materials aim to foster an experience of predictability and continuity. Within this physical setting, the therapist engages in play and playful discourse (Winnicott, 1971) as a way of inviting the child to play, draw and talk about what is at stake in their inner world. In doing so, the therapist aims to attune to the child's preferential ways of communicating, depending on developmental age as well as on images and metaphors that have become meaningful to the child. As such, this setting aims to become the physical and mental space (Blake, 2008) within which the therapist as well as the child can start to feel comfortable enough for therapeutic processes and change to take place. Or as Jenkinson (2001) expressed, 'there must be a place for play, a "sacred space" (no matter how small), and time' (p. 137).

Although this applies to all children coming to therapy, such experiences of predictability and continuity, as well as of willingness to search for a 'language' tailor-made to a particular child, are especially important for children who have had limited experience of having been held in mind, time and space – or for whom such experiences were fraught with emotional and relational conflict. Some of these children will need a long time to test the solidity of the therapeutic frame before they even allow themselves to start trusting the therapist's benign intentions and to start getting in touch with and working through their feelings of distrust or fear of being unimportant or forgotten. In Lisa's case, who according to her foster carers avoids being touched by them in any way, starting to play 'hairdresser' was only possible within the consistent therapeutic frame, which provided her a time and a space to be with an adult who was willing to engage in her world making use of her way of communicating (i.e., through pretend play). This enabled Lisa to use the playroom as a social and emotional laboratory to start practising with taking the risk of 'giving in' to her desire to be touched in a caring way in spite of her intense fear of being cared for badly. With children who have experienced complex trauma, it is the very process of becoming attached to the therapist and (aspects of) the therapeutic frame that affords them opportunities to experiment with deeply rooted feelings and expectations of being seen, contained, forgotten, in- or excluded, well- or badly cared for. As shown in Lisa's case vignette, often, allowing oneself to be cared for immediately evokes myriad mixed feelings. It brings the child in touch with their profound longing for being cared for incessantly as well as with prevailing representations of being cared for badly, as in Lisa's case, the caregiver never doing the right things, requiring you as the child to take a controlling and punitive position.

In and out, with and without: the frame as the stage for feelings of separation

 At the start of therapy, Mei-Lan's extreme anxiety to be separated from her adoptive mother becomes visible and tangible as she remains pre-occupied with Mother's presence or absence in the waiting room while she is with the therapist in the playroom. The therapist observes how Mei-Lan is unable to feel enough at ease that Mother will remain in the waiting room, as she promised: she keeps looking at the door, unable to let her attention and mind drift to the things she could possibly do in the playroom, continuously fearful that Mother might leave her 'like she always does at home'. Considering Mei-Lan's level of separation anxiety and the way this incapacitates her from even beginning to engage in a therapeutic process, the therapist tries to co-regulate by allowing Mei-Lan to check, now and again, whether 'Mummy is really still there'. After a while, the therapist notices that this helps Mei-Lan to settle a bit, yet, the therapist realises that Mei-Lan will probably need this kind of checking for quite some time.

Many traumatised children, through their history of unpredictable or disrupted care experiences, have been sensitised to every small break in continuity or minimal sign of unpredictability and misunderstanding. Moments of entering or leaving the session as well as transitions from caregiver to therapist and vice versa, as 'small' experiences of separation, often evoke feelings of separation anxiety. Sometimes, the therapist may be confronted with a child who does not want to come into the therapy room, often stemming from fear of separating from the caregiver or of being overwhelmed by the therapist or conversely, a child who refuses to stop play-ing and leave the therapy room when their time is up. Often, traumatised children will repeatedly play peek-a-boo in the transitions between parent and therapist. The therapist will need to manage such situations informed by their understanding of the possible meanings of the child's behaviour as well as with the parent-child relationship in mind (see also later discussion). This may mean that the therapist first verbalises – for child and parent – something about the child's need to check whether the parent is really still there, in order to subsequently be able to explore this theme in play or talk.

In the same vein, the small and inherent breaks in frequency and continuity of therapy sessions, whether planned (e.g., holiday) or unplanned (e.g., illness), often trigger profound separation anxiety and feelings of abandonment in children who have experienced complex trauma. In this sense, these relational crises can be seen as opportunities for the therapist to understand what separation has come to mean to this child and to help the child to get in touch with, make sense of and, ideally, work through their feelings.

The child's drawer or box: containment-within-containment

Later on in treatment, Mei-Lan draws about important elements of her inner world: a nightmare, a difficult moment when her adoptive mother went to a conference for some days, her dog and cat. . . . Her drawer easily fills with crafts and drawings. Once in a while, she wants to 'tidy up' the drawer. In doing so, every piece of work gets a lot of attention and evokes thoughts about when she made it and what it was about, for example 'I was so afraid then', referring to the nightmare drawing (see later example).

As part of the therapeutic frame, we provide the child with a personal drawer or box and a sketchbook, in which the child's creative expressions can be held, meant to foster a sense of containment and belonging and of being held in mind (see Chap-ter 5). Every child will make use of this aspect of the therapeutic frame in their own way. Closely observing this will provide the therapist with a window into how the child relates to the therapeutic relationship and the therapeutic process. For instance, a child may want to decorate the outside of the box or not; they may want to put things in for safekeeping or not; they may keep it neat or instead damage it. For Mei-Lan, in the case vignette, the drawer seems to function as a container for the 'bits and pieces in her mind'. Emotional and relational experiences can be felt, communicated as well as processed only as a slow and tedious piecing together of previously unrelated frag-ments. In that process, the drawer seems to play an important role in experiencing how all these fragments belong to her as a person and how, through and in her, these experiences are more connected to one another than she was previously able to feel.

Taken together, for the frame to be truly therapeutic, the therapist will need to think about the possible meanings of the child's signs and communications in relation to aspects of the therapeutic frame offered and respond in a therapeutic way. In general, this will often come down to finding a balance between holding on to (aspects of) the therapeutic frame where needed to safeguard the child's therapeutic process, on the one hand and flexibly accommodating the child's wish, desire or need when the therapist assesses that this will serve the child's developmental recovery better, on the other. Mei-Lan's therapist, witnessing how Mei-Lan is unable to find enough peace of mind about 'Mummy being there' to remain in the therapy room, decides to afford her space to practise being close to and farther away from her adoptive mother. Whereas with a more securely attached child, a therapist could already rely more on the child's capacity to hold their parent in mind as well as on the therapeutic relationship to contain any signs of separation anxiety. Other situations may require the therapist to make similar considerations impacting the therapeutic frame. For instance, when Youri finally finds something he can engage in – making slime out of soap and water and enjoying this in a sensopathic way – he is frustrated when, upon entering the playroom, he discovers that this week the soap has been all used up. The therapist needs to consider whether to focus on helping Youri to process the frustration about not finding what he longs for or rather on meeting Youri's 'need for soap'. As at this stage, Youri's play is so young and fragile, the therapist gauges this as a critical moment to support him in keeping alive this 'feeling passionate about something'. Therefore, she decides to meet Youri's need by allowing him to get some soap from the toilet elsewhere in the practice centre, whereas she would help more mature children to remain in the playroom and make do with the material available. The therapist holds in mind that helping Youri to bear the frustration about not always being able to have what one wants is for later on – when he has had the opportunity to get in touch better with who he is and what he wants. In any case, for many traumatised children, the therapeutic relationship is the place par excellence to learn to know and start to own feelings and thoughts evoked in a new relationship as well as to try out new, more adaptive relational strategies and capacities, which may eventually generalise to their 'real' lives outside the therapy room.

A continuous focus on relatedness: listening with care to stories about care

 After a most enjoyable family afternoon, working in the backyard and having fun, Lisa's foster carers decide to get fries and to have dinner on the patio with the three children – their two biological adolescent daughters and Lisa. Lisa actively participated in and seems to have thoroughly enjoyed the afternoon family activities, but all of a sudden at dinner, she gets mad and refuses to have fries. Talking about it in therapy, she exclaims: 'They didn't want me to enjoy the fries, I could see it on their faces! That's why I didn't want fries anymore, because I could see on their faces they didn't want to pay fries for me!' The therapist – in this more advanced phase of treatment – can rely on earlier work with Lisa on her feelings of exclusion, as well as discussions with the parent worker reassuring her of the 'good' care Lisa's foster carers try to provide. The therapist first validates: 'Oh my goodness, how awful that a pleasant afternoon ends in such a difficult experience'. Encouraged by the relief she observes on Lisa's face, she moves on and asks: 'When looking back now, are you really convinced they didn't want to pay your fries? Or could this perhaps be that voice again telling you they don't really love you?' Lisa shrugs: 'I don't really belong there, why should they want to care for me'. Further on in the session, she sighs: 'Life is so much easier for the others, they are their real children'.

As discussed, children who have experienced complex trauma enter their new family life with previously developed inner representations of caregiving others as unpredictable 'at best' and rejecting/abandoning and/or excessively harsh and punitive at worst. These inner representations drive them to unwittingly experience and perceive new – mostly well-intentioned – caregivers, such as their adoptive parents or foster carers but also their teacher or therapist, in the same vein. Often, these children, like Lisa, are deeply convinced that they see the rejection on a carer's face or that a carer purposely intended to hurt or exclude them. And what's more, in talking about difficult experiences to others, they sometimes 'succeed' in convincing others of their parents' or carers' 'bad' care. The therapist, in direct work with traumatised children, may find themselves faced with such stories about current neglectful or abusive care, like Lisa's therapist did. This may be complicated by the fact that the therapist sometimes does not know (beforehand) whether the child's experiences or stories reflect actual reality or not. All of these situations require the therapist to remain mindful of the child's relationships to significant others in the way they try to manage and respond to these situations.

It seems obvious that unless there are sound reasons to think that new carers are struggling to adequately care for the child, the therapist should be wary of interpreting the child's stories at face value to the detriment of their identification with the carers. As child therapists, it is very natural to first and foremost identify with the child and their suffering. This is also what a traumatised child initially needs from the therapist: to listen to or experience their negative feelings, anxieties and phantasies about significant others, possibly originating in past difficult experiences. This inevitably elicits countertransference feelings towards the child and parents, through which the therapist can resonate with the child's perspective, including feelings of disappointment, anger or indignation towards caregiving adults. Yet, this also makes the therapist vulnerable to over-identification with the child's perspective at the expense of being able to maintain an open mind to other perspectives (e.g., the parents not providing bad care but just like the therapist being subject to the child's transference of negative expectations and representations). In this context, it may be helpful for the therapist to share their worries with and consult the parent worker, as Lisa's therapist did. The parent worker, aware of the foster carers' efforts to provide 'good' care, can help the child therapist to keep thinking about the child's caregiving representations *as representations*. The child therapist may need the parent worker's reassurance that the child's perceptions are indeed not referring to real experiences or, in case destructive interactions are taking place, that these are being worked on in parent sessions. Exchanges with the parent worker to learn about the parents' experiences of their relationship with the child and about the parent worker's perspective on family dynamics can support the child therapist in their direct work with the child. By contrast, if the therapist loses sight of the real relationships, the risk of being drawn into a – mild or severe – splitting process (e.g., 'poor' child vs. 'bad' parents) can become real.

The core task for the therapist is thus to take the child's narrative serious at a representational level, as the child's reflection of their inner truth: of how they experience and perceive others, rather than at a factual level, as if it reflects how they are being treated in reality. In a more advanced phase of treatment, opportunities will arise to help the child to disentangle current actual relational experiences from 'old' relational expectations and blueprints.

In other situations, it may not be so much that the child conveys a story about 'bad' – neglectful or abusive – parental care as such but talks about a situation in which they tried to solve an issue all by themselves, without any notion or idea that perhaps they could have relied on an adult for comfort, support or help. For example, Lisa once told a story about getting completely lost at school because she couldn't find the room the physical education class was moved to and about how she hurt herself trying to find the room (see Chapter 2). In listening to her story, the therapist was struck by the fact that Lisa didn't – at any time during her search – come up with the idea that she might ask one of the teachers or administration staff to show her the way. Some traumatised children, like Lisa, due to early adverse experiences, grow up without any representation of adult caregivers as people you can turn to and rely upon. In treatment, it will be an important task for the therapist to also listen to the child's stories from that perspective and actively foster the emergence of more helpful representations of caregiving adults.

Keeping a mentalizing stance front and centre: a balancing act

Due to the underdevelopment of traumatised children's social and emotional capacities or else the frequent breakdowns therein under duress, keeping mentalizing 'online' in the direct work with such children is not an easy task. It requires the therapist to keep an eye on holding several balances at the same time.

*Making sense of things can wait – start with
making things 'thinkable'*

Mei-Lan repeatedly has nightmares of being abandoned by her adoptive parents but really doesn't want to talk about it to her therapist. In
a joint session, her adoptive mother tells the therapist that Mei-Lan's
nightmares have been really intense this week. Mei-Lan agrees that
Mum can tell the therapist about them but only after Mei-Lan hides
behind the puppet-show screen. Acknowledging Mei-Lan's need not to
be involved directly (yet), the therapist first talks to Mum about how
scary it can be to have nightmares. She says to Mum: 'All those scary
feelings of having a bad dream can be overwhelming and then kids
really need to be comforted at night by Mum or Dad. Talking about
the dream in the day can really be scary all over again. I wonder how
we could help Mei-Lan with all these scary feelings'. Mei-Lan slowly
comes out from behind the puppet-show screen, walks over to the table
where her sketchbook is and takes a seat. She first draws a bed and then
a child in it and says, 'This is when I'm really scared in my bed, and
I want Mummy to come'.

Later on in treatment, Mei-Lan often looks back on this drawing,
saying something about 'those nightmares that really scared me'. Only
after having explored and revisited, many times, the process features
of having nightmares and surviving the accompanying anxiety, can the
content of the dream – being abandoned by one's parents – become a
topic of conversation and exploration in Mei-Lan's therapy.

Children who have experienced complex trauma often suffer from a double
deprivation (Henry, 1974) with regard to their ability to bear and manage difficult
experiences: life circumstances have exposed them to experiences that are more
difficult to bear and process than children on average need to face, and at the same
time, life often has failed to provide them with 'strong shoulders' to cope with
these difficult experiences. In order to enable a child to work through difficult life
experiences in imaginative and playful ways, by going into the content of it, some
help to distance oneself from the overwhelming affective load of experiences has
to be available so as to allow images and words to surface. Similar to wine needing
a good glass, all mental content is in need of images and words to be contained and
represented, and the more affectively powerful the content that a child has to face,
the better the representational skills that are needed to make it bearable. Therefore,
it is important for the therapist, like in Mei-Lan's case, to attempt to attune to
whether process issues should be prioritised above content themes and to move
flexibly between process and content, between fostering mentalizing capacities
and facilitating narratives, between 'the glass' and 'the wine'. For Mei-Lan, words
carefully chosen to address what happens to her when having scary dreams are a
starting point and help her to come out from behind the puppet-show screen to be

able to take in the therapist's words and engage in the 'telling' process about 'being really scared in bed and needing Mummy'.

Walking the tightrope between support and exploration

 Mei-Lan's first attempt at pretend play using the doll house ends in vain. Sitting in front of the doll house, it looks as if she is starting to play out a story about a family that lives there. But once she starts to play, 'bad people' (a massive group of black-clothed Playmobil knights) enter the house, and everybody has to hide. The family members as well as the knights fly through the doll house and even through the therapy room. Mei-Lan is clearly overwhelmed but doesn't allow the therapist, whom she keeps at a distance, in any way to help or even come closer. A second later, all turmoil suddenly comes to an end as Mei-Lan plays that 'everyone goes to sleep'. The therapist cautiously but clearly says: 'Wow, Mei-Lan, what was happening in there? That seemed quite a lot to take in, wasn't it? Good that things could calm down again'. Mei-Lan only nods in affirmation.

Children who have experienced complex trauma are often first and foremost in need of support for developing – or else regaining access to – their adaptive skills to maintain or regain mental balance and to cope with arousal-provoking situations, before any more exploratory intervention can be attempted. The basic premise about balancing support and exploration – 'support when necessary, explore when possible' – is particularly tricky in working with traumatised children (Bervoets et al., 2021). Therapists can generally fall back on an arsenal of interventions and techniques to support the child in managing difficult feelings and thoughts, as well as exploring new layers of their inner life. Each intervention can be situated along both a supportive and an exploratory continuum (de Jonghe et al., 1992): when necessary, i.e., in situations of overwhelming anxiety and/or dysregulation, the therapist more actively supports the child by making use of scaffolding; where possible, the therapist explores the child's inner world, following the child's leads and cues and attuning to the child's metaphors and images in play, drawings and narratives, while remaining alert for potential dysregulation. Lieberman et al. (2015) caution that 'timing, although difficult to define, is essential in clinical practice. The same intervention may be successful or it may backfire, depending on when and how it is implemented' (p. 100). This is particularly challenging in working with traumatised children, as the margin of error is more limited than with other children. The idea 'nothing ventured, nothing gained' is much less applicable to these children. Exploring too soon or too much may threaten their fragile equilibrium. By contrast, offering too much support at the expense of more exploratory interventions may well keep them regulated in therapy but does not foster more substantial developmental recovery. Mei-Lan's therapist, for instance, responding by trying to understand the details of the play content (e.g., by exploring who the people in the house are and what exactly is happening) or rather, by trying to prevent Mei-Lan from playing out such scenes (in an attempt to prevent dysregulation), might have shut down Mei-Lan's therapeutic process. The aim is to create a setting which is 'safe but not too safe' (Bromberg, 2006; Ogden et al., 2006), requiring the therapist to continuously walk the tightrope between support and exploration, while never really being sure that they are providing just 'the right dosage' of both.

Facilitating making sense: actively scaffolding or providing words and images

 Youri was often left unfed as a baby, and although he has no memories of this, his foster family notices that he always wants to have a sandwich by his bedside before he will go to sleep. For his foster carers, this becomes rather frustrating. They feel that Youri is being controlling, and they worry that he may develop unhealthy eating habits. When the foster carers speak with the therapist about this, she helps them to see it not just as controlling behaviour, but as a reflection of very early anxieties that he can't put into words. They think about a way in which his foster mother can respond to these demands with a kind of story, about a small child who might have been so hungry once in his life that only when assured of food, can he fall asleep. In therapy too, the therapist tries to actively provide words for Youri's experiences.

In general, child therapists try to maintain a receptive stance, i.e., actively remaining open to receiving the child's communications and following the child's lead. Yet, for children who have experienced complex trauma, there are often many experiences that have shaped who they are but for which they have no words or images. At times, the therapist will therefore be required to more actively and explicitly provide words or images for experiences. Words and images facilitate meaning-making, which in turn helps to contain unpredictable and 'weird' or 'crazy' experiences and to integrate those experiences into an emerging sense of self. As in Youri's case, trying to find words to capture (fragments of) experiences helps to think about these experiences as having meaning, even when this meaning is not entirely clear yet. Sometimes, this will require the therapist to ask parents or carers for background information. Many of these children further along the treatment trajectory will actively ask their parents to tell the stories about their (past or current) experiences repeatedly, in an attempt to understand some aspect of themselves. In this way, such stories can become shared narratives.

Sometimes, the words or images are found in a process of co-creation between child and therapist. For example, when talking with Lisa about her 'stealing behaviour' – so worrisome to her foster carers (see also Chapter 7) – the image emerges of desirable 'stuff' 'calling' her so loudly, louder than the voice in her head warning her against such 'antisocial' behaviour, that she feels she has no control over her own hands and actions. At other times, words or images originating in trauma literature will seem to align with the child's experience. In such instances, these may be helpful as these put words or images to what has never been captured and represented before about what implications trauma ('having been through a lot') has for development and functioning. For instance, a child may recognise with relief when the therapist talks in age-appropriate language about regulation and re-latedness issues in terms of fight, flight and freeze mechanisms or trauma triggers. The image of the lion that attacks first at any hint of a threat or of the deer that runs off when feeling anxious and threatened – as is used in trauma literature to refer to fight and flight mechanisms, respectively – is often gratefully welcomed by the child who feels prone to such mechanisms. For traumatised children, this is often a first experience of having these inner drives addressed in normalising and empathic words (for images and metaphors, see Vliegen et al. (2023)).

Again, timing and balance of the therapist more actively scaffolding or providing words and images to facilitate meaning-making are crucial. These interventions of searching for or offering 'language' for experiences can only be helpful when attuned to the child's cues as well as developmental age as much as possible.

The trauma- and developmentally informed lens: four domains of intervention

Although the assessment phase should be informative as to the child's functioning and dynamics in different domains of development and life, the case formulation is to be considered 'provisional', as originally conceptualised by A. Freud (1965). In that sense, once we enter the therapy room with the child in the treatment phase, we bracket any previous knowledge in the service of trying to meet the child as they present themselves in the here-and-now. In order to guide the therapist in understanding what may be at stake in a child with complex trauma, the four developmental domains (see Chapter 2) can serve as lenses. In the following subsections, we therefore introduce each domain by questions that the therapist could ask themselves as they closely observe the child in the therapeutic encounter. In doing so, we aim to guide the therapist in considering which of these domains is most at stake at any particular time in treatment. Of course, this is in part an artificial compartmentalisation, as developmental issues influence one another across domains. For example, a child who is dysregulated in some way often will have trouble playing in a creative way, or, vice versa, playing about an emotionally charged theme, such as something difficult happening in an important relationship, may destabilise a child, sometimes up to the point of dysregulation. In this sense, the domains are meant as didactic lenses, to be used to aid the therapist's assessment and clinical decision-making processes.

A rule of thumb *across* domains is that intervening at the level of the process needs to take precedence over any intervention at the content level whenever there are indications that the child is finding content issues too difficult. Such indications may range from a child who suddenly puts all the characters in their play to sleep ('sudden sleep onset'; Robinson & Mantz-Simmons, 2003) – in an attempt to avoid the difficult theme – to a child who actually stops playing or who starts 'playing crazy' or becomes incoherent in another way, to a child who falls prey to a state of real dysregulation. Regardless of the specific content or domain, such situations require the therapist to help the child to regain a sufficient level of emotional balance prior to any exploratory intervention at the level of content can be attempted. Therefore, in the subsections, we discuss different ways in which issues in each developmental domain may become manifest in child therapy and offer guidelines and suggestions about therapeutic interventions and techniques that may be applied to address these issues, both at the level of process (the right side in the tables) and at the level of content (the left side in the tables).

Representational capacities as expressed in play and narrative

Whereas Lisa's as-if hairdresser play (see earlier example) offers a window into her inner world of feelings, longings, anxieties and caregiving experiences, Mei-Lan's activities in the first therapy sessions are focused on sorting pencils (see later). One of the first questions a therapist is confronted with in the playroom concerns the child's capacity to engage in playful interactions and activities meant to represent, express, explore and eventually process aspects of their inner world by means of playing, drawing and talking. In this regard, the therapist can ask themselves the following questions.

Does the child engage in and enjoy play:

1. in a basic positive playful activity? Or is there no playfulness at all?
2. in creative or playful activity as a means of connecting to and/or communicating something (small but significant) about themselves? Or is the play rather repetitive and rigid?
3. in pretend play with a story about non-traumatic as well as traumatic experiences? Or is the pretend play fragmented and vulnerable and easily disrupted?

If a child engages in a form of playful and representational activity, the therapist can help to further consolidate and elaborate on this form of play and help the child to remain connected with an inner world and/or to further explore and communicate the content of it. If these capabilities are absent, the question about their underdevelopment (such as in cases of severe neglect) versus the inhibitive impact of traumatic experiences comes to the fore. Then, the primary therapeutic focus needs to be on scaffolding these capacities and/or to address what taxes them (e.g., when inhibited in order to keep at bay difficult feelings and experiences). Therapeutic intervention in this domain is thus rooted in the understanding of the child's play (content and process) and how it is influenced or changed by traumatic experiences. This understanding underpins the therapist's reflections about how to further consolidate and strengthen the development of play capacities, about how to make use of these play capacities to scaffold emotional and relational development, about when and how to explore content and about when to focus on content versus process of play.

Basic positive playful activity: enjoying playing and playfulness

 At the start of her therapy, Mei-Lan often sits down at a small table that children use when drawing and crafting. It seems like she will start drawing or crafting, but she never really does. Her activity is limited to sorting the pencils over and over again. Any question or gesture from the therapist seems to disturb her and makes her shout 'Stop doing that!' or 'Stop asking questions!' This requires the therapist to engage in tough inner work. There is the continuous question about 'how to give Mei-Lan enough space and control to be in the playroom in the presence of an adult without being overwhelmed by fear and anger' on the one hand and 'where to challenge her world of sorting and organis- ing and help her experience a new kind of being playful' on the other hand. A first 'new experience' emerges when the therapist whispers: 'I think I know a game Mei-Lan may like, maybe, just maybe'. Mei-Lan looks up with a questioning glance and the therapist feels comfortable enough to introduce a squiggle game. 'This is a game in which one of us draws a line – it needn't be straight, it can be curved, or whatever shape you like, and we can try to find out what we see in the lines'. At first, in an attempt to keep things under control, Mei-Lan says what she sees in the therapist's line and how she wants the therapist to complete the drawing: a duck, a balloon, a snake. Gradually, Mei-Lan takes her own pencil to take turns in drawing and is able to only slowly let go of needing to control the therapist and the situation. In later ses- sions, engaging in and enjoying drawing and crafting become her first ways of playful activity (see later example).

Some children who have experienced complex trauma show severe difficulties in their basic capacities to engage in playful interaction. For a child who cannot play, the experience of participating in a playful process – whatever the content – is of major importance and can provide a first step towards recovery. When play is almost absent, the therapist can initiate a playful interaction that is focused on mu- tual playful contact, for example, rolling a ball or a toy to the child and awaiting the child's reaction. The child may explore the toy, merely roll it back to the therapist or start a game that expresses significant content. Or the therapist can start a pro- cess of mutual drawing, such as using a Winnicottian squiggle game (Abram, 2007; Winnicott, 1968), like Mei-Lan's therapist did. Sometimes, beginning to hum or sing a song or read a story can be a starting point.

As long as the child's capacity to engage in playful activity or interaction re- mains vulnerable or when issues of relational distrust or traumatic content tax this capacity, the therapist needs to focus on the process. As children always have good reasons to keep playful contact at bay, inviting them to interact playfully requires active consideration about how to go about this at the child's pace and on the child's conditions. For example, the therapist can give the child a sense of being in charge and having control over the situation by inviting them to choose a safe place in the room. Allowing the child to control the distance to the therapist or to direct the therapist to engage/witness or, instead, look away from their play are other ways to help the child to feel more in control. In sum, when a child is functioning at this very vulnerable level, 'the glass' (process) warrants more of the therapist's attention than 'the wine' (content; see Table 6.2).

Table 6.2 Therapeutic interventions at the level of basic positive playful activity

Basic positive playful activity	Present: major focus on content	Absent, vulnerable or atypical: major focus on process
Baseline observation	The child engages in and enjoys playful activity or interactions	The child shows little sign of being able to engage in playful activity or to enjoy playful interaction, shows tension or anxiety when invited to play or draw, postpones being engaged in play by spending a long time in repetitive activity, sorting things out
Understanding	The child practises and experiments with playful activity or participating in playful interaction, cautiously discovers the benefits and anxieties of participating in playful activity or interactions	*Underdeveloped capabilities:* the child has developed few capacities to engage in playful activity or interactions *And/or inhibited capabilities:* playful activity or interaction evokes anxiety; child feels unsafe when engaging in play and/or child is hovering between engaging in play and repetitive activity
Therapeutic goal	Strengthening of and elaborating on playful activity or interaction and – when possible – focusing on the co-construction of meaning of the play activity	Helping the child to engage in playful activity or interaction at their own pace and on their own conditions
Therapeutic response focuses on	Inviting the child and supporting them in playful interactions through a curious and respectful stance; the content of play may be cautiously elaborated (e.g., by introducing a new element)	Inviting the child to engage in playful interaction by actively considering the child's pace and conditions; scaffolding every initiative of the child towards a playful activity or stance; expressing (e.g., by naming) an understanding of the child's struggle to keep their balance as expressed in holding back from playing

Creative and playful activity: co-constructing meaning

 In a next phase of her treatment, crafting becomes Mei-Lan's go-to activity. She explores all kinds of materials: she tries out pencils and felt pens, works with clay, paints with different brushes, folds paper following origami examples she finds in the cupboard. In an early phase of this kind of playful activity, she demands that the therapist does exactly the same as she does, for example, folding the same box, moulding the same shape of clay. Later on, the therapist must engage in the same activity but Mei-Lan can tolerate that she makes something else, which gives room for more mutual activity: while Mei-Lan moulds a snake, the therapist makes a snail with a shell, hoping to open up a first notion about vulnerability and protection without explicitly naming this. In this phase, Mei-Lan discovers what the activity of 'creating' can mean for her. She draws, paints, sews and builds marble runs.

For the traumatised children with few abilities to make use of creative and narrative playful activity as a means to express elements of their inner world, being able to create drawings, crafts and beginning stories can mean a giant jump forward. Finding preliminary images and words may eventually help to incorporate experiences in a meaningful, coherent narrative. Long before pretend play can be helpful to process traumatic experiences, playful activity is thus an important domain of development in offering opportunities to engage in connecting to inner states and getting in touch with inner impulses, ideas or desires as a source for outer (creative) activity: 'Today, I would like to build a marble run, I love to look at the coloured marbles running downward'. Furthermore, playful activity inevitably is embedded within relational processes (see later – Relational domain): the process of being in the presence of an adult in a calm and non-threatening way and of co-constructing and elaborating meaning within a caring relationship. Crafting a heart for Mum, expressing a reparative intention after having had a fight; moulding a penguin, followed by a warm hat and a scarf and eventually a nest for the penguin family (see later) – these can all be considered creative and playful activities that may become meaningful building blocks of early representational capacities.

A child who is struggling at this level requires the therapist to mindfully try to co-construct meaningful play content (see Table 6.3). For example, in response to the child moulding a penguin out of clay:

Oh, wow! You made a penguin. What do you imagine a penguin like this might need? . . . Yes, of course, what a good idea! He needs a warm hat and a scarf. So how would you like to go about this? . . . Okay, you want to make the hat, shall I do the scarf then? . . . Oh, now they're well-equipped for the cold. Do you think they need something more? . . . A nest?

Or, like in Mei-Lan's case, the therapist found a way to build on Mei-Lan's drawing of a hedgehog, adding a tree and starting to tell a story about the hedgehog and the

Table 6.3 Therapeutic interventions at the level of creative and playful activity

Creative and playful activity	Present: major focus on content	Absent, vulnerable or atypical: major focus on process
Baseline observation	The child engages in creative and playful activity and interaction (even if only in small moments)	The child shows little sign of being able to engage in creative and playful activity, first initiatives break down easily (and drawings end up in the bin), the atmosphere turns negative when the child tries to play or create
Understanding	The child practises with exploring play material as a way to express elements of an inner world in the presence of an adult, cautiously discovers the benefits as well as the anxieties of doing this	*Underdeveloped capabilities:* The child has developed few capacities to make use of playful activities to express something about themselves *And/or inhibited capabilities:* Play activity provokes anxiety, evokes negative feelings or memories and/ or play pleasure is vulnerable
Therapeutic goal	Strengthening of and elaborating on playful activity; co-constructing meaning and elaborating the content of the play activity	Containing the negative feelings that emerge; helping the child to develop or to reconnect to playful activity as a means to express and communicate first bits and pieces about themselves; exploring the possibility to co-construct meaning; being alert for content issues taxing the child's abilities for creative and playful activity
Therapeutic response focuses on	Supporting the child when exploring materials and engaging in early creative or narrative expressions; engaging in the co-construction or exploration of meaning where possible, and helping to manage the anxieties when needed	Sensitively observing the child's activity and scaffolding every initiative of the child towards creative activity; when possible, elaborating on initiatives; participating in and creating opportunities to co-construct meanings and stories and giving words to the observed tensions and anxieties

tree. For children suffering from complex trauma, experiencing the benefits of creating something in the presence of or together with a mindful therapist who tries to elaborate on any small beginning equips the child with an important base. As such, the experience of seeking and finding images and words for feelings and experiences in the playroom and in the relationship with the therapist is part of developmental recovery.

Pretend play: representing and processing facets of an inner world

 After Mei-Lan's first 'clumsy' and fruitless attempts at pretend play in the doll house (see vignette earlier – support and exploration), she dresses up as a kitten and demands that the therapist cares for the small and needy kitten: 'give me a hug', 'bottle-feed me'. She repeats this game session after session. For the therapist, nothing playful can be experienced in this repetitive and claiming play. Any question or attempt to add something new makes Mei-Lan shout 'No no no, you can't ask that!' Sometimes, she orders the therapist 'Go ahead, everything is ready, you start playing', only to comment then that – whatever the therapist does – it's wrong. Her high-pitched voice betrays the inner tension that goes hand-in-hand with this game.

In the following phase, this kitten-play is moved to the doll house. At first, much of Mei-Lan's attention goes to 'setting the scene' with all the adult figures and cats and kittens and removing all the child figures. In the same repetitive way, she plays about adults caring for cats and kittens. The therapist receives orders about where to sit and what to do. Any attempt of the therapist to make a minimal personal contribution, for example, pretend-asking as one of the adult figures 'May I ask you, where have your children gone?' leads to an intense reaction from Mei-Lan: 'No no no, you can't say that, you can't speak like that!' She takes all the child figures and throws them away. At other times, she addresses the therapist in a threatening tone of voice: 'I will be very very angry. I guess you don't realise how angry I can be'.

Later on, new fragmented images emerge in her pretend play: in one session, the kittens are taken to an asylum; in another session, a 'truck full of adopted kids' arrives at the house and the adult figures have to buy a lot of baby buggies for all these children; in still another session, the adults go to a zoo with all the adopted children in buggies, but then there is a snake and all the children are afraid and feel threatened. Only gradually, Mei-Lan allows these themes to be expanded on in pretend play. The 'zoo play' in particular becomes a central stage in the playroom for Mei-Lan to play out themes about children being abandoned, lost and found, threatened and reassured. It becomes a lively scene where difficult themes and emotions can start to be worked through.

As children suffering from complex trauma develop pretend play capacities, aspects originating in traumatic experiences will inevitably pop up and colour their play. In Lisa's play, the therapist-hairdresser feels she will never be able to live up to Lisa's expectations of being cared for: whatever she does, it will never be good enough. In traumatised children, trying to engage in pretend play not seldomly leads to situations of involuntary re-enactment of traumatic experiences. The therapist may find themselves playing a naughty child, doing a difficult exercise, while the angry child-teacher shouts at them. Or the child may make the therapist repeat a discomforting experience, by making the therapist take on the role of an awful doctor who hurts and abuses the child or of an adult caregiver who abandons the child. This requires the therapist to consider carefully when to scaffold the child's play and protect it from hasty traumatic content or intrusive traumatic experiences and when traumatic content comes at the centre of pretend play and needs an alert and sensitive therapist to help the child survive and work through these experiences. For a child who is cautiously trying to find a balance between engaging in and enjoying a growth-promoting way of playing and making space for expressing and processing trauma-related issues and images, the therapist needs to balance between giving words to content and to process aspects. Content themes – as are present in Lisa's hairdresser's play – may involve reflecting about what the child's play may mean, integrating what is difficult to integrate, providing words for themes and content. On the other hand, process themes may involve recognising when the child's narrative suddenly stops or gets absorbed in a theme, reflecting about the fact that this may have meaning, helping to recognise what is happening.

In Mei-Lan's case, there is a trauma-characteristic to her 'pretend play' that is rather rigid and repetitive. It seems that engaging in pretend play immediately brings her in touch with traumatising images (people dying, needy kittens, a truck full of adopted kids, a scary snake that spoils the trip to the zoo), with the accompanying feelings of anxiety and distress evoking rigid and controlling defence mechanisms. Mei-Lan's play is rather 'nightmare-like': images pop up as 'bits and pieces' and immediately bring about intense feelings of anxiety and a need for control. For the therapist, they look like a whole of themes and topics that stand on repeat, as narratives that ought to come but never really come. At this level, pretend play is preliminary and hasn't reached the level from which it can serve as the prerequisite to be able to work through traumatic and overwhelming experiences as part of the therapeutic process. What makes the therapeutic work so hard is twofold. There is the fact that one seems only to be able to witness this painful and anxiety-provoking play, without being given any opportunity to alter it, to bring the narrative in motion, to help to process the traumatising content in a lively narrative with a more coherent and more constructive storyline. Moreover, not only can traumatic content have a disruptive effect on pretend play, but relational anxieties quickly boil up from underneath the surface, quickly becoming too real ('I guess you don't realise how angry I can be'). The child is at the mercy of bits and pieces of a nightmare-like inner world (still) lacking the capacity to bring together or process these pieces. So, before any exploration or working through of traumatic content can be attempted, the therapeutic work often needs to be focused on containing the overwhelming affects – stemming from trauma triggers and/or relational anxieties – and fostering the process of pretend play (see Table 6.4). The therapist may need to endure for a long time to be controlled by the child and not to be able to explore the meaning of traumatic play yet, while at the same time, not to give up on carefully trying to challenge the child's play, for example, by introducing a 'challenging' element such as a caregiving adult

Table 6.4 Therapeutic interventions at the level of pretend play

Pretend play	Present: major focus on content	Absent, vulnerable and easily disrupted or atypical: major focus on process
Baseline observation	The child engages in pretend play in which more neutral as well as trauma-related content (e.g., being left behind, being treated badly) or relational anxiety can be incorporated	The child shows little sign of being able to engage in pretend play, or storylines are fragmented, unclear, jumping from one theme to another; rigid/repetitive; anxiety-provoking or leading to play being disrupted or breaking down
Understanding	The child practises with pretend play, experiences the benefits (e.g., pleasure, humour, relief) as well as the anxieties of this play; the child shows abilities to process and work through (traumatic) life experiences and issues and to bear the accompanying pain, anxiety	*Underdeveloped capabilities:* the child has developed few capacities to engage in pretend play as a means to process (traumatic) life experiences *And/or inhibited capabilities:* the child's attempts to engage in pretend play provoke anxiety or function as trauma triggers, such that the child is easily overwhelmed by pain, anxiety, anger . . .; pretend play pleasure and benefits are yet to be discovered
Therapeutic goal	Strengthening existing capacities for pretend play in order to enable the processing of life experiences	Helping the child to develop or reconnect to capacities for pretend play as a means to represent and process life experiences and helping to bear the accompanying difficult feelings
Therapeutic response focuses on	Helping the child to expand the themes and the circles of communication within pretend play, by making use of an inquisitive stance; affording the child space and providing support to elaborate on (traumatic) content, while remaining alert for moments of being overwhelmed; taking the role the child assigns you in pretend play (role disposition), while maintaining reflective about content as well as process	Helping the child to remain in a pretend mode while helping to manage the anxieties ('safe but not too safe'); focusing on the process of how difficult thoughts and feelings are emerging and helping the child to manage these intrusive or overwhelming thoughts/feelings

figure. Often, this proves quite a challenge, as expressed by Mei-Lan's therapist at a team-meeting:

> She's so extremely controlling, there is not the slightest space for a personal contribution on my part, any attempt to say or ask something results in her trying to silence me. She hasn't the slightest confidence that I am there to help her. Sometimes, it feels as if I should be happy that she tolerates me sitting next to her.

Eventually, both process and content will need to be addressed to enable the child to represent experience in a stable, coherent, integrated and meaningful way. In children who have experienced complex trauma, the development of this ability will take time (Slade, 1994): 'a thought becomes thinkable often by a very slow gradual process, a process which cannot be rushed' (Alvarez, 1992, p. 153), and it will require the support of the therapist as a developmental object (Greenspan, 1997; Hurry, 1998). Re-enactments within a safe and containing relationship with the therapist enable the often gradual, sometimes indirect, expression and mastery of powerful affects and anxieties and overwhelming experiences and thus the working through of traumatic experiences.

Affective development and regulation strategies

Another important domain of functioning that is observable to therapists when working with traumatised children relates to the basic affective mood and range of expression the child is able to show, their state of emotional balance and their ability to regain emotional balance when dysregulated. In working with children who have experienced complex trauma, the importance of helping to develop or restore regulation and regulatory capacities cannot be overstated. Only when the child is able to find a minimal equilibrium of calmness, vitality and regulation can psychotherapy in the sense of being able to engage in a narrative and mentalizing process take place, and child and therapist can start discovering and understanding what is going on in the child's mind, as a basis for finding more adaptive ways of coping. With easily dysregulated children, a therapeutic relationship can grow out of a series of experiences of being held together, calmed down or reclaimed when too far away. . . . The experience of being adequately (co-)regulated by an emotionally available therapist in a way that is attuned to their needs and capacities, that is embedded in language and that gives rise to a shared history between child and therapist can serve as a first therapeutic and healing experience in the child's route to developmental recovery. In Mei-Lan's case, she started to store all her colouring pictures, drawings and craft works in her personal box, which formed the material manifestation of what was going on in her internal world.

With regard to regulation issues and capabilities, the therapist can ask themselves the following three questions.

1. What is the child's current affective mood and state of (dys-)regulation? Is the child calm or, rather, vital enough to be in the presence of the therapist and to focus on content? Or are there signs of current or imminent dys-regulation? And can the child access strategies to regulate themselves?
2. Are affective states and regulation difficulties in actual and recent real life a central topic in the child's stories?
3. Are affective states and regulation issues and processes the core content of this child's (pretend) play or drawing?

When regulation issues are at stake in one of the previously mentioned ways, the therapist can observe to what extent the child manages to stay (relatively) regulated or what they need to regain a regulatory equilibrium. When the therapist has been able to scaffold regulatory capacities, the focus can switch to the content the child is bringing to the fore. By contrast, when a child who has experienced complex trauma is observed to become or be dysregulated, the primary therapeutic focus needs to be on regulatory processes and scaffolding regulatory capacities.

Current affective state: being in a mindful place

Mei-Lan is sitting in the waiting room with an angry face and a de-fensive attitude, saying she doesn't want to be here. Her adoptive mother explains that Mei-Lan has been sleeping badly the past few days, gets angry easily and reacts with much rage. Mum tells about a recent incident in a busy market, where Mei-Lan ran away in anger. The therapist responds by saying that it must be a difficult period for Mei-Lan. Grudgingly, Mei-Lan follows the therapist to the playroom and takes the seat the furthest removed from the therapist. The thera-pist tries to reconnect by asking Mei-Lan what may be at stake at these difficult times, and offering to do something that normally helps her to calm down, like colouring a picture or folding an origami ani-mal. But Mei-Lan only yells angrily: 'Shut your mouth, I don't want to be here! I'll run away and no one will find me'. The therapist, feel-ing unable to reach Mei-Lan, starts feeling uneasy and anxious that Mei-Lan may not be able to regain enough calmness to tolerate being in the same room with her. Realising that she has to prevent herself from becoming dysregulated with Mei-Lan, the therapist takes a sheet of paper and starts to draw. She searches for a regulating image in her own mind, and draws a hedgehog (an image that had become mean-ingful in an earlier phase) in his cosy hole under the ground. She fills the hole with a lot of objects surrounding the hedgehog, all things she knows are important in Mei-Lan's life: a cat, a stuffed dog, a guitar, a picture of her family. . . . While drawing, the therapist keeps an eye on Mei-Lan, who remains silent but seems to be calming down a bit. After a while, the therapist notices that Mei-Lan is trying to see what she is doing, and says: 'I'm making a drawing, do you want to see it?'. Mei-Lan hesitates and then nods slowly. 'Is this a good time for you to come closer to watch?' Mei-Lan nods again. The tension lowers bit by bit, and the therapist – feeling she still has to be on her guard – keeps her gaze fixed on her drawing, in order to give Mei-Lan as much space as possible. Mei-Lan approaches slowly, takes a seat next to the therapist and looks at the drawing. The therapist asks: 'Would you like me to tell something about my drawing?' Mei-Lan responds by nodding again. 'This is Little Hedgehog, he feels restless and disturbed, he tries to calm down. To be able to do that, he needs his room and all the things he loves. Look, this is his doggy, he can cuddle if he wants to; and this is his cat, she is snoring for her friend Hedgehog and his guitar here . . . and a picture of his mum and dad and brother here. . . . Being there among all the things and people he loves helps Little Hedgehog to find some calmness'. Mei-Lan moves slowly to her drawer, takes a princess picture and starts colouring. The rest of the session she keeps colouring in silence. The therapist watches carefully without disrupting the silence. At the end of the session, she says: 'I'm so glad we could be here together today, let's go to your mum now'. Mei-Lan takes the drawing and puts it in her drawer. In the waiting room, Mei-Lan puts her arm around her mother, and they leave together. Luckily, mother is experienced in handling her adoptive daughter's dysregulated states, and understands what she needs now: she doesn't say or ask anything and responds with putting her arm around Mei-Lan and giving her a cautious kiss on her hair. In later sessions, Mei-Lan often looks at the drawing, telling the story of Little Hedgehog calming down when he has the things he loves around him.

Sometimes, a child can be in a state of severe dysregulation in a rather undefined way and aroused 'for no obvious reason', as in Mei-Lan's case or, rather, more specifically anxious and/or angry due to something that happened. Dysregulation may also be about a child who is 'playing crazy', for example, laughing or crawling around or spilling paint 'uncontrollably' so that no meaningful narrative can emerge. Or dysregulation may be about a child who is overly regulated and inhibited or even numb and unreachable. In children who have experienced complex trauma, dysregulation is also often about rapidly fluctuating between different arousal/feeling states.

Moments of dysregulation require an immediate regulatory response from the therapist: the child needs a therapist remaining calm and helping them to regain their equilibrium and understand what is going on in their body and mind. In traumatised children, this often includes (co-)regulating distance and closeness in order to find a safe and anxiety-reducing way of being together. For Mei-Lan, physical and emotional distance is needed to prevent her from getting completely overwhelmed and running out of the room. The therapist is aware of the risk of being experienced as intrusive and overwhelming and tries to hold back and wait. After Mei-Lan was able to calm down a bit on her far-away chair, the therapist observes first signs of interest and a longing to come closer. Being offered as much control over the distance as possible, Mei-Lan is able to re-engage cautiously and allows herself to reconnect with being curious and interested in what the therapist is doing.

Sometimes, (co-)regulation concerns helping the child to engage in activities that help to evacuate tension and negativity and to feel more calm and positive. For Mei-Lan, these are repetitive fine motor activities that slow down bodily processes (e.g., colouring or origami); for other children, these may involve intense gross motor activity (e.g., throwing a ball, rope skipping, sports). Still other children are in need for particular perceptual or creative activities, such as listening to or making music.

Sometimes, imagining a safe place can have a regulating effect on a child in distress. In the case vignette earlier, the therapist's drawing serves a double goal. She first started to draw to regulate the tension she herself was beginning to feel and, also, to divert the focus of attention away from Mei-Lan. But drawing the 'hedgehog in his safe hole with all his precious things' became a way of imagining safety to help Mei-Lan to calm down and to find safe images in her own mind. For children who are 'playing crazy', helping them to recentre their bodily energy, for example by grounding or breathing exercises, can help to regain some calmness. For children whose minds have drifted too far away to be in touch with themselves and their surroundings, revitalising and reclaiming interventions (Alvarez, 2012), such as explicitly addressing the child by their name and scaffolding 'vital sparks', are often helpful.

Interventions aimed to foster affect regulatory capacities may be situated on a continuum from taking over regulation completely when necessary to prevent destruction, harm or a dangerous situation (such as running away) or, rather, to prevent the child from falling into apathetic and numb states; to co-regulating, based on the relationship and mutual expectations that have developed during the therapeutic process. For example, when a child is in such a hyperaroused dysregulated state of mind that it becomes destructive or dangerous, the therapist obviously needs to take over completely until the danger has subsided. Yet, with a child who is not completely dysregulated, who is 'playing crazy' or who has withdrawn in a numb state of mind, the therapist might try to co-regulate the child by verbal (e.g., calling the child by name) or physical intervention (e.g., touching the child's arm to draw attention) without taking over completely. In this regard, the therapist tries to keep an eye on maintaining a level of arousal and tension which the child can experience as bearable, as 'safe but not too safe' (Ogden et al., 2006). Only when the child is regulated enough and their regulatory equilibrium is no longer threatened can child and therapist engage in more exploratory interventions aimed at fostering understanding and reflection (see later). In other words, when current dysregulation is an issue, as illustrated in Mei-Lan's case, we try to address this in the heat of the moment by helping the child to get (back) in a state of mind that is calm enough or, rather, vital enough. However, this doesn't mean that the therapeutic work ends there: in later and more regulated circumstances, we often try to talk about these incidents and/or refer to them as marking experiences in the therapeutic process (see later). As such, (co-)regulating the child in a calm way at times of dysregulation and talking about what precisely was at stake at more regulated times function as complementary processes in fostering the child's affective development and regulatory capacities (see Table 6.5).

Table 6.5 Therapeutic interventions at the level of the child's current affective state

Current affective state	*Calm or, rather, vital enough to focus: major focus on content*	*(Imminent) Dysregulation: major focus on process*
Baseline observation	The child is calm or, rather, vital and focused enough to engage with affective themes and experiences	The child is currently in a state of dysregulation (hyper- or hypo-arousal or rapidly fluctuating between hyper- and hypo-arousal; overwhelmed by aggression, anger, anxiety, flat affect, dissociation)
Understanding	The child is currently able to regulate their arousal and feelings; there are no experiences or feelings too intense to bear here and now	*Underdeveloped capabilities:* the child has developed few capacities to regulate arousal and feelings *And/or inhibited capabilities:* current experiences are overwhelming the child to such an extent that they are unable to access their own regulatory capacities to stay regulated enough
Therapeutic goal	Elaborating narrative content	Regaining a basic level of regulation and getting back to a mindful place
Therapeutic response focuses on	Supporting the child to expand on the content of narrative communication and play	Managing the current dysregulation, taking over or providing co-regulation in order to optimise opportunities for developing or reconnecting with regulatory capacities

*Affect(ive dynamics) in actual and recent reality: talking
and thinking together about real-life feelings and experiences*

 Youri enters the playroom in an agitated state and starts talking incoherently about having been punished unfairly at school. When the therapist, struggling to understand, invites him to tell her what happened precisely, Youri becomes more upset. The therapist proposes: 'Maybe you could try to draw and tell me what happened, so I can really understand what has made you so upset?' Youri, eager for the therapist to understand what happened to him, immediately starts to draw the playground at school. While talking about a fight and him being the only one who was punished, he gets upset again: 'It was so unfair, you know!'

Therapist:	'Youri, let's pause here for a moment. Just to make sure I really understand, could you rewind the movie of what happened just a bit for me? I really want to understand what has made you feel upset and unfairly punished. So, could you tell me what happened first, when you were on the playground?'
Youri:	'Ahmed, Idriss and I were playing with the ball here (draws a circle on one part of the playground) and Kenneth, Alan and Bryan came from over there (points to the other side of the playground) and they wanted to join our play. . . . And I just punched him!'
Therapist:	'So, there was a fight over the ball?'
Youri:	'No, at first, everything was fine. We started playing a match together and we were really having fun'.
Therapist:	'So, at first, you were all playing together, and it was fun. Do you remember feeling when it started not to be so much fun?'
Youri:	'We were going to lose, and I didn't want to lose, I hate losing! . . . And then, I called Kenneth "red head", and then Kenneth pinched his nose and looked at his friends and said "Do you smell the same as me? You can smell the brown apes", and they all started laughing. And then . . . I looked at Ahmed's face . . . and I just punched Kenneth!'
Therapist:	'Wow, it feels like things started happening really fast from when you felt you guys were going to lose the game till you punched Kenneth! Something must have happened inside of you when you saw Ahmed's face and just before you took a swing at Kenneth, I wonder what that was?'
Youri:	'It's just, I know that look on Ahmed's face, he looked so hurt! I knew I had to do something! And then it happened: I punched Kenneth in his face, he was bleeding! He started hollering. And then the teacher only punished me. He didn't hear what Kenneth said about us, and he didn't care when I tried to tell him!'

Sometimes, a child wants to tell the therapist about an emotionally laden event they experienced outside the therapy room. This 'telling' process is often the way for normally developing children to better understand what exactly transpired and, in that sense, to gain mastery over the experience. With children who have experienced complex trauma, the therapist will find themselves confronted with a child who urgently wants to talk about a situation at home or at school but who, while starting to talk about the incident, easily gets upset 'all over again'. This requires the therapist to more actively help the child to regain a calm enough state of mind to be able to try to figure out together what actually happened both in external reality and in the child's internal reality (see

Table 6.6 Therapeutic interventions at the level of the child's affect(ive dynamics) in actual and recent reality

Affect(ive dynamics) in actual and recent reality	*Calm or, rather, vital enough to focus: major focus on content*	*(Imminent) Dysregulation: major focus on process*
Baseline observation	The child talks about a recent incident in real life without getting overwhelmed	The child is trying to talk about a recent incident in real life, but the story is difficult to follow or telling the story seems to upset them again here and now
Understanding	The child is able to find words and images to express and reflect on what happened in the situation as well as on what they were thinking, feeling, etc.	*Underdeveloped capabilities:* the child has developed few capacities to regulate the arousal and feelings evoked by talking about affective experiences *And/or inhibited capabilities:* the child is trying to express and reflect on what happened, but the content of the story raises too intense arousal or feeling, bringing about difficulties to regulate themselves and to continue to find words and images
Therapeutic goal	Elaborating narrative content	Regaining a basic level of regulation that will enable expression of and reflection on the experience
Therapeutic response focuses on	Supporting the child to elaborate, explore and reflect on what happened in external reality as well as in internal reality and how both are linked to one another	Actively helping the child to find words and images that adequately capture their inner experiences

Table 6.6). To this end, the therapist may make use of specific techniques. A 'stop-and-rewind' process, often integrated in a draw-and-tell method (Driess-nack, 2005, 2006; Vliegen et al., 2014), as Youri's therapist applied it or mak-ing use of play props can support the child in the 'telling' process of what happened inside-and-out. To the extent that the child is not yet able to find own words and images, psycho-education may be warranted. Psycho-educational interventions then serve the purpose of offering images that help to put into words what the child experiences, based on the therapist's assessment of what may be at stake in the child's mind. For some traumatised children, the most helpful experience is the fact that difficult experiences *can* be put into words. In this regard, it is important to offer accepting, containing and non-judgmental words about what is happening and what may be helpful. An easily dysregu-lated child is in high need of reassurance that their dysregulation is a normal response to a situation that is too difficult for them to manage. Normalising and reassuring words counter harsh convictions about oneself of being a 'mad' or a 'bad' child, reduce feelings of shame or guilt and facilitate communication about difficult experiences which traumatised children would otherwise tend to ignore or keep to themselves. Hence, psycho-education is always a means to an end: without words or images that help the child understand what is at stake in their inner world, they lack the necessary tools to understand, explore and process the inner turmoil of thoughts and feelings, longings and needs, anxie-ties and concerns.

For children who are easily dysregulated, being able to start talking and thinking together about incidents in their lives with a supportive and reflective adult, like the therapist – striking the iron when it has cooled down (or at least, when it's not so hot anymore) – is important to be able to fall back on in 'hotter' circumstances. This will form the basis for the emerging ability to think about what is happen-ing in one's inner world, to better understand why one behaves like one does, as well as to find more constructive ways to handle difficult situations or relational conflicts. In Youri's case, it was with the therapist's support that he eventually man-aged to disentangle his 'good intention' to protect his friend, on the one hand and his 'fighting-like-a-lion' reaction which got him into trouble, on the other hand. In subsequent sessions, Youri was able to talk and think together with the therapist about what could help him to feel earlier on 'when he's turning into a lion', what or who he could turn to 'to not react like a lion' and what might be better reactions than 'fighting like a lion'.

Affect(ive dynamics) in (pretend) play: representing and processing affective themes and experiences

Mei-Lan is playing one of her zoo scenes rather quietly, in which a baby giraffe is born. Supported by the therapist through a back-and-forth conversation, the play unfolds. Other animals come to take a look, to admire the baby. . . . The conversation about what is happening leads to a new scene: Mum-giraffe asks an elephant to keep an eye on her baby while she searches for food. Then the pace of Mei-Lan's play quickens, with the baby giraffe suddenly disappearing and everyone frantically searching for the baby. Mei-Lan moves the animals around quickly and restlessly. All the animals end up in one big pile. Mei-Lan says: 'I think it's time to clean up this mess'. The speeding-up of Mei-Lan's play took the therapist by surprise. She found no way to intervene and slow down the events or to maintain a more explorative curious stance towards the play content. As stopping the play and cleaning up the scene seems to prevent Mei-Lan from dysregulating completely, the therapist decides to scaffold Mei-Lan's self-protective and defensive move, saying: 'You're starting to know well what helps you most when things get heated and become more difficult. Let's tidy up the animals for today'. While moving closer to the play materials to help Mei-Lan tidy up, she adds as a kind of throwaway remark: 'Maybe some other time you can show me more about what happens to the baby giraffe'.

During a traumatised child's play in therapy, images may emerge that capture an overwhelmingly intense and anxiety-provoking emotional aspect of their representations of prior experiences. For example, a child waking up in the midst of the night, alone and upset because there is a monster in the room; a bear or zombie chasing the child who doesn't know where to hide; the child turning into a snowman and being frozen so that they can't move anymore. Such images are expressions of feeling dysregulated or overwhelmed and may be put to use to help the child to process experiences. Yet, it is mostly only in more advanced phases of treatment that a child is able to make use of the therapeutic context to begin to really process experiences of inner turmoil, dysregulation, too-difficult-to-bear experiences in pretend play. As is clear in the previous vignette, such overwhelming images can be extremely short-lived, quickly evoking imminent dysregulation, as expressed in the speeding-up of the play, the motorial restlessness that can be observed and the 'mess' that is made of the play materials. This, again, requires the therapist to closely observe whether the child is in a state calm enough – or vital enough – to focus on and expand upon the content played out in pretend play or, rather, whether this is to be considered too dysregulating at this time and the child first and foremost needs help to regain a basic sense of emotional balance (see Table 6.7). Some children are able to give indications about when dysregulation is imminent, within their play (e.g., by suddenly putting all the play characters to sleep or giving their story an unexpected turn) or outside the play content, like Mei-Lan, by breaking off their play and stating that it's time to clean up or suddenly wanting to do something else. In other situations, dysregulation completely overwhelms the child, requiring the therapist to decisively co-regulate the child first.

Table 6.7 Therapeutic interventions at the level of the child's affect(ive dynamics) in (pretend) play

Affect(ive dynamics) in (pretend) play	Calm or, rather, vital enough to focus: major focus on content	(Imminent) Dysregulation: major focus on process
Baseline observation	The child is able to represent (in play, drawing or story) an experience of an intensely dysregulating emotion such as aggression, anger, anxiety, flat affect, freezing, becoming crazy or overwhelmed without getting (completely) overwhelmed here and now	The child gets easily overwhelmed or breaks up a play, drawing or story when representing a dysregulating experience or an intense emotion such as aggression, anger, anxiety, flat affect, freezing, becoming crazy or overwhelmed
Understanding	The child is able to process experiences of being dysregulated by playing, drawing or creating stories at a metaphorical level	*Underdeveloped capabilities:* the child has developed few capacities to regulate the arousal and feelings evoked by playing, drawing or creating stories about affective experiences
		And/or inhibited capabilities: the child is trying to process experiences of being dysregulated by playing, drawing or creating stories, but the story evokes highly intense and dysregulating affects that easily threaten the affective equilibrium here and now
Therapeutic goal	Exploring the content of the play, of difficult emotional experiences	Helping the child to remain in touch with the inner experience, by making use of play, drawing or stories while helping to contain dysregulating aspects of the experience
Therapeutic response focuses on	Supporting the child to elaborate, explore and reflect on the emotional experience as part of the child's inner world	Actively helping the child to contain, to find words and images for and to explore difficult affective experiences

Attachment development and relational capacities

A third lens to look through for the therapist working with traumatised children relates to what can be observed in terms of the relational dynamics and attachment issues the child brings into the playroom, based on their inner representations of self and other. In this regard, the therapist can ask themselves the following questions.

1. How does the child relate to the therapist? Are they able to be in the presence of and/or rely on the therapist as a secure base and as a safe haven? Or does the child show signs of insecure attachment representations or relational difficulties towards the therapist?
2. Are relational and attachment issues in actual and recent real life a central topic in the child's stories?
3. Are relational and attachment issues the core content of this child's (pretend) play or drawing?

The first aspect relates to the child's abilities to make use of the therapist as an available and reliable adult. The second aspect concerns the child talking about relationships and relational dynamics and issues in actual and recent real-life experiences. The third aspect refers to moments when the child is able to play or draw about relational dynamics, indicative of a more advanced way of processing relational experiences. For each of these aspects, the therapist can observe the presence versus the absence or vulnerability of the child's relational capacities. If one or more of these capabilities is present, the therapist can help to further consolidate these and elaborate on content. If these relational capabilities are absent or vulnerable, the primary therapeutic focus needs to be on scaffolding these capacities and/or to address relational processes.

The therapeutic relationship: feeling safe (enough) in the therapist's presence to show relational unsafety

In the early phase of Mei-Lan's therapeutic process, her way of being with the therapist is one of complete control, characterised by shouting 'Stop doing that!' or 'Stop asking questions!' (see previous vignette – Regulation domain). While crafting, every once in a while, joy and pleasure are visible; most of the time, however, deep frustration and anger dominate the atmosphere in the room. More than once, the materials Mei-Lan is working with fly through the air, because she can't manage them the way she wants. Often, she remains intensely controlling towards the therapist, ordering her what to do and reacting with rage when the therapist doesn't meet her expectations. 'Sitting next to her, silently or being silenced by her' summarises the therapist's way of being with Mei-Lan. It seems that being near the therapist evokes in Mei-Lan a need to control her.

Nevertheless, it is here that change first occurs, albeit in small steps. The first moments of connectedness become observable when Mei-Lan is working with deep concentration and a big smile on her face to draw 'the perfect heart' (because it is Mother's Day tomorrow). She starts to make use of the therapist to help her at small moments: 'Can you make the two sides of the heart so that the curving is exactly the same?'. Later on, the therapist is even allowed to give words to a frustrating situation without being interrupted brutally: 'Oh, Mei-Lan, you wanted to finish your drawing the way you imagined it, but our time is up for today – how hard is this!' Or when the therapist witnesses the first glimpses of shared pleasure when creating a story together: Mei-Lan drew a hedgehog, the therapist started drawing a tree, Mei-Lan asked what it was. The therapist responds with a cautious and small story: 'This is a tree, and once upon a time, a hedgehog came to take shelter from the rain under the tree'.

As in any therapeutic endeavour, the child's relational dynamics as rooted in their attachment representations become manifest in the therapeutic relationship. A large part of therapeutic growth and development therefore emerges within the therapeutic relationship. In children who have experienced complex trauma, intense relational anxieties, stemming from ingrained core expectations to be treated in negative ways, mostly dominate the way they relate to the therapist. Some children try to keep the therapist very close, by being overly compliant or regressive and clingy (e.g., by asking help for the smallest thing, preventing them from growing in agency and autonomy). In many cases, the child's relational blueprint makes it almost impossible for them to trust the therapist's availability, reliability and benign intentions. When such relational anxieties are unbearably high, a child can get stuck in overcontrolling behaviour, as Mei-Lan did. Other children may revert to primary flight mechanisms in an attempt to reduce the distress they are experiencing in relationship to the therapist, such as wanting to run out of the playroom. Or, like Jemal, holding on to an 'anti-dependent' stance towards adults, trying to solve everything on his own and actively pushing away others when they see him struggle. Such a flight mechanism may easily be mistaken for indifference or even arrogance, further complicating relationships, such as with Jemal's teachers at school. Other children might less consciously or actively keep adults at arm's length, but the mindful therapist can observe how they genuinely do not have any notion that they might rely on adults, including the therapist, for help or support, like Lisa's therapist in listening to her telling the story about getting injured at school while looking for the right classroom (see earlier).

Providing a therapeutic response to such relational dynamics in traumatised children often proves a challenging endeavour because efforts to act as a helpful adult and to reduce the child's stress and distrust may backfire. Words meant to comfort or a gesture of closeness meant to (re-)connect to the child can be experienced as even more threatening and thus can further compound the child's ability to make use of the therapist as a developmental object. Often, as in Mei-Lan's and Jemal's cases, the therapist will need to tolerate for some time being controlled or kept at a distance in order for the child to feel safe and calm enough to focus on an activity or to get in touch with impressions and feelings. Moreover, such a first and fragile layer of basic trust is needed, not only to experience what it is like to feel safe and calm in the presence of another but also to dare to show the relational anxieties and fundamental feelings of distrust which traumatised children often struggle with. This often requires a period of trial-and-error, characterised by quick – often difficult to predict – shifts between good-enough, even harmonic moments in the relationship, on the one hand and difficult moments of relational anxiety or anger, and distrust, on the other hand. It may take quite some time and persistence before the therapist gets the feeling that they are starting to get to know the child and can assess what is bearable and helpful – resembling the trial-and-error process early parents go through with their infant. Actively searching for ways to be in each other's presence without getting overwhelmed by relational anxieties may thus need to be the first objective with traumatised children, long before they will be able to play, draw and/or talk about experiences in the therapist's presence (see Table 6.8).

In this regard, therapy provides ample opportunity for the therapist to get to know the child's relationship patterns and relational issues. Separation anxiety, this is the child's anxiety or conviction that caregivers are going to abandon them, forms part of the relational anxieties of a majority of traumatised children. Hence, the transitional moments from waiting room to therapy room – and vice versa – which may be considered as natural Strange Situation Procedures (Ainsworth & Bell, 1970) and the times of separation due to planned holiday breaks or unplanned absence of the therapist in case of unforeseen circumstances or illness are particularly pertinent windows into the child's separation reactions and relevant opportunities to address the child's relational dynamics. In this regard, some children need help to stay connected across distance. Then, installing a transitional object or phenomenon may be warranted. For example, bringing a parent's note saying 'See you when your therapy hour is up' to the playroom can help to remain there during the therapy hour or knitting a piece of string from the playroom as a bracelet for the child to wear home can help to keep therapy in mind.

Moreover, it can be helpful to articulate observations of implicitly and behaviourally expressed relational expectations in thoughtful words. For example, the therapist might respond to the child struggling with craft material and looking at them with expectation: 'I can see you might want some help with this, okay if I try?' As touched upon earlier, some children may be able to make use of the therapeutic relationship to show how negatively they experience caregiving adults, by a sudden negative reaction or paranoid expectation towards the therapist. Such instances of 'the witching hour' (Dahl, 1982) express a deep layer of negative

Table 6.8 Therapeutic interventions at the level of the therapeutic relationship

(Sufficiently) Secure therapeutic relationship	*Present: major focus on content*	*Absent, vulnerable or atypical: major focus on process*
Baseline observation	The child engages in/makes use of the therapeutic relationship	The child shows little sign of being able to make use of the therapist for personal growth and development; reacts overcontrolling, disavowing or aggressive in relation to the therapist, or rather, indiscriminately and boundary-crossing
Understanding	The child is able to make use of the therapist as a developmental object	*Underdeveloped capabilities:* the child has developed few capabilities to make use of the therapist as a reliable adult
		And/or conflict-laden capabilities: the child's longing to feel connected to an adult evokes anxieties and/ or difficult relational representations
Therapeutic goal	Helping the child to understand their relational patterns and to expand their repertoire of relational skills by experimenting in the therapeutic relationship as a relational laboratory	Helping the child to be in the presence of/connect with the therapist as a reliable adult whose presence can help to grow and address relational issues
Therapeutic response focuses on	Acting as a reflective adult who helps the child develop by attuning to and helping to explore their inner experiences, by inviting to think and talk about the child's relational dynamics	Acting as a controllable and non-intrusive adult, who respects the child's relational anxieties and defences; keeping an active eye on trauma-driven negative or anxiety-provoking experiences and managing the impact of separation reactions and 'witching hours'; keeping an active eye on trauma-driven overly positive/ too close relational behaviour and setting and maintaining appropriate self-other boundaries

caregiving representations which get projected onto the therapist. However challenging it may be for the therapist to be perceived or even addressed as if they are a neglectful ('You never give me what I need') or maltreating ('You're hurting me!') caregiver, helping the child to recognise and 'survive' such moments, without moral judgement, is of major importance to be able to eventually work through these deeply ingrained unconscious relational expectations. In this context, the therapist will need to tolerate and to 'own' to a certain extent the child's projections ('Oh, my gosh! I really gave you the impression that I don't care about you. That wasn't my intention, but I see now how it came across'.). The aim is to grant the child the opportunity to express and explore caregiving representations. Similarly important will be for the therapist to provide a response that does not match the child's relational expectations based on their attachment representations ('representational mismatch'; Horowitz, 1987). This aims to support the child to gradually be able to disentangle what the therapist is like in reality and what is part of their inner world of relational anxieties.

Working on relational issues within the therapeutic relationship is thus often at the core of therapeutic work with traumatised children. And often, it proves to be a protracted process. For example, wanting to come 'too close too soon' often increases the child's relational anxieties and is a step backwards in building a relationship that can be experienced as trustworthy and helpful by the child. Only when a basic level of trust has been established can the therapist carefully start to name, explore or challenge the child's capacity to relate to an adult as potentially helpful and supportive, by asking a question or adding an alternative idea.

The same principles hold for traumatised children who present at the 'opposite' side of the relational spectrum: the children who seem not to discriminate between known and trusted adults, on the one hand and unknown adults, on the other – children who are 'indiscriminately friendly' or 'socially disinhibited' (see also 'epistemic credulity'; Fonagy et al., 2019). Or, at an even more basic level, children who show little ability to differentiate between 'me' and 'not-me' and therefore seem to merge with others, including the therapist, coming too close too soon and crossing self–other boundaries. Such presentations equally point to alarming developments in the relational domain and call for firm though thoughtful management by the therapist. The therapist might, for example, respond by naming the child's desire to cuddle or crawl onto the therapist's lap ('I can see that you want to come really close now') while also setting clear boundaries ('but that's not how we're going to go about this, we could do a high five instead').

Relational themes in actual and recent reality: talking and thinking together about real-life relational experiences

 Around Christmas time, Lisa rushes into the playroom, exclaiming indignantly that her foster carers have purposefully chosen her therapy hour to visit the Christmas fair (which takes place right in

front of the therapy centre) 'without her'. The fact that they – unbe-
knownst to the therapist – already promised to go with her after her
therapy hour cannot counter Lisa's paranoid phantasy that they're
out to exclude her. The therapist first acknowledges Lisa's feeling
of missing out on a time of shared pleasure. Keeping in mind the
relationship with her foster carers, the therapist then tries to explore
whether Lisa has been able to express her disappointment to her
foster carers about not being able to join in. Lisa reacts with a mere
'No! But they should know, shouldn't they!' It is clear that representations of bad care reign her inner world despite the therapist's
efforts to contain her arousal. After the session, when her foster carers come to fetch her, Lisa continues her angry tirade. The therapist
learns about the foster carers' prior intention to visit the fair with
her now but also sees them struggle visibly to go through with their
original commitment, as Lisa continues her verbal attack. It seems
as if Lisa's paranoid anxiety and anger are 'contaminating' her real
relationship with her carers.

Sometimes, a traumatised child will talk about relational themes they are experiencing or have recently experienced in their life outside the therapy room.
Struggling to disentangle actual relationship patterns from 'old' caregiving representations, they are often hypersensitive to the smallest sign of non-perfect attunement within a caregiving relationship or are sometimes even convinced of
being treated in negative ways. For Lisa, not being able to participate in an outing
with her foster carers can only mean one thing: she's not important to them because they don't want her to be with them. Although very difficult to understand
and handle for the foster carers, it makes perfect sense when taking into account
Lisa's 'hypersensitivity' to feelings of exclusion (see earlier – vignette about the
fries for dinner). In other stories traumatised children may share in therapy, the
therapist may be struck by the lack of a notion in the child's mind that they might
have relied on a trusted adult in the vicinity to offer help or support, like Lisa's
therapist when she told her the story of trying to find the room a class was moved
to (see earlier example).

In such situations, acknowledging the subjective 'truth' of the child's experiences (e.g., genuinely feeling excluded or all alone and agitated) by finding words
or images that adequately capture the child's experiences of significant others is
primary (see Table 6.9). At the same time, the therapist is mindful not to equate
the child's representations to actual reality (e.g., not joining the child in talking
about their parents or carers as if they really are bad parents). Only when the child
feels heard will fragile windows open to cautiously challenge the child's relational
representations and help the child to disentangle actual from previous relationship
patterns.

Table 6.9 Therapeutic interventions at the level of the child's relational dynamics in actual and recent reality

Relational dynamics in actual and recent reality	Can be expressed while remaining regulated enough to focus: major focus on content	When expressed, this immediately evokes (imminent) dysregulation: major focus on process
Baseline observation	The child talks about a recent relational incident in school or at home in a coherent way without getting overwhelmed	The child is trying to talk about a recent relational incident, but the story is hard to follow or telling the story seems to upset them again here and now
Understanding	The child is able to find words and images to express and reflect on what happened in a particular relationship	*Underdeveloped capabilities:* the child has developed few capacities to regulate the arousal and feelings evoked by talking about relational experiences *And/or inhibited capabilities:* the child is trying to express and reflect on what happened relationally but has difficulties to remain regulated enough and to continue to find words and images
Therapeutic goal	Helping the child to understand what is happening in actual relationships, in order to find new/better relational attitudes or responses	Helping the child to find words and images that fit with what is at stake in the relationship and that enable reflection on the relational patterns; scaffolding awareness about relational functioning as a theme in psychotherapy
Therapeutic response focuses on	Supporting the child to elaborate, explore and reflect on the relational content	Actively helping the child to regain a basic level of regulation and to find words and images for what happens in relationships

Relational themes in (pretend) play: representing and processing relational experiences

 Encouraged by the containing therapeutic relationship, Lisa elaborates on her hairdresser's play during multiple sessions. Spending a lot of time in the hairdresser's chair, having her hair done, with the therapist-hairdresser touching her hair and taking care of her is at centre stage for quite some time. Core to this play is the image of Lisa – who can't bear being touched by her foster carers – positioning herself to be at the receiving end of 'endless' bodily care by the therapist, who is doing her utmost to offer 'good' care. Sometimes, Lisa is visibly enjoying the care offered and expresses a deep longing for it to be endless – it can't last long enough. At times, this takes a negative turn towards the feeling of 'never good enough', when Lisa looks in the mirror critically, saying her haircut is not short enough or not dark enough. Sometimes, she takes on an even more actively negative stance, when she refuses to pay for the hairdresser's services and runs out of the shop, she herself commenting on it as 'stealing'. At other times, Lisa reverses roles by taking care of the therapist-hairdresser, offering her a chair and a magazine, as well as coffee and 'marvellous biscuits'.

In this vignette, Lisa is clearly experimenting in pretend mode with different roles and positions with regard to (bodily) care – a deeply conflict-laden topic for her, as taking bad care of herself and 'refusing help in self-care' have become important issues at home.

When traumatised children are able to symbolise themes of relatedness and attachment issues in play, a drawing or a story, it is important for the therapist to address these in a metaphorical narrative way. This will help the therapist and the child to better understand how the child experiences and tries to negotiate relationships with significant others while respecting the displacement afforded by play to not talk about these often emotionally charged topics with direct reference to themselves in – past or current – relationships. The therapist might, for example, support the child in exploring different (subconscious and unconscious) aspects of their attachment representations in the context of prior life experiences by encouraging the unfolding of pretend play. Yet, for many traumatised children, this will not be possible until the more advanced phases in treatment, as for many of these children relational themes may have come to function as trauma triggers, destabilising and potentially dysregulating the child's emotional equilibrium. This requires the therapist to remain mindful of any indications of (imminent) dysregulation in the child when playing or drawing about relationships and thus to help the child to regain emotional balance prior to refocusing attention to the relational content (see Table 6.10).

Table 6.10 Therapeutic interventions at the level of relational themes in (pretend) play

Relational themes in (pretend) play	*Can be expressed while remaining regulated enough to focus: major focus on content*	*When expressed, this immediately evokes (imminent) dysregulation: major focus on process*
Baseline observation	The child is able to represent (in play, drawing or story) relational dynamics without breaking up the play or getting completely overwhelmed here and now	The child breaks up a play, drawing or story or gets overwhelmed when difficult relational content arises
Understanding	The child is able to process aspects of relational dynamics by playing, drawing or creating stories at a metaphorical level	*Underdeveloped capabilities:* the child has developed few capacities to regulate the arousal and feelings evoked by playing, drawing or creating stories about relational themes
		And/or inhibited capabilities: the child is trying to process relational dynamics, but the content is so anxiety-provoking so as to destabilise or dysregulate the child's emotional balance here and now
Therapeutic goal	Exploring the content of the play, of particular relational dynamics	Helping the child to remain in touch with the relational content, by making use of play, drawing or stories while helping to contain difficult feelings that arise
Therapeutic response focuses on	Supporting the child to elaborate, explore and reflect on the relational dynamics as part of the child's inner world	Actively helping the child to contain, to find words and images for and to explore difficult relational dynamics

Sense of self and identity

A fourth theme or lens that is crucially relevant in a trauma-informed treatment approach is the child's sense of self and identity. The mindful therapist can get a sense of how the child perceives and feels about themselves, by asking themselves the following questions.

1. Does the child show signs of liveliness and vitality, of being in touch with an inner world of feelings and thoughts? Or, does the child come across as flat and detached, even numb and devitalised?
2. To what extent and in what way does the child experience and process feelings of loss and mourning?
3. How is the child involved in the 'telling' process of their life story? Including coping with the awareness of being a foster or an adopted child?

Some traumatised children present in therapy with a rather 'flat' mood, not really knowing what they want or who they are, lacking a basic sense of vitality. Such children may show difficulties to experience, let alone process, bodily and emotional sensations, whereas others, who are in another stage of life and/or treatment, are aware of who they are now, what they like to do and/or who they want to be in the future. A second important aspect in traumatised children's developing sense of self and identity is the extent and the way they are able to experience and process feelings of loss and mourning in their young lives. A third aspect concerns the child's ability to create a coherent and essentially positive narrative about their life. For foster and adopted children, this includes (though is, of course, not limited to) how they are able to cope emotionally with being a foster or an adopted child and how these elements can be integrated into their life narrative. For each of these aspects, the therapist can observe the presence versus the absence or vulnerability of the child's capacities with regard to a sense of self and identity. If one or more of these capabilities is present, the therapist can help to further consolidate these and elaborate on content. If these capabilities are absent or vulnerable, the primary therapeutic focus needs to be on scaffolding these capacities and/or to address relevant issues.

Vitality and connection to an inner world: feeling alive and in touch with one's inner world

At the start of therapy, the therapist experienced Youri as a 'closed off' child. His standard response to any question or invitation seemed to be 'I don't know'. The therapist gathered that this was his way of blocking every impulse, thought or feeling coming from inside. 'I don't know . . . what I want to do today, how the Easter break was, what happens next in the story'. It required a lot of patience from the therapist who often felt blocked out too. It felt as if it was her responsibility to find openings to connect to Youri and to constantly nudge him to get in touch with his own inner world.

A first feeling of connectedness occurs around making music together. At first, Youri is somewhat surprised when the therapist – sensing that this may be one of Youri's vital sparks – fully engages in making music with him, but soon he allows the game to become reciprocal, work-ing hard to think about questions like 'What rhythm shall we play?' or 'How is the "concert" going to unfold?' Youri starts talking about what he likes so much about making music and allows the therapist to ask what he feels about this or that kind of rhythm or instrument.

In a next phase, activities extend to playing with skittles and darts. During this play, the therapist introduces conversations about what Youri likes, what makes him feel happy or angry. . . . It often seems as if he's asking permission to have a thought or a feeling: 'Can I feel angry when . . . Dad (referring to his biological father) forgets my birthday?'

Youri's foster mother sometimes supports this 'telling' process in bringing him to therapy. She will mention things like 'The music teacher gave you a huge compliment last Saturday, he said you were making great progress. That was nice, wasn't it, Youri?'; or 'Yester-day was a difficult evening, wasn't it, Youri? You were sad when you went to bed, but you didn't want to talk about it'. When the therapist offers 'we can draw and tell about it, if you want', it occurs that Youri nods in affirmation. 'Drawing together' in Youri's therapy means that he gives the instructions and wants the therapist to draw. As she strug-gles to find a fitting image for his experience, first conversations are about what happened exactly, who said what and what was difficult, but gradually Youri is also able to talk about how happy, sad or disap-pointed he felt.

Some children who have experienced complex trauma, like Youri, are so pro-foundly disturbed in the development of their sense of self and identity that they are in a state of numbing and devitalisation, giving little sign of being able to recognise, experience, process and give meaning to bodily or emotional sensations or to be in touch with their own inner world. In such instances, two important foci of therapeutic intervention can be held in mind (see Table 6.11).

First, cherishing the vital spark. When a child barely gives cues about what they are experiencing in their body and mind or are unable to experience and to show what is vitalising in their life, it is important for the therapist to take on a more ac-tive though still non-intrusive stance. The therapist tries to tune into the smallest signs the child provides about their bodily or inner states and explicitly acknowl-edges these ('I can see that your shoes are untied, would you like some help with tying them?'). Core to these interventions is often mirroring and putting into words of presumed sensations or experiences. For example, 'Wow, I can see from your expression that you really love to feel the sand in your hands!' or 'I see you look-ing at the pencils, would you like to use them? Oh, you're smiling! Does that mean you really would love to use them?' Such interventions aim to help the child to become aware of bodily signals and behavioural cues, and the fact that these do not just 'happen to be' yet have meaning, in that these can be linked to inner states or experiences.

Table 6.11 Therapeutic interventions at the level of vitality and the child's connectedness to their inner world

Vitality and connection to inner world	Present: major focus on content	Absent, vulnerable or atypical: major focus on process
Baseline observation	The child engages in (narrative or playful) activity and in the relationship with the therapist, showing to be in touch with an inner world	The child shows little sign of vitality and seems out of touch with impulses, longings, thoughts and feelings, as expressed in apathy or numbing
Understanding	The child is able (to an increasing extent) to remain in touch with sensations and inner states and experiences	*Underdeveloped capabilities:* the child has not been able to develop a basic sense of vitality, or has developed few capabilities to connect to sensations, feelings or thoughts (an inner world)
		And/or inhibited capabilities: bodily sensations and inner states provoke so much arousal and anxiety that the child is reverting to blocking out and numbing
Therapeutic goal	Helping the child to understand, express and further develop their sense of self and identity	Helping the child to become aware of/to get in touch with inner sensations and experiences, while containing the accompanying anxiety and helping to understand what is going on in body and mind
Therapeutic response focuses on	Helping the child to trust and use aspects of their inner world to direct small decisions in life	Actively tuning into signs of vitality and connection with a feeling or a thought (a smile, a gaze); explicitly mirroring and putting words to presumed sensations and inner states

Second, actively helping the child to connect to aspects of an inner world and make use of these to find direction in life and own their life. With children who may often be out of touch with their own inner world, the therapist can support them to (re-)connect and help them to (re-)find which direction they would like to go in and what is important to them to learn or to want to be able to do. In supporting the child to become author and director of their experiences, the therapist helps them to own their life. The therapist may do this by helping the child to trust and give worth and reality value to inner states. Subsequently, these feelings can be used to make choices and direct small decisions in life ('Do I prefer to draw or to paint today?', 'Do I prefer the yellow or the red candy?'). As such, the therapist can help the child to hold on to a perspective for the future, to be able and to dare to dream of the future – a future that is connected to current vitalising and positive experiences as well as to past experiences of loss (see also later).

Loss and mourning as part of life

 In a further phase of treatment, Youri is able to express questions about why his biological parents couldn't care for him. Realising that many of his classmates, even those whose parents split up, still grow up with at least one of their biological parents, elicits questions about why Dad (his biological father) can't take care of him. In talking about his dad's illness, Youri seems able to grasp some aspect of the need for his placement in a foster family. Yet, when his dad, once again, creates expectations which he doesn't fulfil (promising to be there and then not showing up, or promising Youri a Playstation as a birthday gift and then not buying it), it visibly upsets Youri time and again: he withdraws, becoming 'hard-to-reach', also in therapy. The therapist, alert to these signs, patiently tries to re-engage Youri: 'I can see that today talking is hard . . . maybe we can find other ways for you to show me what's happened and what's on your mind?'; after a next disappointing visit to Dad: 'Hmm, today I seem to have the Youri here who I also saw a few weeks ago, the Youri who is really silent and seems to be struggling with something really difficult inside. . . . I wonder whether something in particular has caused this?'. Youri slowly and hesitantly starts to talk about these experiences and share some of his thoughts and feelings.

As children suffering from complex trauma have been subjected to multiple discontinuities in life, they have had to face feelings of loss and mourning, of being vulnerable and injured. Being burdened early in life often exceeded and consequently strained their developing capacities to bear and process feelings of sadness, anger, feeling vulnerable, abandoned or hurt. Sometimes physical scars remind them of experiences they would prefer to forget. Various accounts, both unconscious and conscious and at times incompatible and incoherent, require a sensitive therapeutic stance, in order to foster a healing process and/or facilitate a process of transforming difficult experiences into growth-promoting life events (see Table 6.12). For many children, 'smaller' themes of getting hurt physically or feeling vulnerable psychologically need to be worked through and integrated in their sense of self before any therapeutic work can be conducted on 'bigger' losses in life (such as aspects of being a foster or an adopted child: see later discussion). In this context, typical content traumatised children may bring to the session concerns getting hurt or injured and being dropped (Boston & Szur, 1983): either toys are dropped or the child jumps or falls perilously. By bringing to the fore such themes, they

Table 6.12 Therapeutic interventions at the level of loss and mourning as 'part of life'

Loss and mourning as 'part of life'	Present: major focus on content	Absent, vulnerable or atypical: major focus on process
Baseline observation	The child plays, draws, or tells a story expressing thoughts and feelings about being vulnerable or hurt, about loss or mourning, without getting (completely) overwhelmed here and now	The child disavows any feeling of vulnerability, loss or mourning or, rather, is preoccupied with being vulnerable and hurt in a troubleso me and destructive way (e.g., escalating danger or aggression in play)
Understanding	The child is able to remain in touch with feelings of loss and mourning and is in need of someone who listens and helps to reflect and process	**Underdeveloped capabilities:** the child has developed few capacities to bear or process experiences of being vulnerable or hurt *And/or inhibited capabilities:* thoughts and feelings of vulnerability are so threatening to the child's emotional equilibrium that they get stuck in deep feelings of sadness, anger, feeling abandoned or rejected . . .
Therapeutic goal	Helping the child to come to terms with this particular aspect of their life history and to integrate it in their sense of self and identity	Helping the child to make experiences of loss and mourning bearable and thinkable, while managing the accompanying anxieties
Therapeutic response focuses on	Offering an open-minded, listening and actively curious stance; helping to figure out what it means to be this child with this particular history with regard to experiences of loss and mourning; while remaining alert to and respectful of adaptive moments of 'the need to forget'	Actively attuning to small occasions to raise this topic in a non-intrusive way; being receptive to and help manage intense feelings of being hurt, of sadness, hopelessness; helping the child to (re-)connect to a basic sense of safety and of emotional equilibrium

seem to 'practise' with the topic of vulnerability and loss, regardless of explicit references to aspects of their personal history, within the therapeutic relationship. This often requires the therapist to engage profoundly in listening to stories about smaller and larger injuries – in pretend play or in the child's reality – and to attend to these mindfully. In elaborating on what the small injuries feel like (e.g., 'It seems that [play character] really hurt themselves?', 'Oh, I see the cut in your finger; shall we put a band aid on it? Does it still hurt? What do you need to feel a little bit better?'), we create therapeutic opportunities to explore what pain, discomfort and being injured feel like and what that may evoke; what the child needs to heal; what it feels like to be comforted or, by contrast, to feel left alone with what hurts inside. Practising with being taken care of with these smaller, often physical, injuries, may function as a stepping stone towards also entrusting the larger, mental injuries to the therapist, like Youri was able to do in later phases of his treatment.

Owning one's life story: towards a coherent life narrative

Youri, by now, feels safe enough in the presence of the therapist to voice aspects of his experience of being a fostered child: 'Why am I so different?', 'Why do things go wrong for me so often?', 'I don't really belong there' (in his foster family). Being fostered really makes him feel so different from any of his classmates, to the extent that Youri has never told in class that he lives in a foster family.

In this period, Youri starts to talk more openly in therapy about playing the violin and performing on a stage. One session, Youri brings his violin, giving a short performance for the therapist. The therapist can see that he's nervous and relieved but also somewhat proud when he finishes, saying 'I've never performed for anyone outside our orchestra! Not even for show-and-tell in class!'

A few weeks later, Youri talks all excitedly about a contest organised by the national philharmonic orchestra. The orchestra is planning to hold a series of concerts to raise funds for foster care, and they're organising a contest for musicians in foster care. Five foster children will be selected to perform with the orchestra at the fundraising concerts. Although Youri would really like to enrol in this contest, he also hesitates 'because then all my classmates will know that I'm a foster kid'. Youri's doubts about enrolling and being 'exposed' as 'different' open up conversations and reflections, both at home and in therapy, about what 'being fostered' means to him. One of the first things Youri wants to do is to make two family trees, one of his biological family and another one of his foster family.

For any child or adult person, the (co-)creation of a personal life story is essential to the development of a healthy sense of self and identity. For children whose biological parents were unable to take good enough care of them and/or abandoned them, this developmental domain is severely compromised and sometimes remains fragile and vulnerable well into (young) adulthood. As the creation of a life story is a never-ending process (Wright, 2009) for any child – but for traumatised children in particular – the story needs to be uncovered layer by layer and thus partially re-written, attuned to what a child can face at any particular time in development and/ or treatment. Youri, in the previous vignette, is really struggling with what parts of his identity he wants to share with the world around him: does he want others to see him play the violin and know about his longing to be a musician? And does he want to play the violin in public, when this means others will immediately know he is a foster child, implying his biological parents were unable to take care of him? This requires the therapist to help the child to find their own pace, to find bits and pieces of themselves and framing these in time and space, to help create a sense of historicity and coherence and to help reflect on 'what may others know about you?' When the child is up to it – and in the case of traumatised children, this is often not until the advanced phases of treatment – emerging bits and pieces of narratives may be bundled into a book. Even when a 'sense of history' about real life is still far off, a first sense of containment, historicity and continuity may be experienced with regard to the therapeutic process by bundling drawings, experiences and aspects of play in a sketchbook.

Foster and adopted children in particular have to cope with an aspect of identity that is unique to their lives: the awareness of being a foster or an adopted child. Consequently, what is self-evident for children growing up with their biological parents – a sense of belonging to a family and, more generally, in the world – foster and adopted children have to find at a more explicit level. Often, they need help to get in touch with and to express what they think and phantasise about their concep-tion, birth and the circumstances of their out-of-home placement. As discussed in Chapter 2, for children who have gone through often multiple breaches of continu-ity in (sub-)cultures, this is actually embedded within a broader and deeper process of an – often lifelong – search for a level of integration that affords a sufficient sense of self-continuity and -coherence. For (internationally) adopted children in particular but also for some foster children, this process involves the evolution from feeling as if they don't belong to any (sub-)culture ('falling in between cul-tures'), to coming to terms with the fact that actually they belong to several (sub-) cultures. Unsurprisingly, this is a process which takes (a lot of) time and is in need of (much) revisiting. In Jemal's case, for example, small but important steps were taken when he started to be able to embrace sharing Ethiopian food with his Caucasian adoptive family and really experience the pleasure he derived from that instead of getting confused and upset by it (see vignette in Chapter 2).

The process of developing a sense of self and identity in children who have experienced complex trauma inevitably evokes feelings of anxiety, sadness, worth-lessness and hopelessness, which may compromise adaptive identity development if left unattended. Feeling unloved always implies feeling unlovable. Facilitating the (co-)construction of narratives, attuned to the child's cues (including symp-toms, signs, bodily experiences, parents' observations), while remaining sensitive to cues indicating that the child is feeling anxious and/or threatened in exploring these issues and supporting the child to bear and manage these feelings is part of therapeutic work with these children (see Table 6.13).

Table 6.13 Therapeutic interventions at the level of the child's owning their life story

Owning one's life story	Present: major focus on content	Absent, vulnerable or atypical: major focus on process
Baseline observation	The child expresses bits and pieces of a personal history or becomes curious about who they are and how their life has been shaped (including the given of being fostered or adopted)	The child never expresses aspects of a personal history or shows no signs of being curious about how they came to be the person they are
Understanding	The child is (increasingly) able to face and process aspects of their personal life history	*Underdeveloped capabilities:* the child has developed few capacities to think about their personal life story (including aspects related to being a fostered or an adopted child) *And/or inhibited capabilities:* thinking about their personal life story is so destabilising to the child that they try to avoid it and/or get overwhelmed
Therapeutic goal	Helping the child to experience an emerging sense of personal historicity and continuity; helping the child to come to terms with all aspects of their life history, fostering the development of a coherent and essentially positive sense of identity	Helping the child to make this topic bearable and thinkable, while managing the accompanying anxieties
Therapeutic response focuses on	Actively helping the child to keep together the bits and pieces of their life history from their perspective (including phantasies); offering an open-minded, listening and actively curious stance; helping to figure out what it means to be this child with this particular history; while remaining alert to and respectful of the child's pace	Actively attuning to occasions to think together about small life events in a non-intrusive way; offering ways to start experiencing historicity and continuity in the playroom (e.g., personal drawer or box, sketchbook, naming continuity or, rather, naming observable evolution when this occurs)

Concluding thoughts

Therapeutic work with traumatised children is often a hard and lengthy process, due to the complexity and pervasiveness of the child's developmental difficulties. It therefore requires the installation and the flexible maintenance of a therapeutic frame and relationship that affords the child opportunities to show aspects of their inner life. This in turn should allow the trauma-informed therapist to observe and mentalize the child's mind and to intervene in a way that is conducive to recovery in relevant developmental domains. Yet, it is important to remember that the direct work with the child not only hinges on what the therapist is able to 'achieve' with the child in the therapy room but also – and perhaps, primarily – on how this work is embedded within a network of mentalizing relationships around the child, starting with but not limited to the child's primary caregivers. The establishment and maintenance of such a mentalizing network will then hopefully enable the child to carry forward any therapeutic gains in and through relationships outside of the therapeutic endeavour.

References

Abram, J. (2007). *The language of Winnicott. A dictionary of Winnicott's use of words* (2nd ed.). Karnac Books.

Ainsworth, M. D., & Bell, S. M. (1970). Attachment, exploration, and separation: Illustrated by the behavior of one-year-olds in a strange situation. *Child Development, 41*, 49–67.

Alvarez, A. (1992). *Live company. Psychoanalytic psychotherapy with autistic, borderline, deprived and abused children*. Routledge.

Alvarez, A. (2012). *The thinking heart: Three levels of psychoanalytic therapy with disturbed children*. Routledge.

Bervoets, E., Meurs, P., Luyten, P., Tang, E., & Vliegen, N. (2021). Walking the tightrope: Ego support and exploration with a child with complex trauma. *Journal of Child Psychotherapy, 47*(3), 415–432. https://doi.org/10.1080/0075417X.2021.2014935

Blake, P. (2008). The setting, physical and mental, and limits. In P. Blake (Ed.), *Child and adolescent psychotherapy* (pp. 193–209). Karnac Books.

Boston, M., & Szur, R. (Eds.). (1983). *Psychotherapy with severely deprived children*. Routledge & Kegan Paul.

Bromberg, P. (2006). *Awakening the dreamer: Clinical journeys*. Routledge.

Dahl, R. (1982). *The big friendly giant*. Jonathan Cape.

de Jonghe, F., Rijnierse, P., & Janssen, R. (1992). The role of support in psychoanalysis. *Journal of the American Psychoanalytic Association, 40*(2), 475–499.

Driessnack, M. (2005). Children's drawings as facilitators of communication: A meta-analysis. *Journal of Paediatric Nursing, 20*(6), 415–422.

Driessnack, M. (2006). Draw-and-tell conversations with children about fear. *Qualitative Health Research, 16*, 1414–1435.

Fonagy, P., Luyten, P., Allison, E., & Campbell, C. (2019). Mentalizing, epistemic trust and the phenomenology of psychotherapy. *Psychopathology, 52*, 94–103. https://doi.org/10.1159/000501526

Freud, A. (1965). *Normality and pathology in childhood*. Penguin.

Greenspan, S. (1997). *Developmentally based psychotherapy*. International Universities Press.

Henry, G. (1974). Doubly deprived. *Journal of Child Psychotherapy, 3*(4), 15–28. https://doi.org/10.1080/00754179708257300

Horowitz, M. (1987). *States of mind: Configurational analysis of individual psychology* (2nd ed.). Plenum Press.

Hurry, A. (1998). *Psychoanalysis and developmental therapy*. Karnac Books.

Jenkinson, S. (2001). *The genius of play*. Stroud.

Lieberman, A. F., Ghosh Ippen, C., & Van Horn, P. (2015). *Don't hit my mommy!: A manual for child-parent psychotherapy with young children exposed to violence and other trauma* (2nd ed.). Zero To Three.

Ogden, P., Minton, K., & Pain, C. (2006). *Trauma and the body. A sensorimotor approach to psychotherapy*. Norton & Company.

Robinson, J. L., & Mantz-Simmons, L. (2003). The MacArthur Narrative Coding System: One approach to highlighting affective meaning making in the MacArthur Story Stem Battery. In R. N. Emde, D. P. Wolf, & D. Oppenheim (Eds.), *Revealing the inner worlds of young children: The MacArthur Story Stem Battery and parent-child narratives* (pp. 81–91). Oxford University Press.

Slade, A. (1994). Making meaning and making believe: Their role in the clinical process. In A. Slade & D. P. Wolf (Eds.), *Children at play: Clinical and developmental approaches to meaning and representation* (pp. 81–107). Oxford University Press.

Vliegen, N., Tang, E., & Meurs, P. (2023). *Children recovering from complex trauma: From wound to scar*. Routledge.

Vliegen, N., Van Lier, L., & Borgions, M. (2014). *Naar de kindertherapeut. [My child psychotherapist.]* Acco.

Winnicott, D. W. (1968). Squiggles. *Voices: The Art and Science of Psycho-therapy, 4*(1), 98–112.

Winnicott, D. W. (1971). *Playing and reality*. Tavistock Publications.

Wright, J. L. (2009). The princess has to die: Representing rupture and grief in the narrative of adoption. *The Psychoanalytic Study of the Child, 64*(1), 75–91. https://doi.org/10.1080/00797308.2009.11800815

Chapter 7

Work with parents

As discussed in Chapter 3, parenting a child who has experienced complex trauma is a particularly challenging task. For most parents raising 'normal' children, trying to remain open and understanding towards what one's child needs and being mindful in how one responds to that can go a long way. Yet, in parenting a traumatised child (and here we are referring to the child's primary caregivers, including adoptive parents and foster carers), mentalizing is even more important, though often more strained, as in and of itself this may not be all that is needed to support the child's developmental recovery.

In this chapter, we present a mentalization-based and trauma-informed model of working with carers and parents of children who have experienced complex trauma; the aims of which are to help parents find (more) growth-promoting ways to address their child's particular developmental needs as well as to cope with the trauma dynamics that enter their family life. As stated by Midgley et al. (2017a),

> When we are able to make sense of the behaviors of others (and ourselves), the interpersonal world becomes a more predictable, safe and meaningful place. But when we misread the intentions of others, or struggle to make sense of our own internal states, this can lead to confusion, misunderstanding, and difficulties in interpersonal relating, contributing to escalating conflict or bottled up anger and fear.
>
> (p. 18)

First, as mentalizing capacities in parents trying to support a child's recovery from trauma are at high risk of breaking down, we outline the core of the work with parents as focusing on their mind. Scaffolding parental mentalizing constitutes the cornerstone of parent work in this model that will hopefully allow the parent worker to venture towards two complementary 'poles' of intervention. As such, we frame how parent work in this model requires the therapist to continuously move back-and-forth among these three 'poles' of intervention, which we elaborate on in the remaining sections of this chapter.

DOI: 10.4324/9781003044918-10

Mentalizing processes front and centre

The purpose of this first section is to outline how mentalization-based principles are central to the work with parents in this model (see Table 7.1). To this end, we set out the frame of the parent work, as a mentalizing structure in time and space to allow this work to unfold. Next, we discuss how therapists can continually consider what the work should focus on, which 'pole' of intervention – as we have termed it. We also show how the therapist, by mentalizing the parents' 'small stories of life', can set in motion a virtuous broaden-and-build cycle scaffolding parental mentalizing abilities. All this, of course, requires the therapist (or 'parent worker', as they are sometimes called) to closely monitor their own mentalizing processes.

A solid therapeutic frame and an unconditionally empathic stance

Work with parents concurrent with the direct work with the child is arguably 'what makes [psychodynamic child] therapy work' (Novick & Novick, 2011). This is particularly true for parents of traumatised children, who are facing a highly demanding family life in terms of being frequently and easily drawn into difficult and sometimes even crisis-like situations. Therefore, in the present treatment approach, parent sessions are planned once every three or four weeks,

Table 7.1 Core components of mentalization-based work with the parents

A solid but flexible therapeutic frame	• Provide predictability and continuity through a (relatively) stable frame: time, space and frequency of sessions (i.e., once every three or four weeks); meanwhile thinking about offering flexible accessibility in-between sessions as appropriate • Take into account the balance between family burdens (with regard to the traumatised child as well as to other family members) and resources
Attitudes and strategies	• Acknowledge and validate the particularities of and difficulties in the child's development and what this requires from parents • Be especially mindful of possible re-activation of 'being and feeling judged' • Move back-and-forth among the three intervention 'poles' of helping parents to regain access to their mentalizing abilities, helping parents to understand the vicissitudes of their mentalizing abilities, and helping parents to keep the child's mind in mind • Convey a genuine curiosity and interest in parents' day-to-day experiences with their child ('small stories') • Be mindful of your own mentalizing processes

depending on the phase in treatment and the urgency of the problems. This frequency – and the accompanying predictability and continuity – aims to offer parents a solid external frame, in time and space, within which important parenting topics can be thought and spoken about. It is through the unfolding therapeutic relationship that parents are enabled to talk openly about difficult affects. In this context, it is not uncommon that parents find seemingly obvious solutions during or following a parent session simply because their reflective mind has been rebooted, wondering why they were not able to come to that solution in the heat of the moment at home. This process creates space for new ways of approaching their children's difficulties, which is the vehicle to effect change in family dynamics and life.

Paradoxically, being offered time and space to think and talk about these difficult affective dynamics is seldom experienced as a gift by parents in the early phases of parent work. Parents may initially experience the suggestion of meetings with them as an 'additional' burden, when they are already feeling stretched or overwhelmed. Indeed, the particular combination of being in high need of support in raising a child with severe difficulties and struggling with their own intense and sometimes overwhelming feelings about their child and parenthood impacts the 'setting the scene' of the work with parents of traumatised children. It will thus require the therapist to patiently invest in building and maintaining the working alliance with parents, for them to be able to experience it as beneficial and helpful.

Given this context, the therapist will need to ensure that they validate the extraordinary challenge of parenting a traumatised child from the very start of the work: it requires more than ordinary parenting skills and it confronts parents more frequently and chronically with more-than-usually difficult experiences.

 Mei-Lan's adoptive mother is exhausted by Mei-Lan's severe separation anxiety: she needs her mother to stay with her until she falls asleep, which is only very late; early in the morning, Mei-Lan wakes up, anxiously screaming for her mother, and during the day, at any 'minor' tension or arousal, Mei-Lan starts to scream and yell and needs her mother's support and patience to calm down again.

Prior to any exploratory work with parents into difficult feelings or mentalizing breakdowns, the therapist needs to explicitly acknowledge and validate the particularities of and difficulties in their child's development and what this requires from parents. Some parents have found creative and helpful responses in attempting to find a way to live with their child's deeply disturbed behaviour. Some families, such as Mei-Lan's, are already offering 'a therapeutic environment' to their child, without being aware of it, managing 'unusual behaviour' such as chronic regressive claims with seemingly endless patience and concern. All of this deserves the therapist's validation.

Moreover, the therapist will need to be especially mindful when thinking with parents about parenthood may re-activate aspects of 'being and feeling judged' when this has been part of the experience of becoming a parent. Prior to the child's placement, adoptive parents and foster carers have usually been evaluated with regard to their desire and their skills to parent a child who is not their own, so parent work may re-evoke anxieties and other negative feelings that were at stake during these evaluation processes. As Mei-Lan's adoptive mother expressed: 'People never realise that it isn't just the adopted child who remains uncertain about their position and being loved unconditionally, as an adoptive mother you always feel you have to prove you are worthy of parenting this child'. Being in need of specialist help in raising their child may then be experienced to mean that, in the end, the results of the screening were wrong, and parents are *not* competent in caring for this child. As such, having to consult for therapy almost inevitably compounds the ambivalence and anxiety which even 'normal' parents are likely to feel. This requires the therapist to listen carefully for how feelings of 'being incompetent' or 'being judged' enter the consultation room and may interfere with parents feeling free to talk about the difficulties they are experiencing in parenting their child. The therapist will need to address these by explicitly conveying an authentically curious and non-judgemental stance, as this will hopefully counter a defensive closing off of parents' mind to what the therapeutic encounter may have to offer (see also 'epistemic trust'; Fonagy et al., 2019).

Finally, the therapist working with parents of traumatised children needs to keep in mind that they are attempting to 'move the furniture while the house is on fire'. This means that, often, the therapist will need to help manage crisis situations outside of the consultation room and hours. Knowing that someone is easily available to reflect with them when they are in heavy weather helps parents to feel less alone and less stressed, which in turn can help them to keep their mentalizing abilities 'online'. Furthermore, unblocking a difficult situation rather quickly and in a thoughtful way can sometimes help to avoid more severe problems. Finally, experiencing that they are able to cope with the problematic situation in a constructive way can empower parents in their parental skills and increase the child's confidence in the parents. So in addition to the solid frame based on regular meetings and perhaps different from 'regular' parent work, flexible accessibility to the therapist (and their mentalizing mind) in between sessions (e.g., via email or by phone) may be important to offer to parents of traumatised children (e.g., parents send an email or leave a phone message and will be contacted back within a reasonable timeframe). This is the case when parents are facing crisis situations or volatile situations in which a crisis could potentially be triggered if parents were to react in a non-mentalizing manner. Specifically, when parents are doubtful about the helpfulness of their spontaneous reaction but are not able to come up with a better response without the therapist's help, such as when a child is stealing, running away, expressing suicidal ideation or other endangering behaviour. In our experience, parents are rather economical with – and grateful for – these in-between session contacts and rarely 'take advantage' of this opportunity. Regardless of the specific arrangements relating to 'on-demand' availability, it is important that the therapist establishes and maintains the frame of 'by-appointment' meetings on a regular basis and that parent work does not take place only when a crisis occurs.

Process versus content in parent work: back and forth among three 'poles' of intervention

 Lisa's foster father talks about an embarrassing incident at school. Lisa told her new teacher that she had thrown away her sandwiches because her foster mother used old and mouldy bread (which wasn't really the case; see also Chapters 3 and 8). The young teacher intuitively shared her own sandwiches with Lisa; after school, she approached the foster carers cautiously to offer the school's help when parents can't afford school materials or proper meals. Foster mother felt embarrassed and didn't know how to react. Foster father became angry when the teacher spoke to them and felt he had been made to look ridiculous and humiliated. The therapist notices that even now foster father is getting all wired up in talking about this incident, as he 'cannot imagine why on earth Lisa would lie about such a thing'.

In parenting a traumatised child, specific challenges come to the fore, which require unusually good mentalizing whilst, at the same time, taxing parents' mentalizing capacities more than 'normal' family life. In such circumstances, there is no point trying to talk 'about' a particular issue (e.g., a difficulty parents are having with the child) unless they are in a state of mind where they are able to think together with you.

Parental mentalizing is often 'offline' at the start of treatment, and such breakdowns may re-appear during treatment, when parents face 'weird', aggressive or destructive behaviour making them feel helpless, powerless, anxious, hopeless or angry or when anxiety runs high (e.g., about the child's future being compromised). At such moments, helping parents to regain access to their mentalizing abilities should always come first – this forms the cornerstone of the work with parents in this model, as in other mentalization-based approaches (e.g., Midgley et al., 2017b). The focus, then, is on the processes of mentalizing (i.e., the parents' state of mind as expressed in the way they talk and present themselves) above the specific content of what they are talking about. The aim is to help parents to think and speak mindfully again, about themselves as well as their child. How the therapist can go about this will be addressed in the next section ('Intervention pole 1').

Only when mentalizing processes are 'up and running' in parents does it make sense for the therapist to turn to the 'what' (i.e., the content) of what parents bring to the session. Content may be about how their child's trauma dynamics constitute a particular challenge to parental mentalizing, such as something that happened the previous evening that made everyone upset and ended with lots of shouting, leaving the parents to wonder how things could have escalated like they did. Explicitly discussing the vicissitudes of parental mentalizing, including offering psycho-educational information about this topic, can help parents to better understand and more easily recognise what may be happening inside themselves. For example, the therapist may try to pause, notice and name how upset the parents are sounding now, even as they are remembering what happened, empathising with the situation they found themselves in and reminding them how hard it is to think about things when they are still so upset. This can play an important role in preventing mentalizing breakdowns from negatively impacting the daily interactions between parents and child and, hence, parents' sense of well-being as well as their child's developmental trajectory. How the therapist can support parents to think and talk together about their mentalizing in relation to their parenting of their child will be addressed in the third section of this chapter ('Intervention pole 2').

On the other hand, content may also be about the child's way of being, relating and behaving, which parents struggle to make sense of. For example, parents may interpret their child's aggressive outbursts as deliberate aggression or as an inherited trait for violence or their child's need of distancing themselves from them as rejection of their care or even of them. Helping parents to reframe such behaviours as trauma responses – that is, to consider them as a result of traumatising experiences in early childhood – can help them become more curious about and understanding of the child's experience. Again, sometimes, parents need to be offered psycho-educational information about this. When parents become more curious about their child's inner world, avenues are opened to consider more trauma-sensitive and developmentally promoting responses. How the therapist can support parents to keep the particularities of their traumatised child's mind in mind will be addressed in the fourth section ('Intervention pole 3').

As such, this intervention model discerns three types of interventions in the work with parents: helping parents to regain access to their mentalizing abilities; supporting parents to mentalize themselves in parenting a vulnerable child and, finally, helping parents to keep their traumatised child – with their very particular behaviour and needs – in mind. In thinking about how these interventions are related to each other, it seems rather obvious that helping parents to regain access to their mentalizing abilities takes precedence over any intervention focused on content that may be at stake. In other words, there is a certain hierarchy between process (i.e., mentalization-based) interventions, on the one hand and the two types of interventions focused on content, on the other, which possibly work at a different level. However, the label 'level' might suggest a more linear nature to the work with parents of traumatised children than we mean to convey. Similarly, the label 'type' might be mistaken to mean that these interventions can be used completely distinctly from each other. As in all psychological growth processes, the work with parents of traumatised children does not simply progress linearly from being able keep their mentalizing abilities 'online', to understanding their

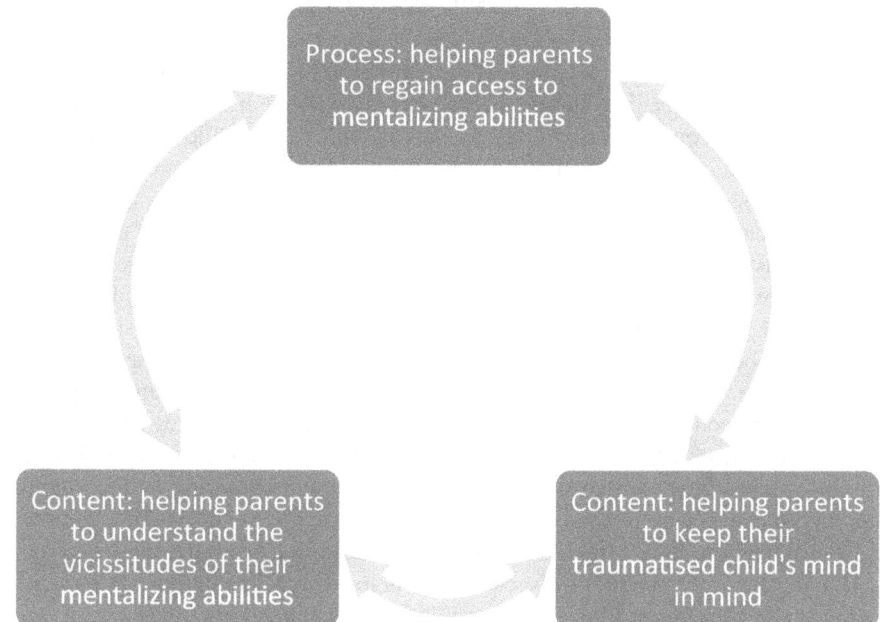

Figure 7.1 Three poles of intervention in mentalization-based and trauma-informed parent work.

own and their child's minds and being able to manage their child's trauma-driven behaviour. In practice, it is a much more iterative and cyclical process, requiring the therapist, for example, to revisit parents' mentalizing abilities when (at risk of) breaking down, or move between talking about mentalizing in parents and focusing on helping parents to reframe their child's behaviour. Therefore, we decided to label the interventions situated at different positions on this cyclical model as three 'poles' of intervention. It is no coincidence that in the depiction of this cyclical model (see Figure 7.1), the intervention pole of helping parents to regain access to their mentalizing abilities is situated at the top. Similarly, the curved double-headed arrows among the three poles of intervention have been chosen deliberately to depict as accurately as possible the therapist's need to continuously and flexibly move back and forth among these poles of intervention, depending on their assessment of what parents are most in need of at any given time within a session.

To aid the therapist in considering which pole needs to be addressed most pressingly, the following sections offer a framework, starting from listening with a sensitive ear to the 'small stories' parents tell to setting in motion the processes needed for opening up parents' minds and supporting them in finding more growth-promoting responses to their child's functioning.

The 'small stories of life': the construction set needed to start 'playing'

In recent years, expert knowledge about complex trauma and its implications for children's development has burgeoned. In working with parents of traumatised children, the temptation to 'simply educate' parents about their child and their child's behaviour from an expert position can be strong, due to the urgency of the family's problems. Yet, merely offering this knowledge from 'top-down', as in separate psycho-educational sessions, seldom leads to the process of change a family needs. Real and sustainable change starts at the heart of a family's experience and dynamics. Therefore, as therapists we attempt to convey a genuine curiosity and interest in parents' day-to-day experiences with their child. We refer to these as 'small stories of life', not because we consider them as unimportant. On the contrary, they constitute the live material we need to talk about in the consultation room, bringing us to the real and concrete yet often unusual, trauma-driven experiences which parents face on a day-to-day basis. Sometimes they have become so used to them that they do not consider them important (enough) to talk about. Marking or highlighting the importance of parents' daily experiences in family life, with special attention to those that seem to have 'stuck' with parents because, for example, they were puzzled by it, they felt 'weird' or disconcerting, helps to validate parents' experiences and provides us with starting points for collaborative reflection.

In being invited to talk about 'small stories', most parents have a lot of daily experiences that come to mind, illustrating what difficulties they face with their child and revealing what parents have on their mind. What parents share about these stories as well as how they do this in particular may provide the therapist indications about the 'status' of their mentalizing abilities. It may, for example, be indicative of an imminent mentalizing breakdown in (one or both of) the parents. As such, it can help the therapist decide how to best meet parents' most pressing needs in terms of mentalizing: help with regaining access to these abilities, with understanding what happens within their own mind when confronted with their child's dynamics or, rather, with keeping their child's particular needs, anxieties and behaviour in mind. Listening to such small stories of life with the three poles of intervention in mind can guide the therapist in considering what is most at the foreground here-and-now and in remaining attentive for shifts from one pole to another during the session requiring the therapist to adapt their interventions accordingly. In the case of Lisa's foster carers (see vignette at the start of the previous section), the therapist – resonating with the overwhelming affective load in the carers' story – first validated their deep feelings of being hurt, embarrassed and angry, naming how hurtful it must have felt to care for a child who is not their own yet as if she was their own child and then being treated as if they are neglectful parents who do not even want to give her good and healthy food. As such, the therapist first uses their mentalizing stance to help the parents regain access to their mentalizing capacities (see also section 'Intervention pole 1').

Later on in the session, once they have had their own experiences validated and experienced a genuine sense of empathy from the therapist, Lisa's foster carers settle a bit and wonder aloud why Lisa does things like this. Now they are no longer stuck in feeling humiliated and angry but are exploring things from a genuinely curious though puzzled perspective. The therapist decides to talk a bit about how these behaviours might be linked to Lisa's early caregiving experiences. She offers this thought in a tentative way, as a possible perspective to think about Lisa's behaviour. In starting to understand how Lisa still expects to be neglected in her basic needs, foster mother asks, 'Does that mean she really believes we don't want to care for her?' And foster father revisits other incidents where Lisa would 'steal' a complete stash of biscuits from the pantry, and eat them in her room, outside of everyone's sight, while 'you know, if she wants to have a biscuit, she knows she can take one from the kitchen cupboard, no one would ever forbid her'.

When parents start wondering about the 'why' of the child's behaviour, like Lisa's foster carers did, mentalizing the child's trauma dynamics can become topic of conversation. The therapist can now bring in thoughts or ideas which the parents are able to consider. In a moment of psycho-education, the therapist discusses Lisa's relational dynamics: her expectation that others won't meet her needs, so if one really needs (sandwiches) or wants something (biscuits), one would better not ask but instead fend for oneself. As such, the therapist focuses on the traumatised child's dynamics, offering help to better understand the child's functioning in order to create a greater sense of empathy in the parents. Once parents can think about their child's behaviour from an empathic position, this can be the basis for parents to find growth-promoting responses to the child's previously 'incomprehensible' behaviour (see also section 'Intervention pole 3').

 Still later on in the session, foster father comes to the conclusion that 'If it's really beyond her control, like that she's projecting "old" expectations onto us but she doesn't realise it, then it actually makes no sense to be angry at her, does it?'. 'But still, it makes me so angry because . . . because I guess, it's hurtful, isn't it: we try so hard, and it seems to no avail?'

Foster father's thoughts and feelings were a good starting point for the therapist to normalise many of the mental states these parents go through in the day-to-day raising of a traumatised child like Lisa. When parents' mentalizing abilities are 'online' but they seem to struggle with making sense of their own feelings or thoughts, the therapist helps parents to understand what is at stake in their inner world and to think and talk together about what they need for a balanced personal and family life (see also section 'Intervention pole 2').

A broaden-and-build cycle in mentalization-based parent work

With the small stories of life functioning as stepping stones and signposts, the parents' therapeutic process can take off. However, contrary to how this process is sometimes thought about (e.g., by some psychotherapy trainees), it is not a swift and linear process from the therapist explaining to parents how they need to treat the child to the parents somehow magically taking these insights home and treating their child differently. In reality, this process resembles much more a broaden-and-build model, as depicted in Figure 7.2, inspired by Lilliengren (2014). This virtuous cycle towards growth of parental mentalizing capacities and positive change in the family starts with listening empathically and mindfully to the family's small stories of life, in which challenging, 'weird' or even disturbing experiences come to the fore. When parents feel heard in the difficulties they face, they start to feel recognised and validated, which can lower their distress and open up their minds

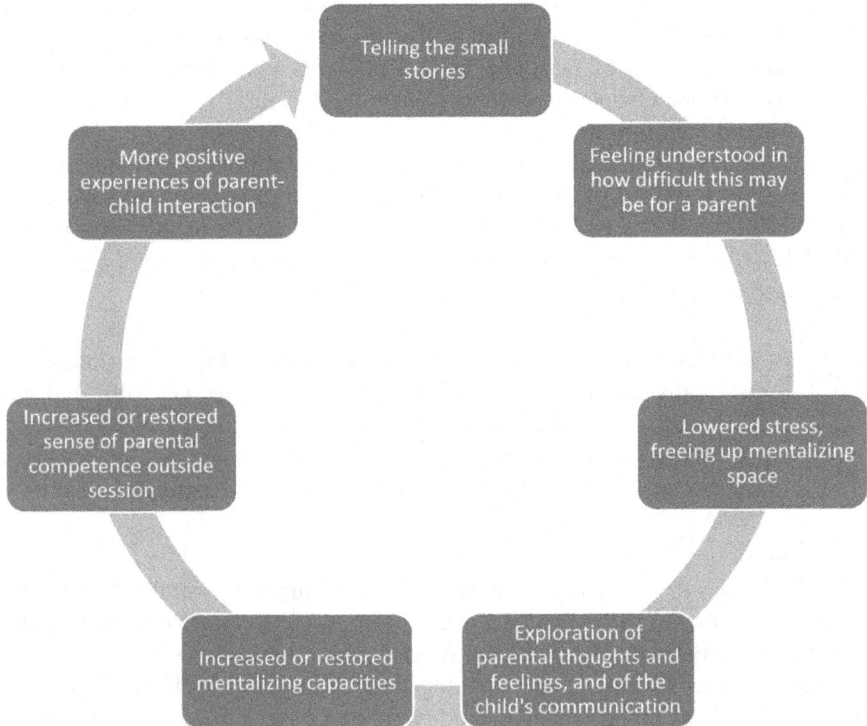

Figure 7.2 A broaden-and-build model of the growth of parental mentalizing capacities and family change.

for further reflection (see also 'epistemic trust'; Fonagy et al., 2019). This forms the basis for further curious exploration of what is happening in their child's inner world, in their own mind as well as in their relationship with the child. It is here that psycho-education may play a role, as illustrated in the case of Lisa's foster carers. As psycho-education is meant to facilitate a new and better understanding of the very particular impact of trauma on the child's development, on the parents' mentalizing abilities and, consequently, on their family life, we aim to provide psycho-educational information in a manner that is directly relevant as well as timely. Provided too soon, psycho-education may close off the processes of thinking and fixate meanings rather than aid in opening up parents' minds in trying to understand what previously had seemed 'incomprehensibly weird or crazy'. As parents' mentalizing capacities grow or restore ('broaden'), they can often find more thoughtful and growth-promoting responses to their child's behaviour and communications ('build'), resulting in increased feelings of being a competent parent as well as more positive family interactions, making family life (more) enjoyable (again).

As the therapist is trying to gain momentum in the parents' therapeutic process, repeatedly going through this broaden-and-build cycle with parents is by no means an even or smooth journey. As we know, in all parents but in parents of traumatised children in particular, mentalizing abilities are often highly transitory across time or situations. A parent may be able to mentalize well when thinking about their child's sadness, for example, but really struggle when their child is angry or aggressive. Moreover, the extent to which the partners within a parental couple are able to keep their mentalizing abilities 'online' may differ substantially at any one moment in time or regarding any one situation. For example, when a mother remains empathic and provides proximity in the face of a child's rule-breaking behaviour, while the father tends to set clear limits, a conversation between them, taking both perspectives into account, can allow for a new shared response to the child's behaviour. Yet, under high pressure, such differences may become more difficult and less negotiable 'breaking points', driving a wedge between parents and leading to a situation in which mother ends up exhausted and burned-out and father reacts increasingly more angrily and even rejectingly to the child. In such circumstances, 'normal differences' can no longer be put to good use as complementary strategies but risk escalating into non-negotiable extreme positions. Such fluctuations within a parent across time and divergences between parents require the therapist to continuously and flexibly adapt their therapeutic response. Sometimes, a small effort may suffice to restore mentalizing, enabling parents to think about their own inner dynamics and/or appropriate ways of managing the child's behaviours and dynamics. At other times, more effort and time will be required to restore parents' mentalizing capacities and/or to address divergent perspectives between parents.

Being mindful of one's own mentalizing processes

As breakdowns in parents' mentalizing abilities are almost inevitable, the therapist is confronted with intense negative feelings about caring for this 'hard-to-care-for' child and/or with parents talking about a child or about responding to the child in a way that seems unmodulated or ill-attuned. This may evoke two kinds of counter-transferential feelings. On the one hand, the therapist may risk over-identifying with the parents' struggles and suffering, thereby one-sidedly colluding with the representation of the child as 'ungrateful', 'bad' or 'mad'. On the other hand, this may lead to feelings of impatience or annoyance towards these 'intolerant' or 'incompetent' parents 'who should just really get their act together'. Both kinds of counter-transferential reactions, however understandable, should alert the therapist that their own mentalizing abilities may be getting strained. Then, the therapist can consider what may be at stake in their own mind and what responses should thus follow. In this context, the parent worker being well-connected (Bevington et al., 2017) to the child therapist and, by extension, to a mentalizing team is a crucial aspect. The child therapist often experiences thoughts and feelings in the direct work with the child that bear similarity to the parents' experiences (e.g., feeling controlled and coerced by the child or inadequate and rejected). Sharing this between the child therapist and the parent worker and thinking together about how such strong feelings in the parent-child relationship may impact upon the parent-parent worker relationship (e.g., the parent projecting their feelings of inadequacy onto the parent worker) may be informative to the work with the parents. It may be helpful in terms of being able to frame one's own counter-transferential feelings and decide from a more mindful perspective how best to respond. By extension, both therapists being able to fall back on a mentalizing team to think and talk together about such issues may aid in getting one's own mentalizing capacities back 'online'. Being able to understand what might have instigated the mentalizing breakdown in oneself in the first place can be helpful, in turn, in understanding the mentalizing breakdown in parents and to support them in responding in a way that is both developmentally appropriate and supportive of the relationship with their child.

Intervention pole 1: helping parents to regain access to mentalizing abilities

As discussed earlier, helping parents to regain access to their mentalizing abilities whenever these have gone 'offline' is paramount. This will be particularly important in the early phase of treatment, when the issue of establishing a firm working alliance with parents requires special attention. Yet, also further along in the work with parents, therapists will be confronted with mentalizing breakdowns, in response to family life experiences that exceed parents' resources. In such circumstances, parent work is more about the process than about content, more 'about the glass than about the wine' as it were.

In the following sections, we discuss therapist interventions (a) to support parents to achieve a safer and growth-promoting relationship with their child and to bring about more positive and pleasurable interactions and (b) to embody ingredients of an inquisitive, 'not-knowing' stance that can help parents to recover their mentalizing capacities (see Table 7.2).

Table 7.2 Core interventions to help parents to regain access to their mentalizing abilities

A continuous focus on facilitating relatedness	• In listening to parents' 'small stories', validate and explore their thoughts and feelings, but refrain from using negative or splitting language • Help parents to manage difficult moments with their child • Help parents to cherish (more) positive moments with their child and to safeguard positive family relationships and interactions
Conveying an inquisitive, 'not-knowing' stance	• Scaffold and mark moments in which parents show curiosity about the child's inner world • Present thinking together as an evident, active way of looking at experiences • Take a position of being 'one expert among others' • Think aloud about what may be at stake in the child's inner world, making use of tentative and playful/metaphoric language

A continuous focus on facilitating relatedness

As soon as parents start sharing the 'small stories' of living with a traumatised child, the parent worker is faced with the challenging task of listening empathically to and managing the parents' suffering while keeping the child as well as the parent-child relationship in mind.

> Whenever Lisa, who just turned ten, is very angry at her foster carers, she goes outside and sits in a chair on the terrace for a long time, even when it gets dark and cold. In doing this, she demonstratively evokes feelings of exclusion in her foster carers and feelings of being neglectful, helpless and incompetent parents. It makes them angry and distant towards her. In talking about this in a parent session, the foster carers first wonder aloud whether they should be stricter and lock the door to let Lisa feel that her behaviour 'is really unacceptable'. 'We already allow and tolerate so much more from Lisa than we would ever from our own children', they comment.

In listening to such stories, it is helpful for the therapist to remind themselves that the extent to which parents of traumatised children have to endure experiences of feeling deeply hurt by the child's behaviour or reactions is often so much larger than what most parents have to go through. Or like in the case of Lisa's foster carers, they have to go through particular experiences which overwhelm them with doubts about their parental competence while previously, in raising their own biological children, they were rather confident and easy-going parents. Or they are concerned about the relationship with their other, 'normally' developing children, wanting them to feel treated equally and fairly but fearing to be blamed for giving the foster child 'preferential' treatment. Of course, when feeling deeply hurt or insecure in one's parental competence, it is extremely difficult to keep a particular child – among the other children – in mind. Such situations thus require the therapist to validate and explore parents' thoughts and feelings, while also being mindful to refrain from using negative or splitting language.

Upon hearing the 'solution' that Lisa's foster carers come up with in the heat of the moment, the parent worker doesn't try to challenge this 'non-mentalizing' response immediately. Instead she responds: 'I can really imagine you feeling shocked and hurt by Lisa's behaviour! We can come back to how we might try to understand what might be underlying her behaviour, but for now, I first want to focus on how you're feeling. It sounds like you're feeling really excluded, and also angry; and maybe also concerned about how taking good care of Lisa could possibly impact the relationship with the older children. Am I right about that? If so, can we talk a bit about that and what you need to feel that you can cope again?' The foster carers start to recognise feelings of being hurt as well as feeling insecure towards their almost grown-up biological children. Being warm and loving parents, they really love to take care of their children, and Lisa's behaviour feels like a rejection of their love and care, and also seems to strain the relationship with their other children.

In offering this kind of empathy and validation, the therapist aims to fully acknowledge parents' experiences and to scaffold their understanding of how an incident impacted them, while at the same time keeping open a future line of meaning-making of the child and their challenging behaviour. As such, the parent worker conveys their efforts to keep both the parents' and the child's mind as well as the parent-child relationship(s) in mind.

In a further step, the therapist will often need to help parents of traumatised children to remain 'good-enough' parents in the face of the potentially overwhelming number of interpersonal misunderstandings and the risk of getting entangled in a vicious cycle of distrust, control and sometimes even violence. Parent work can then focus on how parents can start feeling safe again even in the presence of the child's 'aggressive' outbursts and can feel connected to their child and competent in parenting this child even if the child shows little reciprocity or mutuality.

Talking about their feelings and perspective brings about some relief and enables Lisa's foster carers to gain some distance from and perspective on the situation – their mentalizing comes back 'online'. This creates space for a more empathic stance and a deeper understanding of their angry but vulnerable child. The foster carers become able to explore how Lisa's behaviour might be an expression of her feeling lonely and even abandoned, and her difficulties to accept warmth and love when upset and angry. They decide that being stricter and locking the door won't really address these underlying feelings.

In a following session, foster mother tells about a recent comparable situation, in which she took a warm blanket and left it on the table near Lisa's chair, merely saying 'It's getting colder, I'll leave this here for you, in case you would like to use it'. In doing so, foster mother felt less helpless, more caring and a more competent parent, while at the same time empowered to communicate support and care for Lisa at a level that was bearable and acceptable to her foster daughter. Later on in the session, foster mother talks about how she took home some of the ideas about becoming uncertain towards her older children and how this helped her to open up a conversation with one of them. 'Mia responded in a sensitive way. She said she and her sister had a chat about it, and they sometimes do say to each other "We should never have tried this with Mum and Dad!" But she also added: "We both realise we were never so afraid about where we belong as Lisa can be". What touched me as well was how she said "But honestly, Mum, sometimes we really get annoyed about what Lisa dares to say, you don't deserve to be treated like that!" '

In this context, it is important for the therapist to not only help parents 'survive' the difficult moments with their child but also to help them cherish (more) positive moments with the child as well as to safeguard the other family relationships. In work with parents of traumatised children, these are mostly very challenging tasks that require delicate balancing. Worries, troubles and negative interactions are often predominant in family life with children who have experienced complex trauma. Obviously, the therapist who disavows this by being overly positive is not validating the parents' experiences, as described above. At the same time, bringing positive moments (e.g., sharing pleasure, enjoying being in each other's presence, having a good conversation with a child) back to the centre of experience can function as the highly needed 'antidote' against the burdening difficulties.

Helping parents to cherish positive moments with the vulnerable child may be about scaffolding their reflection about what could be a growth-promoting way of disciplining unwanted child behaviour. Sometimes, parents, when feeling overburdened or out of resources, attempt to structure behaviour by denying the child – and by extension themselves or the whole family – the good things of family life: 'If you don't stop behaving like this, we're not going to the swimming pool tomorrow'. As having fun in the swimming pool can be a good way to have relaxed interactions and repair family relationships, taking away this 'privilege' can add to negative family dynamics. In such situations, it may be worthwhile for the therapist to help parents think about an alternative disciplinary strategy (e.g., doing something for someone, restricting the child's screen time) while also holding on to their initial swimming pool plans, as these can help to break a vicious non-mentalizing cycle ('It was such a difficult week, good that we could also have some fun together').

Helping parents to cherish positive moments may also be about actively searching for and becoming more aware of whatever positive moments child and parents share. Talking about enjoyment and pleasure, about what brings laughter, fun and light in their family, about shared domains of interest, can help parents to more fully experience the good family moments. In Youri's case, these are about playing or listening to music: everyone relaxes, is having fun and feels connected. For Jemal's family, the therapist learns that these are about family vacations and sports activities:

> In parent sessions, it becomes clear that Jemal's adoptive parents struggle with him being hard to reach. But the therapist also learns that when the family is on holiday, Jemal relaxes. Unlike at home, he eats with delight, which helps mother to feel more relaxed, and he is more open and talkative. Although the therapist, much like Jemal's adoptive parents, realises and acknowledges that this way of 'being together' will not endure once home again, the therapist consciously invests time to draw parents' attention to these 'good family times' on holiday, as an anchor for Jemal's adoptive parents to remain positive and hopeful.

Conveying an inquisitive, 'not-knowing' stance

In the face of parents' often intense feelings of helplessness and powerlessness, therapists alike can be drawn into a tendency or 'drive' to act. Although 'immediate action' can sometimes be needed in light of the often intense relational conflicts or crises, the chances of this action being growth-promoting are higher if it goes beyond quick or rash action and it is rooted in a process of thinking together. Therefore, it is of major importance that therapists do not merely succumb to this drive to act but first attempt to actively embody and convey and, as such, model, aspects of a mentalizing mind.

> In the last few sessions with Lisa's foster carers, the therapist can feel their intense concerns about Lisa's recent tendency to 'find' things that don't belong to her: her sister's new t-shirt, a friend's pencil case she likes, even her foster father's mobile phone. They talk about how they've tried to talk to Lisa but to no avail; Lisa's ongoing 'stealing behaviour' is clearly very upsetting to her foster carers. In their minds, it exposes her as a 'thief', raising intense concerns about her future development. 'We've been thinking about taking her to the police station, and making her confess all that she's stolen!' foster father exclaims desperately. Although the therapist can relate to the foster carers' feeling of wanting to 'shock' Lisa into reality, she is also concerned that they may not have thought through the possible judicial consequences of their police station 'action'. Moreover, she's mainly concerned that by not yet understanding fully why Lisa is 'stealing', they may not be taking the most appropriate action.

A most basic way in which the therapist can convey a mentalizing stance is by presenting reflection as an evident, active way of looking at experiences. In the first sessions, when the working alliance still needs to be established, an opening phrase like 'So, what seems important to you to talk or think about together?' may be enough to express a benign and non-judgemental curious stance. Or, when parents seem highly aroused, like Lisa's foster carers in the previous vignette, the therapist might respond: 'I can see that this incident really upset you, would it be alright if we take a moment together to think about what might be happening?' or 'I want to try to fully understand what happened, so maybe later on we can find out together why this happened and what can be done to solve it. Alright if we talk a bit more about what happened exactly?' These kinds of interventions can counterbalance the arousal and the quick-fix attitude parents can be trapped in after a difficult event. Presenting thinking together as an evident first step in managing such events buffers against rash and crisis-like reactions or against a helpless shutting down. Thinking together then can become like the riverbed allowing parents to think about and choose from the stream of parental actions, including appropriate caregiving responses, installing habits and rituals, limit setting.

Presenting these thinking together processes as evident may not always be straightforward in and of itself and may be challenging in working with parents of traumatised children. As discussed, such parents have often tried everything they could before turning to external help. This may lead to the ambiguous situation of expecting better – more professional – solutions from an expert, while at the same time being worried about getting labelled as incompetent parents. Therefore, in parent work, we attempt to find a position that reassures parents that help will be offered in a way that recognises their competences and 'knowledge'. Sometimes, the 'not-knowing stance' (Bateman & Fonagy, 2019) is misunderstood as 'you only listen and don't know anything'. In reality, its essence may be captured more correctly as 'not taking a knowing stance': the therapist is not the one who 'knows everything' but integrates their knowledge about child development, trauma and parenthood as one perspective that is additional and of complementary value to the parental perspective. This attitude – taking a position of being 'one expert among others' – may be phrased, for instance, as

> You are the experts about your child and about your family, I have some expertise in exploring routes and about how (traumatised) children develop, so if we work together, we've got a better chance of coming up with some good ideas/solutions.

The parent worker may share ideas – but they are just that, ideas – so that they can be explored, investigated and seen as the expressions of the processes of one mind working hard to try and make sense of other peoples' minds. In this sense, the therapist is less like the tour guide holding the umbrella showing parents the way, having answers and providing advice but more like a member of a quiz team, whose areas of expertise can hopefully complement that of their team members trying to solve a puzzle together.

This also means that there is always a quality of 'thoughtful uncertainty' to the ideas or understandings that the therapist offers to parents: the therapist shares something with parents which they – based on their knowledge and expertise – think might be relevant and useful but remains open to think together. One way of conveying this 'thoughtfully uncertain' stance is by announcing one's thoughts or ideas as 'thinking aloud': 'I'm just thinking aloud now, so be sure to let me know what you think, okay, but might it be the case that. . . ?' Thinking aloud thus implies offering thoughts about the child and their behaviour, reflecting on possible meanings of behaviour; showing possibilities, making 'mistakes' and taking them back. In this sense, thinking aloud is 'nomadic' thinking (Olthof, 2017): 'essentially an invitation to allow our thought processes to leave the citadel of fixed knowledge and to abandon fixed meanings as far as is possible, creating a free space for' imagination and alternative meanings. 'Instead of reducing reality to the One, reality is made present in its diversity, multiplicity and difference'. Nomadic thinking is an 'as if' mode of thinking, which makes imagination possible and wanders in search of affective wisdom. It needs language that aims to sow and hence is probabilistic rather than aiming to convey expert knowledge. Therefore, the therapist will often make use of conditional, hypothetical, as well as playful or metaphoric language.

After listening to and helping to tease out the feelings and thoughts of Lisa's foster carers about Lisa's 'stealing behaviour', the therapist responds: 'I can really imagine you being worried about Lisa turning to behaviour that could get her into much trouble with the law! I also hear you saying that when you talk to her, she seems to be genuinely remorseful and promising not to take things again which don't belong to her. So, taken together, I wonder whether it might be that, when confronted with an object of desire, the urge to "just take it" in Lisa is too much for her to be able to control?' Lisa's foster carers, having settled a bit, seem to be able to open their mind to the idea offered by the therapist but are, of course, still wondering aloud whether they can 'just let it pass'. Together with the therapist, they can think about alternative responses, less 'extreme' than 'the police station action' or 'just let it pass', that could be more appropriate. Eventually, they reach consensus that they will go with Lisa to return the belonging to its rightful owner so that she will be confronted with the consequences of her actions and will have to make amends.

In sum, conveying a 'not-knowing' stance is less about expressing a fixed idea or interpretation about certain behaviour but rather about modelling an ability to consider a range of possibilities, to change one's mind and to bear remaining uncertain but maybe close to a possible answer.

Intervention pole 2: helping parents to understand the vicissitudes of their mentalizing abilities

As their mentalizing abilities get back 'online', parents of traumatised children can benefit from the therapist's help to understand why and what is happening when their mentalizing capabilities are challenged so heavily in the relationship with the child. This can be helpful to feel more prepared for new difficulties to arise, to try to avoid getting entangled in vicious cycles of negative interaction over and over again and to remain compassionate towards oneself in recovering and repairing relationships when breakdowns do occur. When parents start wondering how come they're losing their patience in relationship to this child while never having experienced this to this extent before with an older sibling or other child, parent work can focus on the content of parents' own mentalizing processes. The therapist will need to support parents to accept, recognise as well as manage the inevitable and frequent mentalizing breakdowns that (will) occur in raising a child who has experienced complex trauma, paying particular attention to situations in which parents' own vulnerabilities get triggered and circumstances that require a diversity-sensitive approach (see Table 7.3).

Acceptance starts with normalising parents' reactions to 'abnormal' circumstances

Work with parents at this pole of intervention often starts with normalising parents' experiences and reactions whatever form they take. Whether it is anger, rage,

Table 7.3 Core interventions to help parents to understand the vicissitudes of their mentalizing abilities

Help parents accept and recognise mentalizing breakdowns	• Normalise parents' experiences and reactions • Provide psycho-education as appropriate • Pay specific attention to 'pseudo-mentalizing', i.e., cognitive 'understanding' that is not rooted in affectively felt experience
Scaffold parents' ability to manage mentalizing breakdowns	• Emphasise the importance of self-care (including care for themselves as a parental couple), and actively explore what self-care may look like for this/these parent(s) • Normalise parents' feelings of guilt for self-care • Promote a genuinely hopeful perspective
Pay specific attention when parents 'get hit where it hurts'	• Help parents disentangle current relationship dynamics and issues from unresolved relationship dynamics and events in their own history • Work towards a referral for individual psychotherapy if appropriate
Actively scaffold mentalizing about diversity	• Actively engage parents in thinking and talking together about possible experiences the child may encounter related to differences in (sub-)culture, including those stemming from being an adopted/a fostered child

bitterness or even cynicism or rejection of the child (in its extreme, increasing the risk of placement breakdown), parents often feel surprised and even ashamed and guilt-ridden by such feelings, like Lisa's foster carers did about their 'harsh' reaction of wanting to lock Lisa out or 'shock' her into reality, after the therapist helped them to settle a bit. Or Jemal's adoptive father who embarrassedly talks about a phantasy he had about their family visiting Ethiopia (Jemal's birth country) and them losing Jemal there.

Repeatedly being confronted with one's own mentalizing breakdowns mostly elicits two kinds of affective reactions in parents. On the one hand, parents may experience profound guilt for not being able to remain a 'good-enough' parent, who is able to 'keep their cool'. On the other hand, parents may also start thinking about their child as the source of all things bad in the family. Although such affective reactions are natural and understandable, they are often not helpful and even counter-productive for parents and the parent-child relationship. A therapist normalising such experiences and feelings can be the first step towards containing and meanwhile countering these non-helpful thoughts and feelings.

Psycho-education about 'what happens in a brain under pressure' can play a role here. Providing relevant images and metaphors for mentalizing processes and breakdowns, for example, the pebble-in-the-pond metaphor (Vliegen et al., 2023), can help parents to find a new and more benevolent 'language' to think about their own experiences in relation to the trauma dynamics brought into the family. As such, the therapist can help parents to better understand and reframe experiences of finding oneself low on energy and internal resources – energy and resources that are so direly needed in parenting a traumatised child. Similarly, the therapist can help parents to better understand and reframe experiences of feeling overwhelmed by strong negative feelings, which no parent might have expected and any parent would prefer to avoid. In foster carers specifically, and even in some adoptive parents, it is not exceptional that the thought of 'we can always send him/her back' crosses their mind in a desperate attempt to 'rid' oneself of overwhelmingly difficult feelings elicited in the interactions with the child – a thought that in turn often evokes equally difficult-to-bear feelings of shame. Finally, the therapist can also help to better understand and reframe parents' experiences of loss and mourning in coming to terms with the fact that good-enough parenting on their part is indeed enough, while even 'ideal parenting' will not resolve all child problems and family life issues.

Mentalizing involves cognitive as well as affective processes

When Mei-Lan, who has previously been 'unable to play' in therapy, starts to enjoy being creative with all kinds of materials, the therapists and adoptive parents are happy to see how she is finding ways to express herself and see this as a major step forward. But this step forward also confronts them with new challenges as Mei-Lan starts to express difficult elements of her traumatised mind. In a parent session, Mei-Lan's adoptive parents talk about how happy they are about her newly discovered creativity: last Wednesday, Mei-Lan was busy with string and nails in her room the whole afternoon. She seemed intensely focused, so parents gave her space to do what she was doing. When she finished her 'craftwork', Mei-Lan was eager to show it to her adoptive parents. Acting as if she was opening an exhibition, she opened the door of her room making theatrical noises, revealing how she had turned her bed into a coffin and used a whole ball of string to craft spiderwebs all around her bed. Her adoptive parents simply praised her for her creativity – at that moment unable to really respond to the more complex feelings this exhibition had evoked.

When a child is taking developmental steps forward, like Mei-Lan in becoming able to 'play', the relief and joy or excitement that parents feel – and that we as therapists often share – may make it difficult to remain open-minded towards troubling aspects expressed in the child's play content. In this context, it is important for the therapist to be mindful of how cognitive understanding needs to be rooted in affectively felt experiences. Genuine mentalizing connects and balances cognitive and affective aspects of experiences, while cognitive 'understanding' devoid of the normally accompanying emotions heightens the risk of pseudo-mentalizing. Pseudo-mentalizing happens when cognitive and explicit mentalizing dominates without being rooted in the felt experience and in intuitive processes (Fonagy & Luyten, 2009). For example, when Mei-Lan's adoptive parents talked to their parent worker about how 'creative' they thought she was when she turned her bed into a coffin and used string to craft spiderwebs all around her bed, they seemed oblivious to the horrible and disturbed nature of their adoptive daughter's 'creation'. Such signs of pseudo-mentalizing – often activated to protect parents against becoming aware of the disturbing meaning of the content – will need to be addressed mindfully by the therapist.

 The therapist working with Mei-Lan's adoptive parents responded by first explicitly validating the relief and happiness they all felt about Mei-Lan starting to engage in play and creativity, as well as the importance of her being able to find images for inner experiences. Following that, she invited the adoptive parents to share what they felt at seeing the content of what Mei-Lan had created 'which seems to have a darker side to it too'. Mother replies: 'Now that you mention it, it did seem a bit . . . odd, you know, the coffin and all of the webs . . . I remember a chill ran down my spine when she opened the door, but she looked so happy and proud'. The conversation turns to what Mother's 'odd' feeling and chill may mean.

Cognitive-affective understanding of why and how mentalizing processes break down can help parents to recognise such breakdowns more easily and thus increase their chances of being able to keep their mentalizing 'online' and draw on these in the interactions with their child (Adkins et al., 2021).

Scaffolding parents' ability to manage mentalizing breakdowns

As well as helping to accept and recognise mentalizing breakdowns, the therapist will also need to scaffold parents' abilities to manage such breakdowns in constructive ways. Prior to any thinking together about 'parenting strategies', this will require the therapist to pay specific attention to certain issues of concern in work with parents of traumatised children. First, in their attempts to stay in touch with their child's inner world, parents may risk losing sight of personal needs and longings. Choosing to do something for themselves, like doing sports in the evening or having dinner with friends, may become burdened with feelings of inadequacy, bad parenting and guilt. As Mei-Lan's adoptive mother expressed: 'I can't go to the movies with a friend in the evening, because Mei-Lan gets completely overwhelmed. As if what is good for me, is neglectful or harmful to her!' Such – understandable though unhelpful – images will need to be addressed by the therapist. Again, after normalising the parent's experience, some psycho-educational information about the pre-condition of self-care (including care for the parental couple) for good-enough parenting may be helpful. For example, the idea that a parent needs to put on one's own oxygen mask prior to being in the position to help one's child, as captured in the image of emergency aeroplane instructions, is a metaphor that most parents can easily understand. In a further step, the therapist can invite parents to explore what such self-care could entail for them personally. For example: 'We've talked about how caring for [this child] is taking a lot of your energy, s/he needs so much care! And at the same time, it's so important that you take care of yourselves first. I was wondering whether we could think together as to what you need as parents to restore some of your energy'. Some parents will require multiple such efforts from the therapist 'authorising' them to explicitly take time for individual and couple activities, away from the needs of their child, which can be experienced as all-consuming. This may include exploring with parents how the caregiving network around their child and family could be enlarged and mobilised.

A second specific issue of therapeutic concern relates to the delicate 'balancing exercise' of engendering a genuinely hopeful perspective whilst also recognising and accepting the real damage that traumatic experiences may have caused. In raising a child who has experienced complex trauma, there are the unmistakable feelings of loss and even despair, that 'more' cannot be achieved in helping their child benefit from good-enough care, on the one hand. There are also the feelings of hope, as parents are supported to also see the small but important positive aspects and progress in the development of their child. In working with parents who are almost continually torn between these seemingly opposing kinds of feelings, it is a challenging though important task to create and maintain a hopeful perspective without being unrealistically positive or avoidant. Generally, this comes down to reassuring parents that adequate help will be offered and will continue to be offered in the face of the pervasiveness of the child's problems. The therapist might, for example, say: 'A lot of parents caring for children like yours struggle with intensely angry or sad moments like you are going through. That's one of the reasons why we are here together, and we will work together on that'. Or: 'we will work hard together to find better ways to handle such difficult moments. We can't predict what the future holds precisely. But we will keep thinking together about how to best support your child's development'. As touched upon earlier, helping to observe small steps forward is another important therapeutic intervention. In this regard, the therapist may invite parents to consider some ideas that may be helpful to keep in mind a perspective on developmental growth. Growth and development take time, and not all problems with the child can be resolved at once. The idea that one may 'choose one's battles' and focus on one developmental domain while tolerating difficulties in other domains may free parents from feeling responsible every second for every single problem that occurs. Moreover, parents often require help to bear that one often cannot solve a problem with one single intervention but that the child will need to 'practise' new behaviours on numerous occasions. A therapist mindfully and timely reminding parents of these ideas can support a realistically hopeful perspective in parents.

When parents 'get hit where it hurts'

The therapist needs to be especially attentive in working with parents whose own vulnerable spots are triggered in interactions with the child. Some child dynamics and issues may trigger and re-activate 'old sores' from a parent's own history without them initially being able to differentiate their child's trajectory from their own.

 For Mei-Lan's adoptive mother, for example, it took a while before she could feel more compassionate towards her adoptive daughter's academic 'underperformance' and align her expectations with regard to school results more to Mei-Lan's vulnerabilities (see Chapter 3). In thinking with the therapist about what made this topic especially arousal-provoking for her, it occurred to mother that her own parents always considered school performances to be extremely important and that, perhaps, she had internalised these high standards. She was, after all, a high-performing student and now is a high-achieving professional.

The work with Lisa's foster carers has been conducted in a very open atmosphere from the start, with the foster carers openly sharing their thoughts and feelings about their difficulties in caring for Lisa and being open to whatever thoughts the therapist has to offer. When Lisa's needs seem to exceed what the foster carers are able to offer, and a network partner suggests to think about sharing the care for Lisa more in terms of semi-residential care for children with special needs, the therapist is somewhat taken aback by foster father's adamant reaction that 'that is out of question and closed for discussion'. In a subsequent session with the foster carers, the therapist returns to this topic by enquiring about foster father's perspective. She learns of his negative childhood experiences with being sent to boarding school. In validating these experiences as the background of foster father's perspective on semi-residential care for his foster daughter as 'unimaginable', the therapist succeeds in opening up some thinking about 'whether shared care will necessarily mean the same to Lisa' as boarding school did to him.

Relational discontinuities or other difficult experiences in one's own personal history can be triggered, interfering with a compassionate and mentalizing attitude towards particular experiences with their child in the present. For example, when a parent lost their own parent and seems barely able to tolerate the child being angry at them: 'He should be happy to have two parents to care for him!'

With regard to being a foster carer or adoptive parent in particular, specific vulnerabilities can also be triggered. For example, there can be the sadness or feelings of mourning inherent to fertility issues ('What if we could have had a child of our own? Life might have been easier then?') or the uncertainty due to not knowing (part of) the child's (genetic) history when facing illness or vulnerability ('If only we knew more about a possible genetic load that could explain these (medical) problems, we could have helped in a better way!').

In all of the cases and situations described earlier, the parent needs some help from the therapist to disentangle current relationship dynamics and issues from relationship dynamics and events in the past which have not been fully resolved, in order to help them to respond in a mentalizing way to current events.

At its most extreme, 'getting hit where it hurts' may happen when a parent's vulnerabilities and issues have remained unresolved to the extent that individual psychotherapy seems warranted to prevent these from (further) compromising their own development as a person and as a parent as well as their child's development. Then, the therapist needs to invest in working with the parent towards a referral for individual psychotherapy.

Actively scaffolding mentalizing about diversity

A particularly delicate though important theme in families with an interracially adopted child – often Caucasian parents adopting a child 'of colour' – is that of cultural diversity in general and racism in particular. In these families, the noticeable difference in skin colour between parents and child often compounds the ambivalent feelings that already exist about (not) belonging together, about (not) being a 'real' family. Adoptive parents are often highly sensitive to their child not being treated differently 'just' because they are adopted, on the one hand, whilst at the same time, wanting others to take into account that their child's being adopted may mean that they have (partially) other needs and thus that others approach their family in an 'adoption-sensitive' way. A difference in skin colour between parents and child makes it so undeniable that the child did not (biologically) start their life with these parents. Often, this may make adoptive parents (and the child themselves) highly sensitive towards indications that others do not consider them a 'real' family. In facing experiences of their skin colour being subject to remarks ranging from teasing to bullying among children as well as in interactions with adults – which in reality happens commonly – the adoptive parents may often not be aware of the child's experiences. For example, when asked about their child's possible experiences with racist remarks, parents sometimes respond that they don't know for sure though they 'guess not because s/he has never told us anything like that'. Sometimes the latter is true, in that children may hesitate to share their encounters with racism or may minimise the incident and/or its impact to protect the parents. There may also be a difficulty for adoptive parents themselves to dare to imagine and thus acknowledge that their child 'of colour' is being teased or bullied *because* of their skin colour. It is important for the therapist not to collude in avoiding this topic but instead to actively engage adoptive parents in thinking and talking about their child possibly being subjected to racist remarks or incidents. Talking about this sensitive topic openly and compassionately helps to contain parents' feelings of being shocked or appalled, which in turn helps them to be open and compassionate towards the child when faced with racism.

 Mei-Lan comes home upset about a children's song she learnt at school about an 'old Chinese man' who ended up in jail. Her adoptive mother first listens to her experience, trying to understand 'from the inside-out' what was so upsetting to Mei-Lan. She then discusses the incident with the parent worker and they decide it might be a good idea to contact the teacher. Mei-Lan's teacher is authentically surprised but also feels embarrassed. She decides together with Mei-Lan's adoptive mother that she will use this opportunity to hold a class discussion about 'being different and being sensitive to differences'. She also removes the song from her repertoire.

A difference in skin colour between adoptive parents and child is, of course, a very noticeable aspect of diversity. Yet, the importance of a diversity-sensitive approach actually holds true also for less visible aspects in which people may differ, or at least feel different, from one another. With regard to raising a child who has experienced complex trauma, this in fact refers to any and all, visible but also less visible, (developmental) impairments that the child may have sustained because of their history of early adverse experiences, such as unpredictably 'underperforming'

at school due to a hypersensitive stress system. Often, adoptive parents or foster carers of traumatised children are not aware of the profoundly detrimental impact that 'feeling different' may have on their child's developing sense of self. It is then part of the therapist's task to also actively scaffold parents' mentalizing about topics and circumstances that require a diversity-sensitive approach.

Intervention pole 3: helping parents to keep their traumatised child's mind in mind

When parents feel safe and secure enough to have access to their mentalizing abilities and show an interest in trying to understand what may be underlying their child's seemingly 'incomprehensible' and 'intractable' behaviour, the therapist can focus on helping parents to take on a (more) trauma-informed and developmental perspective. This third pole of intervention in parent work is equally crucial because the experience of understanding and feeling understood is an essential part of genuine connection and intimacy: 'how we interpret why people are behaving in the way they do, has a huge impact on the way we think and behave' (Midgley et al., 2017a, p. 18). This part of the work is about supporting parents to genuinely understand their child's behaviour 'from the inside-out' (e.g., a child getting into a fight because he genuinely felt threatened or a child 'lying' about not being cared for because she truly felt abandoned and neglected). This may make it easier to not only manage the child's behaviour in a more mindful and growth-promoting way based on that understanding but, ultimately, to more easily accept and love the child despite all the difficulties they bring about. It may help to learn about the peculiarities of raising a child with very specific developmental needs and, as such, to experience oneself as a competent parent able to help and support one's child. From the child's perspective, experiencing one's parents' efforts to understand who one is and where one 'is coming from' may make it easier to feel addressed as a worthwhile person who deserves to be understood and supported, although with children who have experienced complex trauma, this may prove to be a long and winding road.

In the following sections, we first elaborate on the specific challenges parents of traumatised children face to keep mentalizing the child. Next, we discuss how we support parents to explore, starting from the 'small stories', what it is exactly that we're trying to make sense of. Finally, we outline how parents can be supported to mentalize the child's behaviour from a more trauma-informed and developmental perspective, using the four developmental domains as lenses.

Challenges to parents' ability to keep their child's mind in mind

The work with parents at this intervention pole is, although crucial, also fraught with challenges. Thinking about aspects of the child's inner world underlying their behaviour inevitably confronts parents with deeper layers of having to accept their child's functioning and development. First, being willing to keep searching for what a child's behaviour may mean implies staying in touch with the often 'weird' and distorted inner world of a traumatised child. This is the case when parents are confronted with their child's phantasies about small animals being left all alone in the desert or about lying in a coffin covered by spider webs, as in Mei-Lan's case (see earlier vignette). Or when a child – once again – runs away from home because they feel they 'don't belong there anyway'. As therapists working with the parents of such children and used to intensely difficult feelings and disturbed inner worlds, we sometimes forget how difficult, disturbing and even traumatising this can be for parents.

Moreover, it confronts parents time and again with the child's – often pervasive and sometimes even lifelong – developmental impairments, which often seem so removed from what typical development looks like. Coming to terms with this, then, means accepting one's child's development is – and often will remain – so fundamentally different from typical development. And it is the realisation of this thought that is sometimes warded off so forcefully in parents that it inhibits them from accessing the ability to keep their child's mind in mind, as expressed, for example, in avoidance, denial or 'resistance' to the work done in parent sessions.

Therefore, the therapist needs to firmly keep in mind that parents' ability to keep their child's mind in mind is hardly ever a static, accomplished 'position' in parents. Rather, helping parents to access that ability is to be considered a process in motion. For example, we might be working with a parent who just seems to want to stop or eradicate the child's disturbing behaviour as soon as possible or, by contrast, a parent who seems to consider the child's disturbing behaviour as an inevitable part of the child with no need to be understood or addressed. Or, we may notice that parents who have learnt to co-regulate their child when the child is intensely upset become paralysed at the realisation that their child has stolen money from their wallet. But hopefully, the work with parents will also be characterised by moments in which parents allow the therapist to help them 'mentalize their child'.

When parents can experience the time and space and the relationship, offered to them in parent work, as an opportunity to safely think and speak about how best to solve the problems they face with their child, parent work has taken off. Quality time in the parent-child relationship has been said to be best considered as 'problem-solving time' (Fonagy, 2016, November 19), affording the child the opportunity to rely on the parent to help solve problems which they are struggling to solve by themselves. Similarly, enabling parents to benefit from the mentalizing mind and frame offered to them by the therapist in thinking together about what that problem-solving could look like is at the core of the work with parents of traumatised children.

Exploring with parents the 'what' which we're trying to make sense of

So, what is it that parents are trying to solve or at least make sense of? Work with parents at this pole of intervention therefore starts – again – with the therapist listening to the 'small stories' but this time particularly with the developing child in mind. After all, a developmentally informed mentalizing response to child behaviour can only originate from attempting to essentially answer three questions (Oestergaard

Hagelquist, 2018): (a) *why* is the child expressing this kind of behaviour here-and-now? (E.g., why does Lisa keep 'stealing' things that don't belong to her? See vignette in section 'Intervention pole 1'), (b) *what* does the child need to learn? (E.g., Lisa needs to learn to control her impulses when confronted with an object of desire and to first think about the consequences of taking it for herself as well as for her relationships with others), and (c) *how* then can the caregiver best support that? (E.g., how can the foster carers respond in a way that both conveys that taking something that doesn't belong to you is not okay but that also acknowledges Lisa's profound difficulty to refrain from just taking what she needs or wants?)

Trying to answer these three questions starts with a thorough understanding of what precisely transpired. Exploring with parents the 'small story' they shared about their child's difficult-to-understand behaviour or functioning can be done by questions such as 'What exactly happened?', 'What in the child's behaviour or functioning is concerning you?' (E.g., being unpredictable in school achievement) or 'Do you think that the worrisome behaviour is already part of a pattern of behaving?' (E.g., always being demanding when mother is close by.) These and similar questions can help to open up parents' mentalizing of their child.

Supporting parents to find developmentally informed mentalizing responses

After having gained sight on what actually transpired which made things difficult for the child (and for the parents), the therapist may open up joint reflection and discussion about possible answers to the 'why' question, that is, possible meanings underlying the behaviour. For example, the therapist may say: 'Hearing you tell this story about [your child], I'm wondering what would make him/her act/react the way s/he did – what are your thoughts on that?' Such interventions are meant to explicitly invite parents to share their 'knowledge' and thoughts about their child's behaviour as well as to think further together about the meaning of the child's behaviour and perhaps even ways of managing it (that is, trying to answer the 'what to learn' and 'how to support' questions).

Exploring different perspectives can go hand in hand with offering psycho-education about particular aspects or domains of development as these are impacted by complex traumatic experiences. The therapist sharing, in a tentative way, some of their developmental and trauma-informed knowledge to help understand what seemed 'weird' (e.g., a child telling an untrue story about receiving bad food) or what evoked otherwise difficult thoughts and feelings, can help parents to open up their minds again (see later for examples of what psycho-educational interventions may look like).

In attempting to understand the dynamics underlying the child's behaviour or functioning, the four developmental domains (i.e., representational, affect regulation and relational capacities and sense of self and identity) can function as signposts. Similar to the child therapist listening to and observing the child from these four perspectives and tailoring their interventions accordingly in the direct work with the child (see Chapter 6), the therapist in the work with the parents listens with a sensitive ear to indications that one or several of these domains are currently most at stake. In the following boxes, we offer suggestions about aspects in each of the four developmental domains that may become salient at some point in the 'small stories' of traumatised children's parents and which the therapist thus can listen for and address in ways to support parents to respond in growth-promoting ways. For each of these domains, we also present a case vignette to illustrate what the work with parents at this intervention pole may look like in practice.

Themes in helping parents mentalize their child's representational capacities

- How to understand the child's strengths and difficulties with regard to representing aspects of experiences and of an inner world
- How to scaffold the child's ways of expressing themselves in relaxed and small day-to-day moments
- How to help the child express themselves in moments when emotions run higher
- How to respond when confronted with trauma-related content in their child's stories or play

---

Youri's foster carers talk about him being closed-off, unwilling to engage in a conversation. Recently, he had to wait for his siblings in the cafeteria of the sports centre, together with his foster father, and the situation felt awkward. 'Being alone with him, and having time for a father-son chat, you look for something to talk about but without any result. Every attempt to start a conversation felt more like an interrogation of an unwilling interviewee', foster father says thinking back on the situation. 'We can't seem to find something to talk about'. The therapist wonders about Youri's abilities to represent what is absent as she wasn't sure about Youri being unwilling to have a real conversation with his foster father. She decides to raise this question with the foster carers: 'In listening to your story, I was wondering what might be behind Youri's not engaging in a conversation. Do you think he really doesn't want to talk with you, or might it be that he finds it difficult to talk about something he's not in the middle of?' Foster mother, intrigued by the therapist's question, responds that they have noticed that Youri can only talk about school when the event is sufficiently present in his experience. 'Oh yes, like yesterday, when we asked how the birdbox which they are working on in class is progressing', foster father adds. 'Then, you see his eyes light up, and he starts talking about how they finished the carpentry today, and that next week they may choose a colour to paint it. . . . But he would never talk about that spontaneously'. The conversation continues with the foster carers talking about how they've come to think about Youri as being closed-off, preferring to keep things to himself. They never realised that he might find it difficult to talk about things that feel further off for him. This deeper understanding (why) brings about new questions, with foster mother wondering aloud: 'so, how can we help him, because we don't always know something about his day at school?' The therapist, aware of the nearing end of the session, responds: 'That seems like a really important question, let's return to that next time we meet, okay?'

At the start of the next session, foster mother proudly tells: 'Youri was drawing and colouring before we had to leave to the sports centre, and I suggested him to bring along his sketchbook and his colouring pencils. Turns out that was really helpful! He was drawing sports cars, and I started to ask him about cars. He almost became talkative! I didn't know he was so interested in cars and motor cycles! He teased me when I couldn't answer his questions about our own car!' 'You felt really good, and so did he', foster father adds. 'We were thinking about taking along a sketchbook and pencils at occasions like this'.

So, although the initial parent meeting ended without having found a definite answer to the foster carers' struggle in having a real conversation with Youri, the therapist's opening up genuine curiosity in them, making use of minimal trauma-informed knowledge about representational skills, scaffolded more openness and awareness about Youri's potential developmental vulnerability in this domain. Furthermore, it also helped them to find, within themselves, a more creative – and as it turns out, a 'successful' – answer to a difficulty in the relationship to their foster son.

The question 'How can we help our child to have new experiences or to develop new skills or ideas?' can emerge in a parent's mind, as was the case in Youri's foster carers or can be suggested by the therapist: 'So, if we think [your child] acted like s/he did because s/he was feeling . . . could we think a bit further together about what might be helpful to him/her?'

Themes in helping parents mentalize their child's regulation capacities

- How to understand issues of discomfort, pain and anxiety in daily situations and how these influence family life
- How to scaffold language for emotions in daily conversations and interactions with the child
- How to recognise and manage behavioural dysregulation in the child (including trauma-related dysregulations such as trauma triggers and fight, flight and freeze mechanisms)

Mei-Lan's adoptive parents talk about her severe separation anxiety taxing their own resources, with mother on the brink of parental burn-out and father increasingly frustrated by the lack of quality time as a couple. The therapist, sensing both parents' increasingly negative arousal around Mei-Lan's 'clinginess', first created enough room in her work with the parents to validate how heavy the burden of raising their adoptive daughter felt. As this helped the negative arousal in parents to lessen a bit, the therapist could then wonder aloud how it might be that going to sleep still elicited such strong feelings in Mei-Lan that going to bed still remains such a dysregulating event every single evening. The adoptive parents respond: 'It seems as if she just cannot trust that when she closes her eyes to go to sleep, that we and the world as she knows it will not have disappeared by the time she wakes up again!' The conversation turns to how this may have become an almost built-in survival mechanism stemming from difficult experiences of having been abandoned in Mei-Lan's early life. As Mei-Lan's adoptive parents can be helped to reframe this behaviour as less meant by Mei-Lan to intentionally 'keep mother away from the other family members' but more as a genuine fear of loss and abandonment from deep within, space opens up to think together about how Mei-Lan could be helped to go to sleep more at ease. In these conversations, the idea of putting a family picture at her bedside emerges, so that from the moment she wakes up she can be helped to feel reassured that her family and the world has not disappeared. This helped Mei-Lan to open up around the theme of her separation anxiety, as became clear in a series of treatment sessions in this period: she started playing about a baby who cried and cried and didn't know how to stop crying as he didn't know where his mum was.

Themes in helping parents mentalize their child's relational capacities

- Naming and talking with parents about positive moments of interaction
- How to create small moments of warm interaction in everyday activity (meals, bedtime) and to recognise what interactions are growth-promoting (e.g., with regard to distance, bodily contact activity)
- How to meet a child's needs for nurturance, even if these seem regressive or age-inappropriate, for example, helping the child to survive moments of separation
- How to differentiate between emotional versus actual truth when 'old' relational representations influence current relationships ('the witching hour' directing the child's functioning or behaviour)

The previous vignette about Mei-Lan shows how themes from several domains can be intertwined and how one theme can move on to the other. Once Mei Lan's adoptive parents can see the dysregulated behaviour she shows evening after evening as rooted in deep anxieties about being left behind, they can open up their minds and start to think about her relational needs. They can start to reflect on her needs for having her adoptive parents close to her, better tolerate her clinginess and find ways to remind her that they are there for her (e.g., by putting a family picture at her bedside), whilst continue thinking about their own needs and longings. Another example of this has been described earlier in this chapter, about Lisa literally distancing herself from her foster carers (by staying outside) in an 'angry fit', making them feel so excluded that they would consider to really lock her out of the house. It is through acknowledging the foster carers' hurt feelings and exploring the possible trauma-driven dynamics underlying Lisa's 'rejecting' behaviour that the foster carers' could be helped to find a more developmentally and relationship-fostering response (foster mother coming up with the idea to offer Lisa a warm blanket).

Themes in helping parents mentalize their child's sense of self and identity

- How to recognise, cherish and scaffold vital sparks when they occur, as well as to recognise a numb/devitalised state of mind and to help their child out of this state
- How to find strategies that scaffold a child's self-awareness (e.g., recognising bodily experiences or finding words that adequately capture the child's sensations and feelings)
- How to be sensitive to issues with regard to a sense of self and identity (e.g., in the domain of hobbies and interests) as well as with regard to the child's history (e.g., early life experiences, being fostered or adopted, aspects of diversity such as skin colour) when particular occasions arise
- Coming to terms with being parents of a child 'of many parents' and to help their child with their issues (including recognising and containing the child's feelings of loss and mourning and understanding and managing the dynamics of phantasies and cover stories)

Youri's foster mother tells about a moment at the kitchen table: she was cutting vegetables, with Youri next to her drawing quietly and concentrated. He made a drawing of the place where the family lives: he drew the houses surrounding the market place. 'This looks like the market place?', foster mother asked to invite Youri to talk a bit. Youri responded: 'Yes, this is our house, and this one is Tina's and Neil's (neighbours). And in the middle of the market place a rotten egg was dropped and all the people in the houses around the market place became ill of the smell of the egg!' Youri's foster mother, who is rather sensitive to her foster son's expressions, realised he was expressing a part of his self-image, and talks about how shocked she felt and how she didn't know how to react. Afraid of saying something that would be hurtful to Youri, she remained silent, but in the parent session she fights her tears, only now allowing herself to feel the overwhelming sadness she tried to suppress at home.

The therapist first validates foster mother's competence in immediately being able to recognise that she probably witnessed a glimpse of Youri's deepest thoughts and feelings about himself: being the one disturbing others and making them ill. She also normalises foster mother's feelings of shock and sadness in being confronted with such an overwhelmingly negative image her foster son carries with him. In talking about the profound sadness foster mother but also foster father and the therapist now feel in hearing this story, the conversation turns to how this might in part reflect the sadness Youri is living with. Thinking further about this, it occurs to them that foster mother's response at the time might have been the most adequate: showing interest in and listening to the phantasy about himself that Youri shared with her, without making it too conscious or too real but also not trying to minimise or change it (too quickly). The therapist then thinks together with the foster carers about how they can keep open the space at home for Youri to show and share these images, without him and the foster carers getting overwhelmed. She also shares some of the images she knows that Youri is also showing in his own treatment sessions, so as to reassure the foster carers that this is a domain that is also being worked on in therapy.

Concluding thoughts

Although in the present treatment approach, the work with the child's primary caregivers is often less in frequency than the direct work with the traumatised child themselves, the work conducted in this parent track is not less important or less difficult (for the parents and the parent worker alike). Supporting parents of traumatised children to feel acknowledged in what they are already offering their child, as well as to grow as parents in order to foster their child's developmental recovery are the main objectives of this work. The process in which the therapist tries to engage parents is often slow and iterative/cyclical, as mentalizing breakdowns are – understandably – common. Paradoxically, slowing down, taking time and creating mental(izing) space is arguably a key 'antidote' against the urgency and severity of the problems families with traumatised children present with. Therefore, helping parents to regain access to their mentalizing abilities is at the core of this work – the aim of which is to be able to venture with parents towards a more compassionate understanding of their own parenthood and parenting, as well as a more trauma-informed way of relating to a child with specific developmental needs.

References

Adkins, T., Reisz, S., Hasdemir, D., & Fonagy, P. (2021). Family Minds: A randomized controlled trial of a group intervention to improve foster parents' reflective functioning. *Development and Psychopathology*, 1–15. https://doi.org/10.1017/S095457942000214X

Bateman, A., & Fonagy, P. (Eds.). (2019). *Handbook of mentalizing in mental health practice*. American Psychiatric Publishing.

Bevington, D., Fuggle, P., Cracknell, L., & Fonagy, P. (2017). *Adaptive mentalization-based integrative treatment: A guide for teams to develop systems of care*. Oxford University Press.

Fonagy, P. (2016, November 19). *What is mentalization?* Retrieved from www.youtube.com/watch?v=MJ1Y9zw-n7U

Fonagy, P., & Luyten, P. (2009). A developmental, mentalization-based approach to the understanding and treatment of borderline personality disorder. *Development and Psychopathology*, *21*(4), 1355–1381. https://doi.org/10.1017/S0954579409990198

Fonagy, P., Luyten, P., Allison, E., & Campbell, C. (2019). Mentalizing, epistemic trust and the phenomenology of psychotherapy. *Psychopathology*, *52*, 94–103. https://doi.org/10.1159/000501526

Lilliengren, P. (2014). *Exploring therapeutic action in psychoanalytic psychotherapy: Attachment to therapist and change* [Doctoral thesis, Stockholm University].

Midgley, N., Ensink, K., Lindqvist, K., Malberg, N., & Muller, N. (2017a). The development of mentalizing. In *Mentalization-based treatment for children. A time-limited approach* (pp. 15–37). American Psychological Association.

Midgley, N., Ensink, K., Lindqvist, K., Malberg, N., & Muller, N. (2017b). *Mentalization-based treatment for children. A time-limited approach*. American Psychological Association.

Novick, K. K., & Novick, J. (2011). *Working with parents makes therapy work*. Jason Aronson.

Oestergaard Hagelquist, J. (2018). *The mentalization guidebook*. Routledge.

Olthof, J. (2017). *Handbook of narrative psychotherapy for children, adults, and families: Theory and practice*. Karnac Books.

Vliegen, N., Tang, E., & Meurs, P. (2023). *Children recovering from complex trauma: From wound to scar*. Routledge.

Chapter 8

Work with the network

In growing up, most children become surrounded by a network of caregiving adults beyond their immediate carers, including extended family, teachers, the family's GP, friends and acquaintances of the family. For children who have experienced complex trauma, this may also include a social worker or a psychologist or psychiatrist. Despite the many positives that can come from all of these relationships, these caregivers and professionals who are part of a network surrounding a traumatised child and their family may not always be prepared for the particular challenges that come with this group of children and often face emotional and relational issues that exceed their capacities and resources. Through experience and/or formal training, they may be used to managing child issues which make up 'ordinary' life. Yet, when it comes to traumatised children, attempting to create a 'facilitating environment' (Winnicott, 1971) becomes a particularly challenging task. The aim is to create a network of people who are able to keep the child's mind in mind so as to be as conducive as possible to the child's development. Often, the professional network around these children has necessarily become large and, thus, more difficult to organise and manage in a way that fosters mentalizing. At the same time, caring for traumatised children tends to elicit much more complex emotional and relational dynamics, taxing mentalizing capacities to an even greater extent and thus evoking responses that may be little or not conducive to positive relationships or healthy development. Therefore, creating and maintaining a forum where the different actors from the child's daily life are enabled to mentalize the issues they encounter forms the basis of the work with the network as set out in this book.

In this chapter, we present a mentalization- and trauma-informed model of working with the network surrounding traumatised children and their families (Asen & Fonagy, 2021; Fonagy et al., 2021). First, we outline the cornerstone of this work as fundamentally mentalization-based, as mentalizing abilities in adults caring for the child in one way or another tend to be greatly strained. Work at this first 'pole' of intervention – that is, helping the network to (re-)gain access to mentalizing capacities when it gets lost – aims to enable the members of the network to look at the child's – sometimes disruptive and 'disturbing' – behaviour from a more trauma-informed perspective. The latter makes up the second 'pole' of intervention in the work with the network in this model: scaffolding the network's ability to mentalize

DOI: 10.4324/9781003044918-11

the child's functioning, in order to inform decisions about ways of responding to developmental needs. Both poles of intervention will be discussed in the remaining sections of this chapter.

Creating a 'facilitating environment': forging partnerships in the network that foster mentalizing

The purpose of this first section is to delineate how mentalization-based principles are central to working with the network in this model (see Table 8.1). We outline who makes up the network surrounding a traumatised child and their family and discuss the particular challenges faced by the network members. Following that, we outline how the work with the network thus requires a mentalizing frame that takes into account the particularities of complex trauma dynamics. We then, introduce the core of this work as revolving around two 'poles' of intervention, aiming to mitigate any potentially retraumatising interactions around these children and their families.

Mobilising partners: who is or should be in the network

As with all children, children who have experienced complex trauma grow up in social networks that consist – by and large – of two kinds of relationships with adult carers outside of the immediate family. First, there are the formally structured relationships with people who have received formal training in child education, such as teachers at school or coaches in sports clubs or other leisure contexts. For

Table 8.1 Core components of mentalization-based work with the network

A solid but flexible therapeutic frame	• Consider who to include as a partner in the network, and when not yet existing, start to build a network around the family • Organise or participate in network meetings (once a term, three to four times a year) • Make agreements on communication lines in-between meetings, for example, in case of unforeseen challenges or crisis situations
Attitudes and strategies	• Acknowledge and validate the particular challenges of being involved with a child with complex trauma and their family • Move back and forth between the two intervention 'poles' of helping the network to regain access to mentalizing abilities, on the one hand and helping the network to keep the child's mind in mind, on the other • Convey a genuine curiosity and interest in the network partners' day-to-day experiences with the child ('small stories') • Be mindful of your own mentalizing processes

these actors in the child's professional network, each individual child is part of the group of children for whom they carry responsibility. Second, there are the particular, more informal and less structured relationships with people who have often received less or no formal training in child education. This may concern a grandparent or a neighbour whom the child visits daily after school, an uncle whom the child has a closer bond with, a teenage babysitter or a student helping with schoolwork. These actors in the child's informal network mostly meet the child in tailor-made one-to-one interactions. For both groups of caregivers, attempting to be an emotionally available adult who offers growth-promoting interactions to a vulnerable and traumatised child may bring great pleasure and reward but can also be particularly challenging for various reasons elaborated on in Chapter 3.

Considering who to include as a partner in the network is a task of the starting phase of the therapeutic work with a family (see also Chapter 5). Sometimes, this is rather obvious. In nearly all situations, school is represented by a teacher, a special educational needs coordinator or a head teacher, who is involved in helping the child with academic skills and/or behavioural management in classroom and playground situations. For some children, a child psychiatrist and/or residential care worker or a social worker from child protection services is involved. For others, a sports coach or a grandparent plays an indispensable role in keeping the child on a constructive developmental track and/or in keeping parents' and family life liveable. For foster families, it is obvious to include the social worker of the foster care service, who is often engaged in supporting the foster family and who may also be the one who initiates or supports the child's referral for treatment. Then, this social worker forms part of the network from the outset. In this sense, foster families are often rather well-embedded in a supportive societal fabric, particularly when there is a good bond with the key social worker. Then, it will be key for the therapist to try to navigate the already existing network bonds in a constructive way, so as to scaffold the child's and families' existing relationships (Bevington et al., 2017; see also later discussion).

Depending on local post-adoption policy and service organisation, the situation may be very different for adoptive families. Sometimes, adoptive parents can rely on little post-adoption support, making the process of seeking professional help more difficult. Then, the task of helping adoptive parents to build a network around their family becomes even more important. This may include actively searching for and trying to involve people around the child and their family who hold a positive and benign attitude towards a child who proves 'harder to raise', like football coach Michael in Jemal's case (see Chapter 3). Or, as discussed earlier, important adults having a more informal bond with the child and the family may be invited to participate, such as family members living close by and functioning as a safe haven when things get too heated at home. In some cases, a benign and supportive network has been lacking so far or relevant partners have not been mobilised yet. This requires the therapist to address first with parents what their network needs are and who can be asked to help meet these needs. For some parents, this work may entail first and foremost helping them accept and reflect on the importance of a supportive network to keep being able to raise the child in their family on the long term. This happens when families have become rather isolated in trying to handle the child's difficulties within their own family. They will need support in coming to terms with the idea that what they are able to offer the child will not be enough and that sharing care with others does not mean they are incompetent parents. Often, it is not so much a case of families not having people around them whom they could rely on, but of supporting parents in thinking about who they would want to really get involved as a member of this facilitating network. The idea of inviting people like an important member of the extended family to be part of the network is often something that emerges in the process of the work with parents. Or, in other cases, when parents themselves grew up without the need for additional support, they do not always realise that it may be helpful to actively search for people with a heart for atypically developing children.

Beyond 'good intentions': the challenges of partnering up around a traumatised child

Deciding who to involve in the treatment network around a traumatised child and their family is one thing. Subsequently laying the groundwork for constructive and effective work to be accomplished within this group is fraught with challenges when it comes to children who have experienced complex trauma. The reason for this has a lot to do with the given that the more complex a child's developmental needs are, the more network partners are likely to be involved and the more complex the dynamics among them can become. Each of these workers may have a very different view of the child and a very different conceptual model about what kind of support is needed (Bevington et al., 2017). A grandparent or other member of the extended family may be most invested in supporting the child's parents to offer the child a family life that is as good as possible; a teacher aims to teach the child, as part of a class group, the knowledge and skills they need at this age; an educational psychologist might be involved because of apparent learning difficulties, a medical team because of a physical health condition or a child psychiatrist because of ADHD. The diverging goals of their involvement with a particular child may complicate efforts to see eye to eye about the need for a 'network', if any and how then this should work (who should be part of it, who holds what position, when and where to meet, what the aims of meetings should be).

So, aside from the common intention to support the child and their family, the primary aim when difficulties arise for most of the adult carers involved with a traumatised child is for the child's 'difficult' or 'disturbing' behaviour to cease. Unlike adoptive parents or foster carers who can often be supported to reconnect to a genuine curiosity about what is underlying their traumatised child's behaviour, as this is grounded in deep parental commitment of wanting to understand and help the child *because* it is their child, other adult carers' commitments and responsibilities towards the child lie elsewhere.

When Lisa's teacher, Maïté, is teaching new spelling rules to the class, she feels she's about to lose patience when Lisa gets hung up in talking about the conflict in the playground over and over again. Maïté has already had a chat with the children involved and tried to comfort and regulate Lisa. But when Lisa keeps interrupting class angrily, Maïté notices herself thinking 'That's it! I've had it!'

When a child's disruptive and disturbing behaviour interferes with the task at hand and makes one's job more difficult, wondering about the reasons behind this behaviour is naturally *not* the first idea that comes to mind. Adult carers 'just' want to see the child 'happier', 'performing more age-appropriately' or 'functioning better'. In the first instance, this often does not (yet) imply a wish to better understand where particular behaviour or a particular way of functioning comes from. In other words, members of the network around traumatised children do not naturally ask for help 'to better mentalize the child'. In some cases, the child's differing presentation in different contexts may make it even more difficult for particular network members to see the sense in being part of a mentalizing network. For example, a child may behave in a socially desirable and overly adaptive way at school but 'release all breaks' at home, making it hard for the teacher/school to take parents' concerns seriously, as 'there are no problems at school'. Or, as in the case of Youri, for example, who is rather hard to reach and to relate to at home but who adapts easily to a class situation, his teacher sees no point in attending the network meetings. By contrast, Jemal often experiences difficulties in regulating his behaviour in classroom situations, whereas his adoptive parents have learnt how to provide a secure and almost therapeutic home environment thus preventing difficulties at home. This sometimes leads to network conversations in which the school is trying to convince the parents of the severity of the problems, with the parents responding with 'but you could prevent a lot of problems if you would take the time to understand him', leading to the school emphasising even more the extent of the difficulties which they feel the parents are denying. From these perspectives, investing time and energy to meet with other adult carers to 'try to better understand the child' may be easily considered as a waste of – already strained – resources and/or may evoke tension or even disbelief in the relationships between parents and network partners. In other words, it will sometimes not be obvious to members of the network how such meetings will be of any use to them (or to the child for that matter). This makes the task of the therapist trying to forge mentalizing partnerships in the network a particularly challenging one.

Paradoxically, being engaged in a group of people who share the common ground of being involved in fostering the child's development in one way or another can be helpful in several ways. First, hearing that other adult caregivers experience similar feelings of anxiety or powerlessness, anger or rage, embarrassment or shame and guilt in their difficult encounters with the child helps to become more compassionate towards oneself as well as other carers. It helps to acknowledge and validate such difficult feelings and, in doing so, also to be able to move on from these to a more constructive state of mind (i.e., to get mentalizing back 'online'). Following that, discovering that there may be particular patterns in the child's behaviour when considered from a more trauma-informed perspective helps to engender more sympathy and empathy for the child and their family, possibly countering the 'harsher' feelings one also feels. For example, in network meetings, a teacher can learn about the huge efforts parents and other caregivers are putting in to provide the child with a 'liveable life' and the family with a relatively balanced family life. Witnessing the efforts exerted to support the child's development and hearing others talk about the child's suffering underlying the 'difficult' behaviour, can also help the teacher reframe some of the child's behaviour as being trauma-related. This may bring about a more compassionate stance towards the child's struggles as well as engender more curiosity to 'learn more' (see also 'epistemic trust'; Fonagy et al., 2019). It also helps to highlight the important role each of the members of the network really play in their cumulative – and hopefully – positive contribution to the child's developmental recovery. This is an especially important aspect as most traumatised children are extremely sensitive to becoming dysregulated by negative or harsh reactions from caregivers, making already difficult moments even worse, as coach Michael learnt from his experiences with Jemal (see Chapter 3). Experiencing how things really do become easier to manage or get resolved more quickly when responding more from a trauma-informed understanding – and how this really makes a difference to the child's growth and development – then makes it easier to experience the joint 'problem-solving time' (Fonagy, 2016, November 19) as 'time well spent' and thus to continue to engage in the work together.

A time and space to dwell and reflect on challenging situations

In order to establish well-functioning partnerships among the members of the network and to prevent 'good intentions' and 'strong commitments' from resulting in fragmented or even opposing initiatives, work with the network requires a solid frame to safeguard a time and space to reflect together. In case a network has more or less been formed and meetings are organised (and chaired) by another member of the network, the therapist (who in the present treatment approach is also the parent worker: see Chapter 4) seeks to align themselves with the existing partnerships in a way that is respectful of prior – sometimes implicit – agreements whilst also seeking to foster mentalizing in the network. In the case a mentalizing network needs to be newly formed, the therapist initiates – and often, also chairs – the network meetings.

Regardless of who takes the initiative or chairs the meetings, mentalization-based work with the network requires agreements about the frequency of network meetings as well as about how to keep communication lines open in between meetings. A workable rhythm is to hold meetings once a term, three to four times a year, irrespective of whether there are pressing problems at that moment or not. Meeting each other and learning to know each partner's mandate and perspective, as well as discussing ways of managing demanding situations at more quiet times, is important to be able to act united when crisis situations do emerge. For similar reasons, we aim to establish a more or less set group of people attending the network meetings, which may in and of itself be a challenge due to the often long-term follow-up needed for traumatised children and the reality of personnel turn-over in education, social care and child mental health services.

Like in parent work, network members need to know who is available and may be contacted where and when in-between meetings when faced with unforeseen challenges. As introduced in Chapter 4, aside from planned meetings with the whole group and ad hoc contacts at moments of crisis, it may be important to consider holding more frequent meetings – in person or by phone or video-conferencing – with one or several members of the network who have a particularly important or close – or by contrast, an especially strained – relationship to the child. For example, Lisa's social worker and the special educational needs coordinator at Jemal's school, who were more intensely involved, were conferred with more frequently in-between the meetings with the larger network, so as to ensure sufficient continuity.

Ultimately, such a collaborative reflective network aims to form a mentalizing and trauma-informed team around the child and the family, in which relevant information about how the child is doing in different contexts is exchanged, and consistent, coherent and continuing care for this child can be coordinated. This is the ideal, aiming to foster growth and development in the child as well as facilitate (more) positive relationships with peers and adults beyond the immediate family, but the reality may often not match this. In the remaining sections of this chapter, we will explain what the specific challenges to this work with the network are, as well as outline the principles of how these challenges can be tackled by the therapist.

So, similar to how the work with parents is aimed at providing them a time and space to think and talk together about what happens in family interactions and situations, both the professional and the informal actors surrounding traumatised children can benefit from a forum that affords them opportunities to pause and try to understand what happens in their encounters with the child. This means that, similar to parent work, the work with the network requires sharing of the 'small', daily experiences which have puzzled the participants or 'stuck' with them in another way (e.g., because it surprised or annoyed them or made them feel concerned, scared or angry) as starting points of conversation and reflection.

Process versus content in network work: back and forth between two poles of intervention

Meeting with members of the child's network is thus meant as a frame within which caregivers can regain access to their mentalizing capacities and are provided with trauma-informed knowledge about child development and developmental

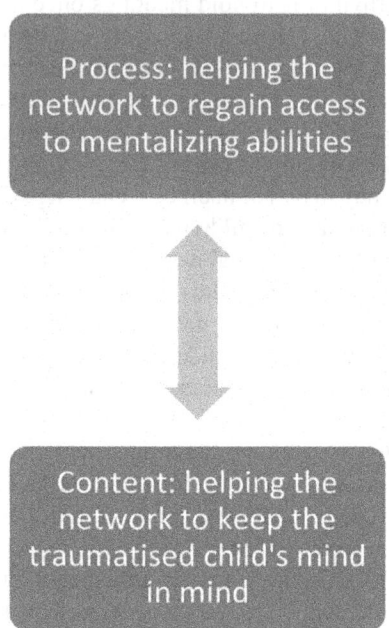

Figure 8.1 Two poles of intervention in mentalization-based and trauma-informed work with the network.

problems. These two foci of intervention form the core of the mentalization-based and trauma-informed model of working with the network set out in the present treatment approach. In line with the concept of 'poles', as has been introduced in the previous chapter on parent work, we refer to these two foci of intervention as 'poles' of intervention (see Figure 8.1).

Similar to the work with parents, work at the pole of intervention depicted at the top of Figure 8.1 takes precedence over focusing on the other pole. Indeed, there is no point in trying to talk 'about' a particular issue or situation (e.g., the child throwing a fit in the middle of class) as long as the teacher and the other members of the network are not in a state of mind where they are able to think together with you. Mentalizing breakdowns in one or more members of the network surrounding a traumatised child and their family are commonplace. So, helping them to recover from these breakdowns should be a recurring focus of intervention. On the other hand, being 'able to think' will not necessarily translate into behavioural responses that promote developmental recovery in the child, unless these thinking processes are informed by knowledge about how complex trauma impacts development in terms of patterns of feeling, relating and behaving. As such, this model of the work with the network requires the therapist to continuously and flexibly move back and forth between the two poles of intervention.

Intervention pole 1: helping the network to regain access to mentalizing abilities

As discussed earlier, bringing together a (large) group of people coming from – sometimes very – different backgrounds around the shared objective of 'thinking together' about a particular traumatised child and their family is often a challenging endeavour in and of itself. When trauma is at stake, adult carers' mentalizing abilities may be taxed severely because of the emotional intensity of trauma-related dynamics in which not only parents but also other caregiving partners surrounding the family may get entangled.

 When invited to share 'some things about Lisa at school to think together about', Lisa's teacher, Maïté, attending the network meeting for the first time, talks with visible embarrassment about 'the mouldy bread incident' (see also Chapters 3 and 7), during her very first week at school. After the children had left the classroom for lunch break, Lisa had returned and told Maïté that she didn't have any sandwiches to eat for lunch because her foster mother used old and mouldy bread, so she had thrown her sandwiches in the bin. 'She looked so sad and I felt so sorry for her. I wanted to help her, so I shared my sandwiches. I remembered the headmaster talking about a fund the school has for families that can't afford school materials or meals'. Turning to Lisa's foster carers, and remembering the expression of disbelief and shock on their faces when she had approached them, Maïté says: 'I really didn't mean to embarrass you! I just never imagined that a child would come up with such a story if it wasn't true'. Foster father has already been able to put most of his indignation and anger aside by having processed this incident in their parent sessions with the therapist (see Chapter 7). He responds compassionately: 'Don't worry about it too much', and while winking at the teacher, he adds: 'Didn't you know? We neglect all of our kids'. The therapist, in an attempt to validate and normalise Maïté's embarrassment, responds by saying: 'I get it completely – I think if I'd been in the same situation I'd have done exactly the same! And I hope I'd have been as brave and honest as you to come and talk about it in a network meeting like this!' In the more relaxed atmosphere, others in the meeting share how Lisa has asked them too for food or money (to buy food or 'stuff'). The therapist then invites the people around the table to explicitly mentalize about these incidents: 'Has anyone got any thoughts about why Lisa might do this?'.

After several network members share their thoughts about potential motivations underlying Lisa's behaviour, the therapist shares some of her trauma-informed knowledge about children 'lying' as a way to keep fending for themselves even if the current caregiving circumstances are not neglectful anymore. Maïté responds frankly about how she didn't know about this kind of relational dynamics as being trauma-driven.

This, in turn, opens up the conversation around the table that others too have not realised that Lisa's 'lying' is part of a pattern of behaviour that could be better understood when considered in light of the early adverse experiences she had suffered.

In the face of the continual (risk of) mentalizing breakdowns in the network, the therapist initiating and/or participating in the work with network partners can rely on several interrelated ways of facilitating the re-emergence of mentalizing (see Table 8.2).

Minding the intense trauma-related emotional dynamics in the network

Forming a mentalizing network around a child and their family challenged by the consequences of complex trauma is only partially about knowledge about the impact of trauma on child development (see 'Intervention pole 2'). It is as much about intense emotional dynamics stirred up within and among people. The people involved with a traumatised child are, in the first place, confronted with the emotional and relational consequences of severe trauma. They witness the compelling deep suffering of both child and parents, become involved in situations in which a turmoil of positive and negative feelings are at stake and get entangled in intense conflicts and crisis situations (e.g., school suspension or expulsion). In this regard, it is not hard to imagine the child's needs and difficulties exceeding caregivers' resources. When adult carers feel their efforts only have limited success or when they become involved in too many intensely negative interactions, a tendency to become controlling and punishing or, instead, to withdraw and disengage may

Table 8.2 Core interventions to help the network to regain access to mentalizing abilities

- Convey a benign, active curiosity in what is on the other network partners' minds
- Make use of the network partners' 'small stories' as 'windows of opportunity' to reflect together on what is happening
- In listening to network partners' 'small stories', validate them for staying afloat amidst emotional turmoil
- 'Stubbornly' model a stance of benign, active curiosity about why the child would behave the way they do
- In trying to co-create an image of the child from different perspectives, convey being 'one expert among others' and scaffold the child's relationships with important others, by validating each network partners' perspective (e.g., school/class versus home, one-to-one versus group context) as contributing to a more comprehensive understanding of the child's functioning and dynamics
- Be mindful of and search for ways to address the intense trauma-related emotional dynamics in the network (e.g., by thematising the 'contagiousness' of stress and offering psycho-education as appropriate)

emerge, compromising the ability to remain thoughtful in their approach to the child. It is important to be mindful of the fact that this influences not only the relationship between the child/the family and the caregiver within the network but also the relationships *among* network partners. When arousal is high, models of the mind easily become simply black or white, solutions are seen in quick-fix action-reaction sequences, and different perspectives are experienced as one view being correct and the other one wrong and thus as a source of dispute, conflict and possibly disintegration (Bevington et al., 2017). In other words, the network is confronted with the double challenge of not only to keep mentalizing in the network (about the child and the family) but also to keep mentalizing (about) the network itself.

When these emotional dynamics can become subject of joint reflection and conversation, as illustrated in the vignette earlier, mentalization-based work within the network can take off. However, scrutinising situations in which one felt embarrassed, anxious, powerless or angry and manipulated is mostly not what network members expect from the meetings at the outset. For example, a teacher expects to report what happened in class without expecting it to become food for thought, or a special educational needs coordinator is commissioned to offer their diagnostic assessment of a child to convince the network that the child would fit in better at a special education needs school or in residential treatment. It requires courage, an open mind and a certain degree of trust in others to 'admit' one's assessment of a situation was wrong and to become aware that one's best intentions to help a child has brought about an embarrassing situation in one's relationship with the child's foster carers, as in Maïté's case. Time and effort need to be put in to create a safe and reflective atmosphere in a network to enable its members to share in such an open and honest way. Helpful ways to accomplish this will be described in the following subsections.

Part of the intense emotionality of the dynamics in networks around traumatised children stems from the confusing mix of profoundly positive and negative feelings which these children tend to bring about in their close relationships. On the one hand, it is not uncommon for caregiving adults to experience strong feelings of warmth, compassion, and even phantasies of rescuing the child from bad or hurtful others. When a child has suffered neglect or abuse, it is very natural that everyone around the child wants to avoid this from being repeated. This may make caregivers highly vigilant towards any signs that the child is being badly cared for and even suspicious towards others. In some cases, those suspicions may be justified, but often, they are expressions of a deep fear that an already vulnerable child may be retraumatised (as may have been part of Maïté's unconscious anxieties in being confronted with Lisa's story of only having mouldy bread to eat). On the other hand, there can be feelings of anxiety and distress, distrust and even intense anger towards a child, partially evoked by the primary defence mechanisms these children tend to fall back on to maintain their fragile affective equilibrium. In an attempt to find a way to live with overwhelming needs for love and support as well as feelings of anxiety, distrust and rage, traumatised children sometimes treat one member of their environment as entirely good and caring and another as bad and inadequate. In Lisa's example, the foster carers are portrayed as neglectful (not providing her with healthy food), while Maïté will probably have been experienced as a good carer, as she shared her own lunch with Lisa. Whilst the possibility of inadequate care must always be taken seriously, it is also essential to understand how the child's tendency to distrust (some) caregivers can easily seep through in the relations among the network partners. The child's different presentation in different situations/contexts can raise questions about how safe, well-understood and well-supported the child is at home, at school or in 'that sports group', sometimes reflecting aspects of the child's inner truth rather than the actual quality of care provided. In the vignette about Lisa, it isn't hard to imagine how Maïté might have – and indeed, did, at first glance – consider the foster carers as bad providers and how the foster carers might have perceived the teacher as incompetent because of taking Lisa's story at face value. Working with the network surrounding a traumatised child thus requires a continuing alertness for early signs of splitting mechanisms or otherwise destructive dynamics unwittingly 'infecting' the relationships among network members and a particular competence to address these as early and constructively as possible. How this 'risk of disintegrating forces taking over' (Bevington et al., 2017) can be countered will be elaborated on in the following subsections.

Fostering mentalizing in networks: a case of 'grasping windows of opportunity' and 'stubbornly holding on'

In light of the 'contagiousness' of (relational) stress and thus mentalizing breakdowns in a social system around traumatised children, the therapist's ability to grasp any window of opportunity to foster the (re-)emergence of mentalizing in members of the network is of prime importance from the outset. Modelling a mentalizing stance may start with the therapist conveying a basic and benign curiosity in what is on the other's mind. An opening phrase of a meeting may be: 'So, what's on our minds today? What are the things we have to think about together?' Or, as in the vignette about Lisa: 'Are there things you (Maïté) want to share about how Lisa is doing at school?'. The teacher's subsequent open-minded response, in the way she dared to put herself in a vulnerable position, may be considered as an important window of opportunity. This kind of 'small stories' about (relational) 'mismatches' are crucial opportunities to learn (more) about Lisa, how to understand different aspects of her functioning and, eventually, how to approach her in a way that fosters developmental and relational recovery. In the vignette, the therapist's previous work with the foster carers on this 'small story', enabling foster father to regain his ability to approach the topic with a sense of humour, without becoming too blaming towards the teacher who took Lisa's story at face value, was an important first element. In the work with the network itself, the therapist's explicit normalisation of the teacher's spontaneous reaction helped Maïté to feel less embarrassed. Moreover, the therapist's explicit validation of the teacher's courage and appreciation for her openness were extremely important not only for Maïté but also for the other network members in becoming more mentalizing, as expressed in their willingness to share similar stories.

The therapist's continually capitalising on these windows of opportunity can thus profoundly support thoughtful exchange and reflection and strengthen further collaboration. It can also help to lower the threshold to get in touch with one another when 'odd things' seem to emerge. Indeed, the partnerships created through this work can also be put to good use at the many moments in which mentalizing is (at risk of) caving in in one or more members of the group. In such instances, it can be helpful to remind the network of the meeting's purpose and the shared objective:

> We are sitting together because everyone here wants to offer Lisa as safe and growth-promoting an environment as possible. So, it would be good if we could keep sharing the moments that felt 'odd' or 'off', or in which we felt really anxious or angry, so we can puzzle out together how we can manage such moments with Lisa.

As mentalizing is interpersonal by nature – a highly interactive activity (Bateman & Fonagy, 2016) – it can not only be hampered but also fostered by the social group in which it takes place. Collaborative partnerships, such as the ones aimed for in the work with the network in the present treatment approach, can function as a social environment in which mentalizing is 'contagiously' spread.

Almost 'stubbornly' holding on to a stance of active curiosity (Borenstein, 2002), of expressing a willingness to understand and validating the different perspectives (e.g., 'That sounds important, how did you experience that?') are central to a mentalizing stance yet by no means an easy endeavour. In this regard, one cannot overstate the value of the workers surrounding a traumatised child feeling heard and validated in what they are experiencing, feeling seen in the major efforts they invest in caring for a child as well as feeling acknowledged for staying afloat amidst the intense emotional turmoil they have been caught in. Even if a therapeutically trained mind can see the worker's role in having contributed to the difficult interactions, this can only be addressed in a next phase of the meeting, after the worker feels heard, seen and validated and has become more at ease and relaxed and so able to reflect with more distance and even some humour about what happened, as illustrated in the case of Lisa's network. Understanding and validating Maïté's experience of the strong appeal coming from Lisa who 'had no sandwiches for lunch' and her caring intentions both in sharing her own sandwiches with Lisa and her approaching the foster carers with the possibility of school support can contain the embarrassment and prevent the accompanying arousal from interfering with mentalizing.

This mentalization-based approach to working with the network is not an easy task, and in an early phase it can even feel almost ridiculous to ask again and again how the person experienced the event, what it may mean and what it can teach us about the child's functioning. 'Are you really going to tell us we have to try to understand what this means?', Lisa's foster father sighs, glancing at the therapist, when different network partners around the table share stories about Lisa going around 'telling lies', appealing to everyone to give her food or money (to buy food). In such instances, courageously and stubbornly holding on to thinking aloud needs to be delicately and thoughtfully balanced with validating carers' concerns about disconcerting behaviour: 'I really agree with you that her behaviour is worrisome. In suggesting to try to understand what is going through Lisa's mind, is by no means meant to justify her behaviour, but it can help us to decide on what would be a good response'. Such an intervention can open up a new train of thoughts about how to understand Lisa's behaviour more from the inside out, based on the different – and sometimes, divergent – perspectives around the table, and how to 'best' respond 'unitedly' to this behaviour.

Putting Humpty Dumpty together again whilst scaffolding the child's relationships

As introduced at the beginning of this chapter, a particular challenge for network partners around a traumatised child often lies in putting together different – and sometimes, seemingly opposite – perspectives on the child's functioning. Some children are at their best, reflecting on and talking about experiences in a mature way, in a one-to-one contact, whereas in a group context, they dysregulate easily. For example, in class where the teacher affords her enough individual time and attention, Mei-Lan presents as a rather easy child whereas in the playground, she doesn't seem to be able to play together with classmates and frequently runs off. Other children, like Jemal, are more at ease among peers but become closed-off and anxious, distrustful or hostile towards adults. Still other children seem not at all comfortable in any close relationship, like Youri who presents like a rather silent, compliant but hard-to-reach child at home as well as in relation to teachers or other adults at school. Sometimes, a child such as Lisa adores one adult and tells stories about being treated badly by another. It is not uncommon for uninformed caregivers, like Maïté, to take a child's stories of neglectful or even abusive parents at face value: not only as the child's expression of an inner world of experiences and perceptions but as factual reports of actual events in external reality. Although it is always important to check out the reality of these stories, it is also important to be curious about the reasons why a child may be saying such things.

In this context of work with the network around traumatised children, the therapist acknowledging being one expert among others and taking a not-knowing stance takes on a particular meaning and function. Among the different partners, the therapist guiding and/or participating in the network holds but one particular perspective on the child (i.e., the child within a therapeutic context). So, even more than in parent work, the therapist needs to act as a member of a 'quiz' team: guiding reflection and offering potential directions based on their knowledge about mentalizing processes on the one hand and about child development and trauma on the other yet explicitly conveying an openness towards different perspectives. This may be phrased, for instance, as

> We all know Lisa in different contexts and from different points of view. If we can put all these perspectives together, we can learn to know about different aspects of her functioning and developing. If we puzzle out together how we can understand her, we've got a better chance of finding ways to support her development.

As such, the therapist aims to validate the different questions and feelings that arise in the network partners as valuable and informative contributions to understanding the child and their particular situation. Lisa's therapist inviting the different members of the network to give their thoughts on the possible reasons underlying Lisa's need to resort to 'lies' about being badly cared for by her foster carers was meant as an attempt to put together the different parts of Lisa to better understand who she is as a whole person. This, in turn, is meant to find enough common ground to be able to agree on a shared plan of care and to prevent premature actions or ill-considered decisions from being taken (e.g., merely resorting to punishment – or the threat thereof – to curb Lisa's 'lying').

In attempting to 'put Humpty Dumpty together again' in collaboration with the different actors in the child's network, scaffolding these existing relationships forms an important part of the work, enabling the network to intervene in multiple domains of the child's life (Bevington et al., 2017). As introduced at the beginning of this section, this requires the ability to recognise and acknowledge how one – unwittingly – can get drawn into particular trauma-related relational dynamics. This can help to transition from feeling embarrassed or ashamed ('I fell into the trap') or from blaming the child (as setting out the trap consciously and intentionally) towards accepting and understanding this as part of the trauma-related dynamics, as a basis for future change. When the experiences shared among the network partners can be used as a starting point of reflection about what kind of responses the child needs from caregiving adults to develop a more mature relational functioning and to grow as a person, the network work is doing what it is meant for: making use of the child's significant relationships to scaffold development.

In this regard, a remark like 'It really touches you and several of us, doesn't it, what's going on with her now?' can sometimes help to acknowledge how these children 'get under our skin'. Or, remarking 'It really moves all of us around the table, everyone wanting him to grow up as good as possible' can help network partners to remain in touch with the child's vulnerabilities as well as with one's caring intentions towards the child. Sometimes, as therapists, we may witness trauma dynamics also eliciting dynamics and straining vulnerabilities at a more personal level in a network member. For example, a residential care worker struggling more intensely with the child's relational dynamics because of their own issues regarding proximity/closeness and distance. Sometimes, as therapists, we are in a position that affords the opportunity to open up a one-to-one conversation by remarking, for example, 'She really gets under your skin, doesn't she?' But often, we are not in such a position so as to guide the work on personal vulnerabilities in individual network members, leading to this being more out of scope in the work with the network compared to the work with parents. Most of the time, one can only hope that the network member can rely on other relationships where they can discuss and work through personal issues being triggered in caring for traumatised children. Even if the network meetings are not the place to do this work, the mentalizing stance carried forward from these meetings may be a helpful vehicle.

Another element of this relational focus in the work with the network is the challenge to keep positivity at the centre of relational experience, in spite of the myriad misunderstandings and conflicts which often characterise traumatised children's relationships. Relationships are the place par excellence where children who have experienced complex trauma can start to experience other, more adaptive ways of being related to. The hope is that this will perhaps eventually help them to start to try out other, more adaptive ways of relating *to* others as well and that these more positive relationships will be conducive to further developmental recovery and growth. In this perspective, scaffolding relatedness can be considered a treatment objective as well as a treatment process – a mechanism of change through which more adaptive developmental outcomes become attainable for traumatised children.

Intervention pole 2: helping the network to keep the traumatised child's mind in mind

Similar to what is ultimately at stake in parent work, members of the network may benefit from a better understanding of what may be underlying a traumatised child's 'incomprehensible' and 'intractable' behaviour. This second pole of intervention is about supporting network partners to understand the child's behaviour 'from the inside out' in the particular situation in which they are responsible for the child and using this understanding to consider how to manage the situation further. The football coach may be puzzled by and even respond angrily to seemingly contradictory behaviour, for example, a child who seems to love being part of the sports club but continues to 'freak out' in the dressing room, where closer observation reveals that such situations trigger early adverse experiences. Or, the arts teacher becomes impatient about a child often complaining that the other children are 'out to get me' but suddenly realises that racial aggression is taking place upon hearing the child being called 'filthy Chinese' by his peers, inciting her to take appropriate action with the peer group. Or, a teacher wonders whether the child 'really lacks the capacities or is just not motivated' in witnessing the child's extremely unpredictable school performances but opens up his mind to the idea that this might be rooted in a hypersensitive stress system. Understanding the trauma dynamics can make it easier to predict and to manage the child's behaviour in more constructive ways.

Similar to what happens in parent work, the therapist when working with the network listens with a sensitive ear to indications that one or several of the four developmental domains (i.e., representational, affect regulation and relational capacities and sense of self and identity) are currently most at stake. With these domains functioning as signposts or lenses, the therapist can help guide the joint reflection and discussion towards a more trauma-informed way of mentalizing the child's behaviour and, ultimately, to find new ways of responding which are constructive and growth-promoting. In this regard, the three guiding questions (Oestergaard Hagelquist, 2018) in parent work may be similarly helpful in the work with the network: (a) *why* is the child expressing this kind of behaviour here and now? (E.g., why did Lisa tell an untrue story about only getting mouldy bread from her foster carers?), (b) *what* does the child need to learn? (E.g., Lisa needs to learn to open her mind to new experiences of relying on her foster carers to take good care of her and facing her feelings of anxiety and anger about not having been taken good care of in past caregiving relationships.), and (c) *how* then can the teacher/network partner support that? (E.g., how can they respond in a way that both conveys that telling untrue stories is not okay but that also acknowledges Lisa's profoundly fearful and distrustful feelings around care?) In this context, exploring different perspectives and emotional reactions can go hand in hand with offering psycho-education about particular aspects or domains of development as these are impacted by complex traumatic experiences. For example, the therapist in the case of Lisa's network (see previous vignette) sharing some of her knowledge about how in some traumatised children 'lying' gets triggered as a trauma-related primary fight mechanism. Offering psycho-education may, for example, be helpful in situations in which network members' thinking seems to get stuck on a quick-fix 'solution' that seems rather little trauma-informed and that thus risks exacerbating rather than alleviating. This may be the case when a school starts to think 'she's becoming a delinquent, we can't tolerate this as a school, she needs to be punished, we'll have to suspend her'.

In the following boxes, we offer suggestions about aspects in each of the four developmental domains that may become salient at some point in the 'small stories' of traumatised children's network and which the therapist thus can listen for and address in ways to support the network to respond in growth-promoting ways. For each of these domains, we also present a case vignette to illustrate what the work with the network at this intervention pole may look like in practice.

Themes in helping network partners mentalize the child's representational capacities

- How to understand the child's strengths and difficulties with regard to representing aspects of experiences and of an inner world
- How to scaffold the child's ways of expressing themselves in relaxed and small day-to-day moments
- How to help the child express themselves in moments when emotions run higher
- How to respond when confronted with trauma-related content in their child's stories or play

Teacher Maïté talks about Lisa entering the classroom in complete distress last Monday morning: 'She was crying and sobbing, with some of her classmates hovering over her and trying to comfort her. When I asked what happened, one of the classmates said that Lisa's (biological) mother is going to die. And Lisa exclaimed how much pain she was in, already missing her mum terribly. I was shocked, and tried to understand what was going on. The children told me that Lisa's biological mother has cancer and is going to die. Lisa had shared that with them earlier that morning in the playground'. Maïté talks about how she consciously approached Lisa with extra patience and deep consideration for the remainder of the day, and how she learnt at the end of the school day, when Lisa's foster mother came to pick her up, that none of it was true.

In the network meeting, Maïté further shares how she felt manipulated, betrayed and angry and how she – at that moment – wanted to disengage entirely from 'such a manipulative child'. Lisa's foster carers join in the conversation by sharing other experiences of Lisa telling and upholding stories with such conviction while none of it is true. The therapist wondering aloud what might have preceded such 'incomprehensible' behaviour helps Lisa's foster mother to recall that Lisa was supposed to visit with her biological mother the previous weekend but that her mother had an appointment at the hospital and completely forgot about Lisa visiting. Thinking together about how having been forgotten by her mother might have impacted Lisa softens the tone of the conversation at the network meeting. The therapist decides to share something about what she knows about traumatised children turning to 'cover stories' as a way of simultaneously expressing as well as surviving unbearable feelings of abandonment and rejection. She explains that for traumatised children, this kind of 'lies' can simultaneously function as an expression of profound feelings of sadness, anger and confusion which they know no other way of expressing as well as a way of ensuring themselves of the support and comfort they so desperately need from others. In considering what has been said around the table, Maïté – less indignantly now – responds: 'I can imagine it being more bearable for Lisa to have her mother dying of cancer than to have to deal with feeling abandoned and rejected by her'.

This vignette can be situated at the crossroads of several developmental domains. Within the representational domain, it can be helpful to think of 'lies' or 'cover stories' as attempts to express elements of an inner world that cannot be expressed in other, more constructive ways. Lisa isn't equipped with the nuanced language or other representational capacities that one needs to express difficult experiences as being forgotten by one's mother. One can imagine that the phantasy 'Mum would only forget me if she is so ill that she's almost going to die' is more bearable than the thought 'I am of so little importance to my mother that she just forgets about me'. At the same time, this is also about the relational and identity domains (see later discussion), because it inevitably also relates to Lisa's relationships with her biological mum as well as what her stories bring about in other relationships (with peers, teacher, foster carers).

Themes in helping network partners mentalize the child's regulation capacities

- How to understand issues of discomfort, pain and anxiety in daily situations and how these influence interactions with the child
- How to scaffold language for emotions in daily conversations and interactions with the child
- How to recognise and manage behavioural dysregulation in the child (including trauma-related dysregulations such as trauma triggers and fight, flight and freeze mechanisms)

Oliver is Mei-Lan's first grade teacher. Thanks to his warm dedication, Mei-Lan has been able to feel calmer and become better regulated in classroom situations, and this has enabled her to develop more academic skills and make scholastic progression. At the network meeting, Oliver shares how lately regulation issues seem to predominate again, with Mei-Lan getting upset about the 'smallest' issues, running out of the classroom, sometimes even slamming the door. And 'what is most disconcerting', Oliver continues, 'is that all progress we had made seems to be lost again!' Talking about Mei-Lan's difficulties at school is clearly upsetting to Oliver. 'I'm just wondering why we keep doing all of this! We've worked so hard to help Mei-Lan get to a place where she feels at ease enough to actually be able to learn things at school, but there's nothing left! I really don't think we can help her any further; maybe there are better and more suitable schools for children like Mei-Lan'. In trying to somewhat contain Oliver's feelings, the therapist says: 'it must be very hard to see what has been built up torn down again'. Oliver responds intensely emotional, with a clearly breaking voice: 'You sound so "professional"! It seems as if it doesn't really touch you. How can you remain so calm, when a child has to go through this! Can't we find better ways to help her? There must be better places for a child with her needs'. Therapist: 'I'm sorry if I came across as cold or stand-offish, that wasn't my intention. It does touch me, as I can imagine it touches all of us. And I can also imagine, it touches you in particular, as you've invested so much and are now witnessing it apparently all disappearing'. Oliver affirms: 'it's so hard to watch!'. Therapist: 'the fact that you and all of us are so moved by Mei-Lan's suffering also attests to how involved and dedicated we feel towards her. At the same time, I think it's important to remember that traumatised children may frequently fall behind again on some developmental domain or another, after a period of progression, sometimes without us knowing what may have triggered this. We can certainly think about this further together. But, staying on board, as you and we have been doing, may be the most important help we can offer right now. I think Mei-Lan is showing us in her behaviour how difficult it is for her – for whatever reason – to hold herself together in class. Helping her to survive her difficult emotions and to regain some sense of emotional balance seems to be the most pressing thing we can do to help her get through this difficult period'. At this, Oliver settles a bit, feeling his concerns are shared by the group, and he asks, with genuine curiosity: 'Of course, I don't mean that Mei-Lan needs to be shipped off to some other school! But what can we do at school to help her?' The therapist replies: 'Okay, let's think a bit together about what might be helpful to prevent Mei-Lan from dysregulating so severely in class, and what we can do to help her get back on track with learning and thriving. I don't want Oliver to leave here today without feeling he's got something to work with!'

Incidents of behaviour or changes in behaviour that seem to come out of the blue are often subject of conversation in networks around traumatised children, because of the 'contagiousness' of unpredictable dysregulation. As expressed in the pebble-in-the-pond metaphor (Vliegen et al., 2023), parents, siblings, adult network partners and peers often 'feel' and are drawn into/'infected' by the child's distress before they can think about and mentalize what is at stake. Mei-Lan's teacher, in the vignette, clearly becomes distressed at having to witness all her scholastic progress disappearing seemingly for no apparent reason. Exclaiming to transfer Mei-Lan to another school is probably an expression of feelings of powerlessness and perhaps even failure and the intuitive reaction of wanting to rid oneself of these feelings. Or, in Jemal's case, football coach Michael's observations of Jemal's waning motivation at trainings and him sharing these observations with Jemal's adoptive parents was disconcerting enough for these parents to consult. In the work with the network, the therapist can offer time and space to distance oneself somewhat from 'the heat of the moment' (the spot where the pebble hits the water and makes the biggest splash) so that mentalizing abilities can get back 'online' (see 'Intervention pole 1'). This can be done by explicitly validating a network member's experience and distress, like the therapist did towards Oliver in the vignette. In a second 'move', the therapist can help network partners to consider possible meanings of the child's behaviour. Sometimes, this involves reframing of the child's behaviour in case trauma-related dynamics may be at play, such as is plausible in case of Mei-Lan's sudden underperformance at school. Again, it may be helpful for the therapist to share some trauma-informed knowledge, as the therapist did in the vignette. This, in turn, may spur further thoughts and discussion on how 'best' to proceed.

Themes in helping network partners mentalize the child's relational capacities

- Naming and talking with network partners about positive moments of interaction
- How to create small moments of warm interaction in everyday activity (e.g., in class or other groups, in the playground) and to recognise what interactions are growth-promoting (e.g., with regard to proximity and distance)
- How to meet a child's needs for nurturance, even if these seem regressive or age-inappropriate, for example, helping the child to survive moments of separation
- How to differentiate between emotional versus actual truth when 'old' relational representations influence actual relationships ('the witching hour' directing the child's functioning or behaviour)

When invited at the network meeting to share 'things from your perspective that you want to think or talk about together', Dave, the social worker working with Youri's foster family, turning to the foster carers, says: 'actually, I was wondering whether we could schedule future home visits during school hours? That might make things easier . . . for everyone'. In a throwaway manner, Dave adds 'I don't think it would matter to Youri if I would visit when he's not home'. Foster mother, clearly taken by surprise, reacts: 'Of course, if you think that would be better'. Yet, the therapist, sensing that there could possibly be more to Dave's question, invites him to share some of his thoughts about his impression of his home visits 'not mattering' to Youri. Dave responds: 'Well, for starters, when I come in, Youri doesn't greet me, right? And when I try to engage him by asking him how he's doing, he only says "okay" and continues playing with his cars, or colouring or drawing. . . . He just goes on doing what he was doing when I came in. He doesn't ask me anything . . . I don't want to force him, or to make him feel uncomfortable by me being there . . . I can imagine he has other people that he relates to more easily and could turn to if he wants to talk about stuff'. Foster mother joins in the conversation saying: 'Oh, Dave, is that really the impression you have? You can't imagine how your visits do matter to Youri! At bedtime on the evening before he knows you will visit, he will ask a ton of questions. Sometimes, it's about whether he will stay in our family forever, or about how his dad is doing. And the evening after your visit, he will talk about what he heard from you. Once he asked "My dad really wants me to be here with you, doesn't he?" remembering you talked about how ill his father was and how he was starting to accept his son growing up in our family'. Upon hearing this, Dave's initial question quickly disappears and the conversation turns to what could be behind the discrepancy between how Youri presents himself during and outside of Dave's visits.

Youri's rather distant and stand-offish style of relating – and his difficulties in expressing himself – may easily be experienced and interpreted as if relationships don't really matter to him. The social worker's seemingly straightforward request to schedule the home visits when Youri is not home seems to be rooted in feeling uncertain about what these visits actually mean to Youri and contribute to Youri's well-being. It is the therapist picking up on a potential deeper layer of experience underlying Dave's request – and inviting to explore what this experience is about – that helps to start making sense of it. Foster mother sharing her observations and experiences before and after Dave's visits helps to gain a broader perspective. This, in turn, helps Dave to not further disengage from Youri but, instead, helps him and the other members of the network to become genuinely curious about Youri's experiences.

Themes in helping network partners mentalize the child's sense of self and identity

- How to recognise, cherish and scaffold vital sparks when they occur, as well as to recognise a numb/devitalised state of mind and to help the child out of this state
- How to find strategies that scaffold a child's self-awareness (e.g., recognising bodily experiences or finding words that adequately capture the child's sensations and feelings)
- How to be sensitive to issues with regard to a sense of self and identity (e.g., in the domain of hobbies and interests) as well as with regard to the child's history (e.g., early life experiences, being fostered or adopted, aspects of diversity such as integrating elements of their culture of origin) when particular occasions arise
- How to help the child with being a child 'of many parents' (including recognising and containing the child's feelings of loss and mourning and understanding and managing the dynamics of phantasies and cover stories)

Lisa's tendency to fall back on 'lies' and 'cover stories' when confronted with stressful relational dynamics (e.g., her biological mother forgetting about her visiting) and accompanying difficult feelings (e.g., of being abandoned and left all alone; see earlier example), has sensitised the adult carers around her to be especially mindful to how she experiences the visits to her biological mother. Sophie, Lisa's social worker from foster care, is present during these visits as this allows for careful monitoring of these visits as well as for preventing interactions from becoming too negative. At a network meeting, Sophie shares some of her observations of how Lisa treats her biological mum, as these have been puzzling her: 'One moment, she's extremely positive to her mum, all sweet and loyal; the next moment, she looks all anxious and distrustful. . . . Then, I see her mum getting anxious, and withdrawing from Lisa, which only adds to Lisa's distress and distrust. It's really difficult to witness and not get entangled in, especially because I feel so responsible for "fixing" things between them! Last time, I even had to cut the visit short, because things were getting out of control! In the car on our way back to the foster family, Lisa whisperingly asked me: "Mum's really sick, isn't she, in her head, I mean?"' In an attempt to validate Sophie's experience, the therapist responds: 'I can imagine how hard it must be, you feeling stuck in between a child and a mum whom you're both trying to support! I also really appreciate you sharing what has been puzzling you about Lisa's seemingly contradictory approach to her mum'. The therapist then invites the network partners to share their perspectives: 'Could we spend some time to share our thoughts on that?' The group comes to a shared understanding that Lisa seems to be testing the solidity of her mum's commitment to her, with her mum having little or no skills to fall back on to 'survive' Lisa's testing. As the group agrees that there is little margin for progress with Mum, the conversation turns to how Lisa can be helped to start to grasp some of her mother's vulnerabilities and how this can be done in light of Lisa's feeling that she is somehow responsible for her mother's difficulties and her anxieties that she might end up just like her Mum.

For children in long-term foster care, like Lisa, the bond with biological parents is often an arousal-provoking and difficult topic. It confronts them with the loss of the 'idealised' biological parent(s) and the subsequent struggle to somehow balance and integrate the different aspects of their 'biological self' and of their 'fostered self'. The latter requires, for example, one to come to terms with – sometimes overwhelming – feelings of responsibility or even guilt for being 'the cause' of the parent's difficulties ('I must be a really bad child'), and/or profound anxieties that they are doomed to end up in the same way ('I'm mad too'). Although placement in a foster family is, of course, meant to afford the child a better environment to grow up in, it also confronts foster children with what could have been, might have been, or should have been, 'if only'. Successfully negotiating the mourning processes of such profoundly existential nature requires active and mindful support from the adult carers surrounding traumatised children, like in the case of Lisa's network.

As discussed throughout this book, an active awareness of and sensitive approach to all aspects of (sub-)cultural diversity is of particular importance in working with traumatised children in (intercountry) adoptive or foster care placements. This is not only the case in direct work with the child (see Chapter 6) or work with the parents (see Chapter 7) but is equally important in the work with the network. Becoming more aware of and hopefully mitigating instances of (sub-)cultural misattributions or misinterpretations or even systemic racism is a task for any adult carer encountering a child. These instances may involve, for example, not paying sufficient attention and effort to pronouncing the child's – foreign-sounding – name correctly or sighing, 'He's Ethiopian, he can't accept authority' or 'Given her background [referring to the child's mentally ill parent], we can't expect her to be a stable person'.

Concluding thoughts

This chapter on work with the network is the last of three chapters in which we elaborated on each of the three tracks of the present treatment approach to children with complex trauma. Perhaps this order reflects in part our 'natural' inclination as child psychotherapists to first and foremost identify with the child and their suffering. Moreover, network meetings are generally organised at a lower frequency than the direct work with the child and the work with the parents, which may be misinterpreted as this track being less important. Yet, as we hope has been made clear throughout this book as well as in this chapter in particular, in reality this is not the case. In many cases, work in and with the network needs to be done prior to or at least parallel with the work in the other two tracks. In other words, the establishment and maintenance of a mentalizing network is a prerequisite to enable a traumatised child and their parents/carers to make optimal use of the work conducted in both other tracks.

Setting out a frame of regular meetings for the group of network partners, complemented by one-to-one contacts 'on-demand' or when difficult situations occur, is thus of major importance to prevent getting stuck in negative, destructive or even retraumatising interactions. Keeping mentalizing front and centre requires that network partners are kept in mind so as to help them remain open-minded to include trauma- and developmentally relevant information in the way they respond to traumatised children's behaviours and needs.

References

Asen, E., & Fonagy, P. (2021). *Mentalization-based treatment with families*. Routledge.

Bateman, A., & Fonagy, P. (2016). *Mentalization-based treatment for personality disorders: A practical guide*. Oxford University Press.

Bevington, D., Fuggle, P., Cracknell, L., & Fonagy, P. (2017). *Adaptive mentalization-based integrative treatment: A guide for teams to develop systems of care*. Oxford University Press.

Borenstein, L. (2002). The impact of the therapist's curiosity on the treatment process of children and adolescents. *Child and Adolescent Social Work Journal, 19*(5), 337–355. https://doi.org/10.1023/a:1020218413598

Fonagy, P. (2016, November 19). *What is mentalization?* Retrieved from www.youtube.com/watch?v=MJ1Y9zw-n7U

Fonagy, P., Campbell, C., Constantinou, M., Higgitt, A., Allison, E., & Luyten, P. (2021). Culture and psychopathology: An attempt at reconsidering the role of social learning. *Development and Psychopathology*, 1–16. https://doi.org/10.1017/S0954579421000092

Fonagy, P., Luyten, P., Allison, E., & Campbell, C. (2019). Mentalizing, epistemic trust and the phenomenology of psychotherapy. *Psychopathology*, *52*, 94–103. https://doi.org/10.1159/000501526

Oestergaard Hagelquist, J. (2018). *The mentalization guidebook*. Routledge.

Vliegen, N., Tang, E., & Meurs, P. (2023). *Children recovering from complex trauma: From wound to scar*. Routledge.

Winnicott, D. W. (1971). *Therapeutic consultations in child psychiatry*. The Hogarth Press and the Institute of Psychoanalysis.

Chapter 9

Working towards ending

For any child, ending a therapeutic process touches upon the separations and endings in other significant relationships. For example, a child going to kindergarten for the first time, requiring them to separate from parents in the morning, to be reunited at the end of the afternoon but, also, a child losing a grandparent who passes away. The way the child has been able (or not) to negotiate and come to terms with such experiences will impact their abilities to negotiate the process of ending therapy. For children who have experienced complex trauma, ending therapy may be highly emotionally charged and therefore challenging. For these children, having to say goodbye may trigger the feelings and memories that they have built up in reaction to the – sometimes multiple – relationship breakdowns which they have been confronted with earlier in life. As such, the work towards ending as conceptualised in the present treatment approach is to be considered as a new opportunity to work through an ending in better circumstances or, as so aptly phrased by Lanyado (1999), 'so that [a point is reached where] ending therapy acquires the quality of "a page in life" being turned' (p. 375). The ending phase also plays an important role to foster further growth in the child and their carers as developmental catch-up in children with complex trauma may take considerable time, often stretching far beyond the ending of therapy (Fonagy et al., 2021). Although most children will have developed a basic capacity for epistemic trust at the end of treatment, issues with trust in general and epistemic trust in particular may continue to play a role in the child's further development, particularly in contexts that trigger epistemic vigilance. Hence, successful treatment also implies that the child and their carers have sufficiently developed the capacity to deal with these new challenges after the end of treatment.

In this chapter, we first discuss how the work towards ending, as a core element of a time-limited approach, actually starts from the outset of treatment and needs to be thematised throughout the treatment. Following that, we describe the considerations therapists may make, together with the other adult carers around the child, in deciding on and preparing for ending treatment. We then outline how the therapists may shape the ending sessions with the parents, the network and the child. Finally, we formulate some thoughts about options for support after therapy has ended.

DOI: 10.4324/9781003044918-12

A time-limited approach: the ending phase as a core element of treatment

Ending as part of the frame from the outset

As set out in Chapter 4, the present treatment approach has been developed as a medium- to long-term time-limited approach, spanning about 40 to 60 sessions in the direct work with the child. Bringing into motion deeply ingrained patterns of relational and emotional functioning and working through difficult experiences with traumatised children takes time. When, for example, a child has learnt that closing down one's mind and distrusting others are 'good' strategies to survive difficult (relational) experiences, only in small and cautious steps a process can unfold of opening up to engage in the relationship with the therapist, of being able to take in the new relationship as 'holding' and safe (enough) and to share what's on their mind. In this regard, a duration spanning 40 to 60 sessions seems an essential time frame. Moreover, for most elementary school-aged children, bridging the transition from one school year to the next (40 sessions) or approximating two school years (60 sessions) resembles their experience of adult carers entering their life (e.g., teachers at school or coaches in hobbies) and after a year or two, saying goodbye to the 'old' carer and transitioning to new ones.

The nature of a time-limited treatment approach helps all parties involved to keep the finiteness of the treatment in mind. Building in the ending as part of the frame from the outset invites everyone involved to reflect on the theme of ending at set moments. For example, the therapists will need to explicitly discuss this theme at the start of treatment or in the run-up to 40 or 60 sessions. But also throughout the process (e.g., at intermediate assessment times), it will be important to explicitly talk about and refer to the ending theme as it relates to therapeutic gains that have (or have not) been observed. Explicitly thematising 'endings' throughout the treatment offers the opportunity to observe the traumatised child while they practise in one of the most vulnerable domains of life for children whose early life has been marked by separation and loss. In this regard, we aim to help manage such separation experiences in a way that offsets retraumatisation. Moreover, in the work with the child's primary caregivers and with the adult carer network around the family, thematising 'ending' helps in keeping focused on observing growth and development throughout the treatment trajectory.

Therapy as a lab to practise with separation and loss in a non-traumatising way

The ending phase is considered a new phase of treatment, though one that is inherently connected to the prior phases in treatment. Whereas the ending phase can be seen as a more definite experience with separation and loss, a rather long-term treatment such as the one described in this book affords myriad opportunities to practise with surviving and coping with 'smaller' separation experiences. First, there is the transition from waiting room to playroom and vice versa at each session that can be considered as small but continual windows into a child's and a carer's ability to manage the movements in and out of significant relationships. Furthermore, a 40- to 60-session trajectory rarely proceeds without any planned (e.g., holiday) or unplanned (e.g., illness or other unforeseen circumstances) breaks. As described in Chapter 6, such breaks in treatment continuity often evoke attachment and separation issues in children who have experienced complex trauma and thus require careful attending by the therapist. The same holds for supporting parents (see also Chapter 7) and other adult carers (see also Chapter 8) in their abilities to help the child to 'survive' and manage moments of separation which occur in daily life at home, at school or in another context. As such, carefully observing how child, parents and network partners practise with coping with all the small moments of separation and loss that a therapy process naturally offers informs the therapists on how to scaffold relational capacities in the child and in the people surrounding the child and the family. Moreover, it is also informative towards considerations about ending treatment (see later discussion). In this sense, working on and towards ending with a traumatised child is about facilitating a natural and a growth-promoting separation experience (Wittenberg, 1999), that is, offering the child a new and profound life experience of coming to terms with the painfulness of bringing an intimate relationship to a close without this being the most intimate relationships with their primary caregivers.

In the work with traumatised children, where the fear of new traumatising events is particularly present in the mind of the child, their parents and other adult carers in the network, including the therapists, actively attempting to avoid retraumatisation is a particular issue of concern. As discussed earlier, the built-in time frame of a time-limited treatment approach aims to safeguard the child's unfolding of and engaging in the therapeutic process. As such, it increases the opportunity for the ending phase to function as a critically growth-promoting event for both child and parents alike that can help to consolidate the gains that have been made in therapy (see later). For traumatised children in particular, it also aims to decrease the risk of this ending becoming yet another retraumatising discontinuity in their lives.

Embedding ending as a significant theme in the therapy process reduces the risk of premature termination (Ogrodniczuk et al., 2005) – an ending dictated by other circumstances than the assessment that treatment has reached its goals. The risk of such impingements from other factors is much greater in psychotherapeutic treatment of children compared to therapeutic work with adults. This is not surprising, as the child is part of a family, resulting in parents having a major voice in any important family issue, including starting and ending treatment. Parents' views on problems in the family and how best to 'solve' them, as well as different family pressures in terms of financial or time constraints, can play an important role in deciding when therapy should stop (Lanyado, 1999). Moreover, both more and less conscious beliefs, expectations, feelings and opinions parents may hold about the treatment might lead to an unexpected premature termination of treatment. Other situations may relate to the child wanting to end therapy in reaction to a – planned or unplanned – break which they are having trouble coping with, or parents may want to end therapy because they are disappointed at the perceived lack of progress. Of course it is important for therapists to be open to questions about whether the therapy is helpful and whether it is the right option for the child at this particular moment. But with children who have experienced complex trauma, the therapist also needs to be especially mindful about preventing a premature or unplanned ending, because the retraumatising impact on the child is potentially great.

Helping parents and other carers to observe and understand growth and change

A time-limited treatment approach with a planned ending, such as the one presented in this book, is based on the assumption that change and growth are probable and feasible to take place within this set framework. This, by no means, exempts therapists from their responsibility to assess whether growth and change in child and parents are sufficient to end treatment or, rather, not sufficient, requiring to consider what else may be needed. So, again, working towards a timely ending does not start in the ending phase but needs to take hold already during the course of treatment both in the therapists' minds and the support the therapists can offer parents and other carers in becoming good observers of developmental change in the child (see also Chapter 5). The work with parents and the network, if conducted well enough, offers myriad opportunities to reflect together on the child's ways of being and behaving and any growth or changes therein. A good understanding of what growth and change may look like can help parents and network members in thinking about the therapeutic processes and thus be crucially important to inform any decision about continuing or ending therapy. For example, for some children, the ability to show that they are upset when a separation occurs might be understood as an important marker of emotional growth, even if such upset may be hard for the adults to cope with. So, how do therapists help parents and other carers think about and decide when treatment has been enough?

When has treatment been enough? Considering growth and change in light of further development

In general, an 'increased readiness and a capacity to change, to grow in relationships, to be more open to life' (Lanyado, 1999, p. 365) and to keep mentalizing abilities 'online' in the face of new challenges (Midgley et al., 2017) are important indicators to consider with regard to ending treatment. One could say that 'when child and parents are able to get on with life in an ordinary way' (Ryz & Wilson, 1999, p. 401) or the child is now able to make use of the help available to them in their ordinary life, then the overarching aim of treatment has been achieved. But what does this translate to specifically in the work with children who have experienced complex trauma, and how can we support parents, network members and the child in making the relevant considerations?

 Mei-Lan seems to have made good progress in therapy: she is less at the mercy of her inner turmoil, better able to control her own impulses; consequently, the relationship with her adoptive parents is less turbulent. Yet Mei-Lan is still moody and temperamental at times

– 'Mei-Lan remains Mei-Lan', her adoptive father says with a mix of warmth and resignation. In this phase, ending therapy has become a theme in the work with Mei-Lan and her adoptive parents. In talking and thinking together about perhaps letting the treatment come to an end in the near future, the therapists agree with Mei-Lan and her adoptive parents that a joint session to further discuss this would be a good idea. In preparing for this session, the child therapist invites Mei-Lan to talk about which things Mei-Lan feels have already improved. She also talks with Mei-Lan about what she still struggles with – also in relation to her adoptive parents – and how she would like others to support her with these things. Having begun to explore this with her therapist, Mei-Lan decides she wants to share some of her feelings about being a child 'of two countries' with her adoptive parents. To-gether with her therapist she makes a drawing of two countries: one in Europe and one in Asia. In the joint session, making use of the draw-ing and supported by her therapist, Mei-Lan can share something of her feelings of 'not really belonging anywhere'. Her adoptive parents listen carefully and respond that they really want to give her space to be who she is and to become who she wants to be and that they want to help her where possible. Mei-Lan says: 'I know, but you don't always have to ask so many questions; sometimes, I want to figure things out on my own'. Her adoptive mother replies warmly: 'What I've learnt here, Mei-Lan, is to really look at you more when I want to know how you're doing, instead of always asking you how you are'.

Returning to the focus formulation: considering change in the relevant developmental domains

A first important consideration for therapists to make, together with parents and carers, is whether the treatment has brought about change and movement in the child in terms of several of the developmental domains as agreed upon in the focus formulation (which ideally has been adapted throughout the treatment; see Chapter 5). In addition to therapeutic growth in the child, it is also important to consider whether parents and the network have grown in supporting the child with their difficulties and scaffolding their development in these domains. In Table 9.1, we summarise some general signs of growth in each of the four developmental domains, in which we keep in mind aspects of both process and content.

In the sessions described earlier, Mei-Lan shows her abilities to express important aspects of her inner world. She is able to represent an essential aspect of 'being Mei-Lan' as being a child of two countries, and she is able to express her longing for space to find out who she is 'on her own'. Her adoptive parents and the therapists, remembering how things were with Mei-Lan – very 'clingy' and controlling – at the beginning of treatment, consider this as a huge leap forward.

Table 9.1 Signs of therapeutic growth in child and carers in the four developmental domains

Therapeutic growth in the child's development	Therapeutic growth in the carers' development
1. The child has developed or regained an ability to play and to express and represent aspects of their inner world in more mature ways (process). The child is able to engage with themes, images or stories that fit well with how they feel and think about themselves, others and life experiences, facilitating sharing and feeling connected to others (content).	Parents and other carers have developed a trauma-informed understanding of the child's difficulties in expressing and representing aspects of their inner world and an ability to support the child in this domain (process). They can understand the child's inner experiences, can communicate with the child about thoughts and feelings and can mirror what they understand about their child (content).
2. The child has developed or regained an ability to regulate their arousal, affects and emotions in a more age-appropriate way and/or is able to make use of a mature adult to do so. The child is able to recognise and manage trauma-related dysregulations (e.g., fight, flight and freeze mechanisms; process). Particular feelings of warmth and love, as well as of anxiety, anger, sadness or mourning (content) can be contained and processed.	Parents and other carers have developed a trauma-informed understanding of the child's difficulties in regulating arousal and expressing affects and emotions in appropriate ways and skills to co-regulate the child when needed (process). They can understand and contain the particular dynamics of the child's world of feeling and thinking (content) and can be growth-promoting partners with regard to these dynamics.
3. The child has developed a broader range of capacities to relate to adult carers and peers in new, more mature/ flexible/positive/reciprocal ways; process). The child can bear and even enjoy relating to others and starts to understand how they feel within relationships and think about relational experiences (content).	Parents and other carers have developed a trauma-informed understanding of the child's difficulties in relating to others and skills to support the child's relational functioning (process). They can understand the child's particular relational dynamics and can support the child in feeling and thinking about how they experience relationships (content).
4. The child has developed better ways of recognising inner (e.g., bodily) experiences, a better (more positive and coherent) sense of self and identity and better ways of coping with questions about their life history (process). The child goes through life in touch with what makes them feel vital and content and discovers and explores these important domains of life (in particular hobbies and interests; content). The child is able to engage in discovering who they are, what they dream about in life, and what it means to have their particular life history.	Parents and other carers have developed a trauma-informed understanding of the child's difficulties with regard to a sense of self and identity and abilities to support the child in different aspects of this domain (process). They understand the child's particular interests and dreams, take a curious and interested stance towards the child's drives and dreams and support the child's choices (content).

It is important for therapists to remember that therapeutic growth is not to be equated to 'curing the whole of the child, once and for all'. In working with children who have experienced complex trauma, therapeutic gains are to be defined in terms of dynamic movement, rather than in terms of absolute and well-established progress in every domain of development. Progress is about being able to keep travelling on the route without the therapist's presence, not about having arrived at some 'final destination' where the impact of early trauma has been erased. When treatment has helped the child to make substantial progress in one or several domains in which the child's development had previously been stuck and the child is mostly able – often with support of the parents or another carer – to access these new abilities even in the face of new challenges, then treatment can be considered to have been 'effective'. In Mei-Lan's case, for example, we can see the largest improvement in her capacities to convey aspects about her inner world. We also see improvements in terms of abilities to regulate arousal and emotions and to relate to others. Yet, Mei-Lan's regulatory and relational 'attainments' remain vulnerable under stress, although moments of dysregulation are less frequent and last less long, as her adoptive parents have been able to experience at home. As to Mei-Lan's sense of self and identity, all adults involved realise that there is still a long way to go.

This also means that it is important not only to look at whether changes for the better have occurred but also to assess the extent to which these changes have been somewhat consolidated. Have the changes been acquired rather newly and precariously, or has the child had time to practise these new acquirements at several occasions? Have changes been 'owned' by the child; does it feel that these are 'theirs' yet? Sometimes, changes occur in the playroom before they can be observed in the family or the family relationships. Then, we can infer that the child is still experimenting with new ways of experiencing, relating and behaving (e.g., asking for help, thinking about being a fostered or adopted child) within the therapeutic relationship and setting before they are ready to try out these skills outside the therapy room. In such instances, the child therapist's assessment and collaboration with the parent worker will be of particular importance. At other times, the child will first show emerging change in the home environment or in another context of their daily life outside the therapy room (e.g., doing better in school). Then, the work conducted by the parent worker with the parents and the network will be particularly informative in considering ending or continuing treatment. In any case, the importance of a close collaboration between both therapists, conducting the work in all three tracks, throughout the treatment (see Chapter 4) thus extends to the work towards ending (and possibly beyond: see later).

The sessions described above also show how Mei-Lan's adoptive mother has become better able to respect Mei-Lei's wishes to do things at her own pace and not be too intrusive in her desire to be reassured that she is 'okay'. From the parent worker's perspective, remembering how Mother anxiously wanted to know everything about what was in her daughter's mind and wanted to help with each minor problem, this is to be considered a huge change in her attitude towards her adopted daughter and her vulnerabilities.

In mentalization-based trauma-informed work with parents and the network, we aim to foster and facilitate growth in the child's carers in a way that supports adult carers in better meeting the child's developmental needs. In other words, we ideally want to see growth in adults happening, affording them the skills and resources necessary to stand side-by-side with their children as they develop (see Table 9.1).

In this context, parental growth has a lot to do with the growing abilities to contain and to live with their own parental concerns and anxieties, for example, in facing behaviour that attests to 'other-than-normative' development. The emerging awareness that the child being in treatment and the parents being counselled does not result in a carefree family life often sets in motion a process towards a more profound acceptance of the reality of being parents to a more vulnerably developing child, as well as a more adequate containment of the child's particularities. This changed perspective and attitude is a prerequisite for a new and more appropriate balance between 'loving and holding their child in heart and mind' and 'letting go' of the child (Lanyado, 1999, p. 358) who needs to learn when to seek the parent's presence and help and when to rely on themselves, as in Mei-Lan's case.

Looking ahead: assessing the capacities for further growth and change beyond therapy

Aside from assessing whether the anticipated changes in the child's and family's functioning have taken hold to a sufficient extent, therapists will also need to consider whether parents and other important carers have been able to develop enough capacities to scaffold further growth in the child (in ways they possibly could not at the time of referral). This is important so as to increase the chances that therapeutic gains can be sustained and built upon even when therapeutic support has ended. This may be about carers' ability to observe the child (e.g., noticing when stress becomes too high and difficulties will probably emerge), to reflect on what the child needs and to be able to observe what is going on within themselves, in response to the child or possibly due to their own issues. For parents in particular, this also includes their ability to keep mentalizing 'online' even in the face of relational difficulties with the child and to manage mentalizing breakdowns on their own. Are they able to manage misunderstandings and to repair the relationship when a disruption has occurred? Are parents still in need of the therapist's mentalizing mind when new events or challenges emerge, or rather, do they feel confident in responding to new challenges and are they able to find own creative solutions?

Especially important in this regard with traumatised children is the child's ability to benefit from the positive and constructive caregiving relationships. Therefore, the therapist will need to consider whether the child is better able to draw on the support offered by parents and other carers in the service of further recovery and growth. In Mei-Lan's case, for example, her adoptive parents' accepting and warm approach was an important foundation, but their increased curiosity and openness to Mei-Lan's own thoughts and feelings attested to their ability to keep her mind in mind. In the same vein, Mei-Lan's openness to share vulnerable aspects of her inner world with her adoptive parents bears witness to her growing sense of trust in her relationship with them.

When life events happen: transforming an unanticipated ending into a more or less planned one

Aside from the processes of change and growth that take place *within* treatment, it happens that external factors in the life of the child, the family or the therapist play a role in thinking about and shaping the ending phase. Child development does not always unfold as expected, and life is seldom completely predictable and plannable. This means that we sometimes have to negotiate an ending phase that we experience as 'not the best timing' when viewed from the child's point of view, yet taking the whole family circumstances into account, ending therapy may still be a wise decision. For example, parents may be satisfied with the progress the child has already made and feel burdened by the prospect of continuing the treatment, while the therapist feels that the child is still intensely engaged in the therapeutic process. This may be the case when the most difficult issues with regard to behavioural regulation have subsided at home, resulting in a smoother and more enjoyable family life, but in therapy, the child only recently and cautiously started to express difficult feelings about being a looked after child. After having discussed pros and cons, parents decide to end therapy because of the demanding combination of busy family and professional lives. In some cases, it may be better to respect the parents' decision and agree on an ending, in order to preserve what has been achieved, rather than insist on continuing, at risk of losing the parents' real engagement as well as the developmental gain that has been achieved. Nonetheless, the child therapist can rationally agree but emotionally face feelings of sadness or disappointment, meanwhile having to contain the child's complex feelings about this kind of ending. Other situations of having to end therapy at a time that was unanticipated at the outset may have to do with the therapist themselves, for example, the therapist moving house and/or changing jobs.

Regardless of the source of the unanticipated ending, this 'may forcibly remind the therapist of the vulnerability and helplessness of the child patient in determining his or her own life' (Lanyado, 1999, p. 363). Moreover, when therapy has to end at a time which feels 'too soon' in terms of the child's therapeutic process, the child may also try to cope with the feelings of powerlessness and helplessness by projecting these feelings into the therapist (Lanyado, 1999). These processes may be particularly powerful in working with traumatised children, whose repeated experiences of lack of control over what happens to them in life may be strongly empathised with by the therapist. This may, in turn, further compromise the therapist's ability to support the child and the family in negotiating an ending to the therapeutic process in a way that can be experienced as 'good-enough'. Paradoxically, in such circumstances, it will be an especially crucial task for the therapist to transform, to some extent, an unplanned ending into a more planned ending (Lanyado, 1999). In practice, this often comes down to the therapist(s) trying to convey to parents the importance of some sessions – even if it is just one – to end the work both with the child as well as with the parents themselves. This will help to somewhat soften the blow of an abrupt ending, making it possible to have some sense of closure, by touching upon important themes that form part of a 'normal' ending phase (see later discussion) but in an necessarily accelerated time frame.

Working towards saying goodbye

When the natural processes of ending become realistically imaginable

As touched upon earlier, thinking and talking about ending mostly form part of the work with parents much earlier than it comes to the fore in the direct work with the child. In the work with parents and with the network, changes and growth in the child which carers are able to observe and experience are often subject of conversation as treatment progresses. As such, questions about ending, or rather, about a potential need to proceed and what can be expected from further work, often follow naturally in such conversations. This is rather different from the direct work with the child. When a child becomes attached to their therapist and starts to experience things going better in life, this does not always translate promptly into an awareness about 'no longer needing therapy' or 'wanting to end'. Considerations and decisions about ending are often made in conversations among the caregiving adults (parents and network, including the therapists) before the child therapist introduces this topic to the child. In working with children who have experienced complex trauma, it is particularly important for the caregiving adults to have reached a shared perspective on ending, so as to avoid any disagreements from negatively impacting the child's experience of ending treatment.

This shared perspective mainly concerns it 'being a good time to consider ending treatment', based on the considerations described in the previous section. The specific modalities of the ending phase (how much time, how many sessions, etc.) can still be thought and talked about, also informed by the child's perspective. In our experience, in thinking about when precisely to let the treatment come to an end, parents and other carers often make use of rather 'natural' transitions in the child's or the family's life. Sometimes, someone suggests to end 'around the coming summer (Easter/Christmas) break' or 'at the end of September, once the child has got used to the new school/teacher'. There are no rigid rules to let the end of treatment coincide with another ending or, rather, to continue for a bit to help the child across the transition, but offering these possibilities as 'food for thought' may help adults and children feel and think about what would fit their needs best. For example, a child may just want to take the leap: 'I want to make a new start, and I want to do this alone and all at once', and the adult carers feel quite confident that this may be within the child's abilities, while another child may feel rather anxious about making several transitions at once and feel supported by the idea of having the therapist to fall back on until the new situation feels familiar enough before letting go of therapy. It is often only when the theme of ending treatment has become 'real' in the minds of adult carers that reflection turns to the more concrete aspects, such as the timing and the number of sessions to end treatment.

Helping parents to have confidence in their relationship with the child, to trust in themselves as parents and to rely on the network

For parents, once ending treatment becomes a real possibility, myriad mixed feelings are likely to come to the fore. For example, there may be a sense of relief that the child 'is doing well enough' to end treatment and that the child's weekly treatment sessions will no longer burden the family's time and (where relevant) financial resources. On the other hand, there are mostly also concerns or even anxiety about whether the child and the family will be able to sustain the growth and change that has been observed when the therapist will no longer be at their side. Creating space for and supporting parents to work through these feelings is an important task for the therapist in their final sessions with the parents. It may be helpful to revisit parents' experiences of 'knowing the child better' or of 'feeling more connected to and having a better relationship with the child'.

As treatment has progressed, Youri and his foster mother have been able to find better ways to relate to each other. What was very helpful and reassuring to his foster mother was to observe Youri's growing abilities to express what is on his mind and what troubles him. She refers to his ability to talk about a sense of 'being different' from other members of the family, even though everybody wishes for him to 'just be part of the family'. Youri's foster mother adds that she thinks that being better able to express what is occupying him has helped Youri to feel and act less angrily and to have fewer tantrums.

While Mother seems reassured, Youri's relationship with his foster father remains more difficult. Youri holds huge expectations towards his foster father and reacts deeply disappointed when his foster father cannot manage to fetch him from school, for example. Fortunately, they share a big passion for cars, which provides the foster father opportunities to have his own positive moments with Youri. Being able to find their own ways to feel connected to Youri, both foster carers can cautiously start thinking about ending the treatment.

As endings approach, it may be helpful to remind parents how they too have grown as parents, for example, in helping their child to calm down again in moments of dysregulation or in their ability to remain calm and respond in a mindful way even in the face of very stressful situations. Such experiences of having been able to find solutions for problems in the absence of the parent worker can very much empower parents of traumatised children. It helps when the parent worker explicitly validates this. In this regard, it may also be reassuring to parents that they will not really 'be without' the therapist's support, as they will be able to rely on the things they've been able to take away from the meetings with the therapist. In the same vein, it may be important for the therapist to explicitly talk with parents about the network around their family that will remain available to them when needed or to think with them how they will manage things if the network does not provide the support they would ideally want.

In these final sessions with parents, moments of looking back and looking forward often alternate. Looking back may involve revisiting positive as well as difficult or negative moments during parent work, as a way of marking them. What, from the parents' perspective, has been helpful? And what have they found lacking? Which objectives that parents had hoped for or that were agreed upon do they feel have not been achieved? It is important that therapists are able to explore such disappointments in a non-defensive way, in order to help move towards a more realistic ending. Looking forward, in turn, may involve thinking and talking about what will be gained in ending therapy as well as what parents feel will be lost. Moreover, looking forward with parents of traumatised children should also include thinking and talking together about the possibility of 'old' problems being re-activated or new difficulties emerging in a later phase of life. Which people or services are available to the family to reach out to? How will they respond? What therapeutic support can look like for families of traumatised children after treatment has ended will be discussed in a later section.

In the shorter term, it may also be important to alert parents as well as the network that the child may temporarily exhibit more symptomatic or problematic behaviour again in reaction to the news that carers 'are thinking about whether it would be good to end therapy'. This will hopefully help parents or other carers not only not to panic should this happen but also to feel invited to bring this to the conversation.

Negotiating the concrete timing of ending with the child

As discussed earlier, when the theme of ending treatment forms part of the adult conversation and agreement about a possible 'good' timing is growing, this topic is also introduced in the work with the child, so as to allow the child to actively participate in thinking about what feels like a 'good' time from their perspective. Once everyone agrees on a concrete moment or period to let the treatment come to an end, the therapist invites the child to give their perspective on how the final sessions should be organised and shaped.

Children may have different ways of reacting to the idea of ending the therapy (see later discussion), but as a rule of thumb, the present treatment model adheres to three to five sessions with the child, on average, in the ending phase of therapy. The rationale for this is to, again, afford the child enough time to work through the feelings and tasks at hand in having to say goodbye to a person who has become significant in the child's life, at a pace that will allow these processes to take hold instead of stretching these in an unfruitful way. This being said, the therapist can think and talk together with the child whether three sessions would be a 'good' amount of time to have left together or, rather, whether five sessions would seem better and why. The therapist also tries to gain insight into the child's perspective on the interval of these final sessions. Some children may prefer to keep the weekly frequency, so as to hold on to a familiar rhythm and perhaps also not to 'unnecessarily' stretch the inevitable painfulness of the process of ending. Other children may indicate a wish to lower the frequency of the final sessions compared to previous phases in treatment, so as to 'phase out' more gradually. The therapist may also need to touch upon the topic of whether the child feels that 'booster sessions' (see later discussion) would be helpful.

As with parents, thinking and talking about ending treatment may trigger many mixed feelings in the child, which will colour both the content and the process of expressing their perspective on ending therapy. In inviting the child to share this perspective, the therapist will thus not simply follow this blindly but will try to consider what the child's underlying motivations are to prefer one 'format' of ending over another or to want one way and discard another. Often, such considerations will require the child therapist to confer with the parent worker and the network so as to increase the chances of following the child's proposal in the aspects that are growth-promoting and to decrease the risk of colluding in a child's avoidance, for example.

 When invited by the therapist to share his perspective on ending treatment, Youri gets rather anxious. He 'really wants five sessions, not just three!' and asks to come fortnightly instead of weekly 'to have more time'. Having been reassured by the therapist that that could be an option, Youri's mind wanders to how coming to therapy has been for him: he talks about 'how it was to be here'. He surprises his therapist when he hesitantly starts telling her about the very first time he entered the treatment centre: 'It was such a strange and large building; I thought it was a kind of an "institution" or an orphanage, and that I had to stay and sleep here'. The therapist is touched by the way Youri has kept these thoughts and anxieties to himself, leaving him to grapple with them alone for all this time. Nevertheless, she is glad that he is able to share them with her now.

Looking back on his therapy, Youri refers to it as 'the place where I've learnt to talk', and his 'artwork' (see later discussion) is a drawing of the small table in the playroom where he often sat down when he wanted to talk about something. 'Do you know I went to Mary (the school psychologist) when I felt scared in the playground? It was my own idea, and I did it completely on my own!' Youri says, underlining his acquired capacities to talk about experiences.

In these last sessions, Youri seems to savour how it was and is to 'be here' and experiment with how it will be to 'no longer be here'. Unsurprisingly, Youri explicitly embraced the idea of holding 'booster sessions' (see later discussion) every six months for the coming two years.

In appealing for and being granted 'more time', Youri is afforded some sense of control over the end of treatment. This helps to contain his anxiety in the face of the therapeutic relationship coming to an end. He is able to show what is happening inside him and even to process some of the initial anxieties when he was taken to this new place (the treatment centre) and a new adult in his life (the therapist). Keeping a line open to his therapist by making use of booster sessions seems helpful for him to transfer what he has learnt from her to other relationships as for instance with the school psychologist. His 'having learnt to talk' and being able to transfer that capability to other situations is to be considered an important achievement, which the therapist wants to validate by agreeing to Youri's 'terms' in ending treatment.

Shaping the ending sessions with the child

When therapist and child have found agreement on the timing (number and interval) of the final sessions, the therapist invites the child to think and talk about how they would like to spend these final sessions together. The child's response, again, provides a window into what 'saying goodbye' means to the child. For example, a child may want to 'have a party' with the therapist, suggesting that they may prefer to keep positive feelings at the centre, perhaps in an attempt to keep more negative feelings (e.g., sadness, anger) at bay. The same child may then be quite insistent that the therapist should be the one organising the party and bringing all the goodies. Or by contrast, the child may present as quite collaborative in thinking about how to organise the party. It is up to the therapist to listen with a sensitive ear to how such expressions reveal something about how the child is trying to make sense of the impending separation so as to inform a therapeutic response.

In taking into account the child's perspective, the therapist tries to balance this with also sufficiently marking the significance of bringing an important relationship to a close. The therapist may do this by inviting the child to consider what coming to therapy has meant to them (looking back) and what no longer coming to therapy means to them (looking forward), as Youri's therapist did (see previous vignette). A helpful way to do this can be to invite the child to craft something that expresses something that has been central to them in their experience of therapy.

When invited by the therapist to craft something about therapy, Jemal initially responds with rolling his eyes in an exaggerated way. The therapist has come to know this as Jemal's way to show his difficulties in expressing his feelings as well as engaging in an emotionally charged activity. She warmly but firmly holds him to the task: 'I know and can see that it's not your favourite activity, but I think it really is important to think a bit about what therapy has meant before we say goodbye'. Jemal decides to draw 'The Game of Therapy', after the boardgame 'The Game of Life' which he often played in the course of his treatment. In this game, each square a player lands on requires them to make a decision about their life (e.g., go to college or start a job, get married, have a baby). Jemal copies the boardgame and names the squares of his therapy boardgame as phases in his relationship with the therapist: 'being together without talking', 'playing together', 'daring to ask something', 'having fun together', etc. It is an intense work for him. The therapist is surprised at the accuracy with which Jemal expresses how the relational dynamics between them evolved. It takes Jemal two sessions to craft the boardgame; when the work is done, he seems to decide that therapy has finished. During the three final sessions, Jemal wants to play his boardgame, yet is rather stand-offish towards the therapist. Unsurprisingly, given how Jemal manages difficult feelings, he doesn't want to make use of any 'booster sessions' (see later discussion).

In his typical avoidant style, Jemal manages to express in an image how he gradually started to trust and became attached to his therapist as a new adult caregiving figure in his life. In his personalised 'The Game of Life' boardgame, Jemal expresses how he experienced the relationship develop, from distant and silent, towards feeling safer and daring to ask the therapist questions and towards a warm and positive bond in which they could have fun together. The therapist's notes of these sessions read: 'Jemal struggled with this task, but during the two sessions we worked on his game, there was an authentic and positive contact between us'. Becoming attached to an adult carer seems to have become a more natural and positive experience to Jemal. On the other hand, Jemal's way of saying goodbye also shows his remaining difficulties with experiencing a sense of closeness, as he feels the need to distance himself again from difficult feelings as the end nears.

Similarly, the final sessions are a good time for the therapist to invite the child to think and talk together about what they want to happen to the contents of the child's personal drawer or box. What does the child want to take with them? What do they want the therapist to keep and care for? What does the child want to discard of? Again, in listening with a sensitive ear to what the child expresses, the therapist can try to discern the child's feelings and experiences of having to say goodbye.

In the final sessions, Lisa expresses intense mixed feelings about ending therapy. She starts 'negotiating': 'No, no, we don't have only three sessions left, we still have five', 'No, I don't want to stop at the Easter break, I want to stop when it's summer holiday', as if trying to keep in control of the impending loss. At the same time, Lisa also proudly talks about looking forward to the new school she will attend and expresses with excitement the new plans she is making and events that are ahead. Moments of regression, during which she lies on the floor not knowing what to do, alternate with browsing through her well-stocked box, to choose what she wants to take home and what she wants to leave behind.

When invited to craft something about her therapy experiences, Lisa immediately knows what she wants to make: a jigsaw puzzle with each puzzle piece referring to a part of herself. Other moments get filled with going through her 'book of life' which she put together in the course of treatment with the therapist. 'It is as if we are puzzling together Lisa in these sessions', the therapist noted afterwards.

It seems as if for Lisa, the prospect of ending triggers the intense mixed and overwhelming feelings at referral; as if all the stormy feelings overwhelm her again in the nutshell of the five final sessions.

For Lisa, the phase of ending therapy is characterised by browsing through mixed experiences and 'sorting things out'. Feelings of 'missing' and sadness about loss are mixed with feelings of profound confusion, of being proud about doing things alone or about proceeding towards a new phase in life, as well as of enduring feelings of connectedness and warmth about feeling seen, heard and understood.

In the same realm, the therapist should consider whether it may be important to give the child something tangible that refers to the therapy, to function as a 'transitional object' (Winnicott, 1958). This may be something from the playroom, that symbolises something that has become highly significant to the child in the course of treatment or a picture of it. It may also be a card with a personal message from the therapist to the child, or a card to remind the child of the agreed upon 'booster sessions' (see later). As mentioned earlier, sometimes, the child will want to leave behind something tangible for the therapist. For example, a work from their personal drawer or box or something they crafted during the final sessions. In all these cases, it will be important for the therapist not only to acknowledge the child's 'gift' but also to try to explore with the child what it means to them and to also acknowledge what the work with the child has meant to the therapist. With regard to the latter, the therapist may, for example, share something about how she got to know the child or about how she experienced working together. What is shared touches upon positive experiences (e.g., 'I'm glad we've got to work together') or on what one wishes for the child in the future (e.g., 'I really hope and am confident you will do well at home and at school'). The therapist may also refer to difficulties that have been overcome (e.g., 'Remember how anxious you were any time your mum left? I'm so glad to see how confident you are now') or to the help available when the child faces new challenges (e.g., 'I'm sure your mum and dad will know when you need help'). Finally, it may important for the therapist to explicitly voice something about the mixed feelings about saying goodbye (e.g., 'I'll miss our sessions together, but I'm glad you and your family are doing well enough that you don't need to come anymore'), especially with children who struggle to acknowledge one or both ends of the spectrum of feelings.

Therapeutic support after therapy has ended

In the most ideal situation, therapy did not merely help the child and their family to overcome the difficulties they were referred for but also helped them to develop or re-access the skills necessary to face new challenges and to make use of the help available in their day-to-day lives. For some children, this will be the case. Yet, with children who have experienced complex trauma in particular, therapeutic gains and attainments are often of a more precarious nature, particularly given that new challenges may act as trauma triggers and activate non-mentalizing modes (see Chapter 2). Therefore, therapeutic support after therapy has ended often needs to be considered, as it 'may play a crucial role in "augmenting the gains" of the work – providing a secure base to return to both in times of need and quite simply in terms of confirmation of the importance of what has taken place between them' (Lanyado, 1999, p. 366). In general, post-therapy therapeutic support as conceptualised in the treatment model set out in this book can be offered in three possible ways: 'prolonged' work with the parents and/or the network after ending the direct work with the child, a period of 'booster sessions' built in as part of the ending phase or a renewed phase of treatment later on. For some traumatised children, something other or more than the three-track approach may be indicated.

'Prolonged' work with the parents and/or the network

Sometimes, the direct work with the child comes to an end but the work with parents and/or the network continues for a while. This may happen when parents still feel a bit uncertain as to their ability to sustain the therapeutic gains in the absence of the therapist's mentalizing mind. The therapist may then offer additional sessions to parents to follow up on how the child is evolving after ending treatment, to support parents with any potentially regressive behaviour or other symptomatic deterioration in the child in reaction to the ending of treatment and to follow up on whether things are going well enough. Continuing the work with the parents for a bit may also be a good option for families with a child on the threshold of a life event (e.g., changing schools) or entering secondary school/adolescence, where new (emotional) challenges for both child and adults are to be expected. If parents are doubtful about their abilities to handle this new step and to meet the challenges of this new phase in their child's and family life, it may be helpful to remain in sight for a while.

Booster sessions as a safety net

The option of booster sessions as a 'safety net' is a consideration the therapist has in mind when talking about ending treatment. Particularly when a child or a family expresses that ending – however agreed upon – seems to imply that things are 'going too fast' or 'beyond control'. Booster sessions can then help to make 'saying good-bye' more gradual and in that sense seem more 'controllable'. With families who, according to the therapist's assessment, may benefit from such a safety net, booster sessions may be agreed upon as part of the ending phase. Booster sessions with a child may take the form of three or four sessions, once every three or six months or of a 'five-rides pass', offering the child the opportunity to request a booster session when they feel they need one. In Youri's case (see vignette earlier), it seemed important to him to be able to come see the therapist twice a year, bringing his sketchbook and talking about 'how things have been' and 'how his life has been going' since he last saw her. Similarly, booster sessions for parents may be scheduled once a school term for the next year or so or may take the form of five sessions 'on-demand'.

A new phase of treatment in the face of new developmental challenges

Taking into account the severe developmental problems some traumatised children struggle with, new developmental challenges or life events may destabilise the child and/or the family again – temporarily or in a more enduring way. The reassurance offered to parents that services will be available to their family in the future when 'old' or new issues emerge can be particularly stress-reducing for parents of children whose development remains vulnerable. Moreover, a new phase of treatment may be indicated when the parents and/or the child feel that the problems are exceeding their skills and resources.

This may be the case when the child's developmental level only allowed them to work through particular aspects of trauma and developmental problems and the working-through of further aspects and problems and/or at more advanced levels will require further psychotherapeutic work when the child has acquired more advanced developmental capacities. Developmental problems and traumatic experiences can be worked through to the extent of the age- and developmentally appropriate abilities of the child. A seven-year-old child, like Mei-Lan (see earlier vignette), can have been working hard in psychotherapy on regulation and attachment issues, to the extent of her seven-year-old cognitive and emotional abilities. Children often reach a plateau in their therapeutic process and may need time to integrate what has been accomplished. At a later stage in life, issues may present themselves related to the child's early traumatic experiences, causing inappropriate behaviours or symptoms to (re-)emerge, calling for further therapy tailored to their current developmental level and needs (e.g., identity issues).

Another – sometimes intertwined – indication for a renewed phase of treatment may be when the extent of the child's continuing developmental vulnerability will likely severely compromise the successful negotiation of new developmental tasks. This may be the case in adolescence, with its developmental challenges particularly taxing to the young person with a complex trauma history as well as to their family. For example, the high demands with regard to self-regulation and autonomy needed to comfortably negotiate secondary school may give rise to a renewed request for therapeutic support.

> In early adolescence, about two years after treatment ended, Jemal's adoptive parents reconsult, because of difficulties in secondary school. Jemal rebels against authority, leading to difficult relationships with teachers and refuses to do homework, resulting in repeated detentions. In elementary school, Jemal's teacher knew him very well and always seemed to find ways to reconnect with him, again and again, and to overcome any difficulties. At his new secondary school, Jemal's conduct has made him lose any and all credibility with the different teachers, who expect much more autonomy and lose patience quickly. He gets caught in cycles of behaving badly, getting punished and behaving badly again justified by 'everybody always being angry at him anyway'. This re-enactment of traumatic experiences leads to his parents feeling overwhelmed by a sense of losing control over Jemal's behaviour and of helplessness in their attempts to 'negotiate' between their adoptive son and the school. At this point, Jemal seems to be almost unreachable stemming from the re-activation of profound epistemic mistrust.
>
> Meetings with the parents and the school are set up, in which Jemal's academic trajectory can be reconsidered. The school psychologist succeeds in gaining Jemal's trust, and he tells her about experiencing the current set-up to be too demanding and difficult and about the feeling that 'there's no point' to being engaged in school and doing homework since he will 'fail anyway'. Everyone agrees that transitioning to a more technically oriented training may be the most helpful way to unblock and move forward from this crisis situation. Jemal feels as if he has been offered 'a new chance', and he experiences the new teachers' approach to him as 'strict but just'. Although there is some discussion about Jemal returning to therapy, a decision is made to 'wait and see', with his adoptive parents offered some booster sessions to support them through this challenging period.

Beyond the three-track approach: when something more or other is needed

For some traumatised children, it may become clear during treatment that what can be offered in the three-track approach is not sufficient or the 'best' treatment option. This may be the case when the child shows severe (symptomatic) deterioration in reaction to significant changes or stressors in life or when the child's severe vulnerability comes to light triggered by new developmental challenges. In such cases, it is important to pick up on these signals in a timely way and to be able to fall back on the mentalizing network formed around the child and the family to think things through. When a shared decision has been made, an important task for the therapists will be to support the child and the family to transition from this treatment to the new 'plan', which may in some cases involve (semi-)residential treatment or long-term/open-ended treatment.

Concluding thoughts

The work towards ending as conceptualised in the present treatment model for traumatised children and their carers is considered important though complex, much like the work throughout the entire trajectory. We aim for an ending phase in which the therapeutic process can be brought to a close in a way that the therapeutic work conducted and the therapeutic gains achieved, in both children and their adult carers, can be consolidated in the best possible way. Working collaboratively towards an agreed ending is especially important for children who have experienced complex trauma. In this way, the chances of the ending process being experienced as both a natural and an essentially positive experience in the service of growth can be maximised, offsetting the risk of retraumatisation. Even if the actual process of ending is not always as clear as this, having these aims in mind can be helpful in order to provide a basis for the difficult decisions that sometimes need to be made about what is 'the best thing to do'. This actually requires all adults involved – the parents but also the network members, including the therapists – to carry the therapeutic work through from the outset until the moment of saying goodbye (and with some of these children, beyond that).

Due to the complexity and often intense emotional arousal that comes with engaging in treatment with a traumatised child and their adult carers, we might sometimes tend to 'forget' the great value of and reward in doing this kind of work. Being part of a child's raw wounds healing into scars (Vliegen et al., 2023) – however sensitive these may remain – and of supporting parents and other adult carers to regain a sense of mastery and enjoyment in living and working with a traumatised child is what is at the core of 'transforming despair to hope' (Lanyado, 2017). Even if all issues have not been resolved through treatment and many of these children and families will not live a 'carefree' life, the more realistically hopeful perspective of a more liveable and enjoyable life will have been gained and, with that, an essentially positive experience of mental health services, which may help lower the threshold to professional help in years to come, if needed. The latter may be considered an 'achievement' in and of itself in light of this group of children and families still being underserved to date.

References

Fonagy, P., Campbell, C., Constantinou, M., Higgitt, A., Allison, E., & Luyten, P. (2021). Culture and psychopathology: An attempt at reconsidering the role of social learning. *Development and Psychopathology*, 1–16. https://doi.org/10.1017/S0954579421000092

Lanyado, M. (1999). Holding and letting go: Some thoughts about the process of ending therapy. *Journal of Child Psychotherapy*, *25*(3), 357–378.

Lanyado, M. (2017). *Transforming despair to hope. Reflections on psychotherapeutic process with severely neglected and traumatised children.* Routledge.

Midgley, N., Ensink, K., Lindqvist, K., Malberg, N., & Muller, N. (2017). Moving toward goodbye: Endings in time-limited MBT-C. In *Mentalization-based treatment for children. A time-limited approach* (pp. 185–200). American Psychological Association.

Ogrodniczuk, J. S., Joyce, A. S., & Piper, W. E. (2005). Strategies for reducing patient-initiated premature termination of psychotherapy. *Harvard Review of Psychiatry*, *13*(2), 57–70.

Ryz, P., & Wilson, J. (1999). Endings as gain: The capacity to end and its role in creating space for growth. *Journal of Child Psychotherapy*, *25*(3), 397–403.

Vliegen, N., Tang, E., & Meurs, P. (2023). *Children recovering from complex trauma: From wound to scar.* Routledge.

Winnicott, D. W. (1958). *Collected papers: Through pediatrics to psychoanalysis.* Tavistock.

Wittenberg, I. (1999). Ending therapy. *Journal of Child Psychotherapy*, *25*(3), 339–356.

Index